Pharmaceutical Practice and Policy

Pharmaceutical Practice and Policy

Edited by John Jensen

hayle
medical

New York

Hayle Medical,
750 Third Avenue, 9th Floor,
New York, NY 10017, USA

Visit us on the World Wide Web at:
www.haylemedical.com

ISBN: 978-1-63241-898-2

Cataloging-in-Publication Data

Pharmaceutical practice and policy / edited by John Jensen.
   p. cm.
Includes bibliographical references and index.
ISBN 978-1-63241-898-2
1. Pharmacy--Practice. 2. Pharmacy. 3. Drugs. 4. Pharmacology. I. Jensen, John.
RS92 .P43 2020
615.1--dc23

Table of Contents

Permissions

List of Contributors

Index

Preface

It is often said that books are a boon to mankind. They document every progress and pass on the knowledge from one generation to the other. They play a crucial role in our lives. Thus I was both excited and nervous while editing this book. I was pleased by the thought of being able to make a mark but I was also nervous to do it right because the future of students depends upon it. Hence, I took a few months to research further into the discipline, revise my knowledge and also explore some more aspects. Post this process, I begun with the editing of this book.

Pharmaceutical policy is a field which deals with the development, use and provision of medications within a healthcare system. It encompasses biologics, drugs, vaccines and natural health products. Patent laws apply to all pharmaceutical products. Thus, the interpretations of these made by government patent granting agencies can have significant impacts on the incentive to drug development. These also have consequences on the availability of lower-priced generic drugs. Another important dimension of pharmaceutical practice is licensing. A recognized national agency is mostly responsible for reviewing a product and approving its sale. Quality, safety and efficacy are the chief determinants of drug regulation. Once the safety and clinical benefits of a product have been established and its pricing has been determined, a drug manufacturer submits it for evaluation by a payer. This book provides comprehensive insights into pharmaceutical policy and practice. It outlines the varied aspects of pharmaceutical regulation, legal issues and administrative dimensions of pharmaceutical practice in detail. As this field is constantly evolving, the contents of this book will help the readers understand the modern concepts and developments in this domain.

I thank my publisher with all my heart for considering me worthy of this unparalleled opportunity and for showing unwavering faith in my skills. I would also like to thank the editorial team who worked closely with me at every step and contributed immensely towards the successful completion of this book. Last but not the least, I wish to thank my friends and colleagues for their support.

Editor

Trade agreements and drug access: assessment of the impact of the 2009 Peruvian new drug policy on anti-infectives registration and availability

Lita Araujo[1]*[iD] and Michael Montagne[2]

Abstract

Background: The United States-Peru Free Trade Agreement required changes in the Peruvian pharmaceutical legislation that resulted in the National Drug Policy (NDP) of 2009. This study evaluated the registration of brand and generic anti-infectives before and after the agreement and implementation of the NDP and assessed the availability of anti-infectives in community pharmacies located in Arequipa-Peru.

Methods: Anti-infectives registration database, provided by DIGEMID (Peruvian Drug Regulatory Authority), was evaluated from January 2005 to August 2014. Registration status included: new registrations, re-registrations, awaiting registration; or expired, denied, suspended, canceled and disregarded registrations. In addition, ten retail pharmacies located in different socio-economic areas in Arequipa were sampled in August 2014. Descriptive statistics and chi-square test were used for the analysis.

Results: A total of 6112 anti-infectives registrations were categorized (5007 = antibacterials, 340 = antimycotics, 143 = antimycobacterials, and 622 = antiviral drugs). New registrations for brand and generic anti-infectives decreased from 2005 to 2013 (311 to 60 and 164 to 20 respectively). Re-registrations were from 121 (brand) and 115 (generics) in 2005 to 6 (brand) and 5 (generics) in 2013. Anti-infectives awaiting registration increased from 0 in 2005 to 351 (brand) and 137 (generics) in 2013.
The retail pharmacy survey included 1105 anti-infectives. These pharmacies carried 647 (58.6%) products awaiting registration, 74 (6.7%) expired (mostly combination of sulfonamides and trimethoprim followed by penicillin with extended spectrum, and fluoroquinolones), 4 (0.4%) suspended, and 2 (0.2%) denied registrations. Pharmacies in the low socio-economic area of the city had the highest proportion of generics (59.0% vs. 16.1%) from foreign origin (mainly India), and brand anti-infectives from Peruvian manufacturers (68.8% vs. 48.1%). High socio-economic areas had highest proportion of branded anti-infectives (83.9% vs. 41.0%).

Conclusions: The new NDP reduced the number of brand and generic registrations; generics had the largest decline in registrations. Anti-infectives found in pharmacies located in low-income areas were more likely to be generics, and less likely to be currently registered by DIGEMID. The potential reduction in generic registrations resulting from the implementation of the NDP as a consequence of the bilateral trade agreement could result in lower availability of low cost medicines, but may increase the safety, efficacy and quality of marketed medicines.

* Correspondence: lita.araujo-lama@mcphs.edu; lita_araujo@hotmail.com
[1]Pharmaceutical Business and Administrative Sciences, MCPHS University, 179 Longwood Avenue, Boston, MA 02115, USA
Full list of author information is available at the end of the article

Background

Free Trade Agreements (FTA) are controversial for threatening important aspects of health especially access to affordable medicines. Multilateral, bilateral, and regional FTAs, as part of economic globalization, have included trade in health insurance, pharmaceuticals, and health services making health care reform no longer just a matter of national policy. FTAs make it difficult for countries to transfer from market-based health care systems to publicly funded health care programs once health care markets are opened to competition [1]. Many FTAs include provisions such as government procurement, competition policy, intellectual property (IP) rights protection, e-commerce, and more [2]. The IP rights about patent protection (explicitly the length of patent protection and second use patents) and data exclusivity are the provisions that could restrict the most access to generic medicines, and unfortunately, they have become the norm in the US [3, 4] and European trade agreements [5].

FTA between Peru and the United States

On April 12, 2006, the United States of America and Peru signed the Trade Promotion Agreement. The FTA became effective on February 1, 2009; it aimed to improve the overall commercial and investment activity by eliminating or reducing tariffs on many goods including pharmaceuticals, accelerating the customs clearance process for US imports, and fortifying the protection of IP rights [6]. The IP chapter includes, among others, stronger protections for patents and test data as well as tough penalties for piracy and counterfeiting. The agreement restricted the grounds for invalidating patents and set up rules for protecting test data submitted for marketing approval of medicines (article 16.9 and article 16.10.2) [6].

Patent provisions were not changed, maintaining the 20 years of a patent's life as with the World Trade Organization and the Andean Community agreements where Peru is a member. The amendment made to the FTA with respect to data exclusivity kept the 5 years of protection as it was proposed by the US (article 16.10.2(a)(b)) but added a modification: If the medicine is approved by the FDA (marketing registration) the term of protection starts running from the time of the first approval (article 16.10.2(c)(d)), thus reducing the protection period in Peru [6]. According to Rangel [7], this would provide better access to medicines while maintaining strong protection for innovation. However, according to Roca [8], Peruvian law does not require foreign companies to register first abroad, therefore they can register directly in Peru gaining the 5 years of data exclusivity.

New drug policy and its connection to the FTA

The US-Peru FTA involved substantial changes in the Peruvian regulation to meet the requirements stipulated in the treaty. Law 29316 Amending, Incorporating and Regulating Miscellaneous Provisions on the Implementation of the Trade Promotion Agreement signed between Peru and the US of January 2009 sole purpose was initiating the FTA. The most important modifications related to the pharmaceutical sector were included in Article 5 that regulates data exclusivity, and Article 6 that replaced the requirements for the registration of pharmaceuticals, medical devices and sanitary products previously contained in Article 50 of the General Health Law 26842 of 1997 [9]. The General Health Law approved a simple procedure for the registration application process of pharmaceuticals that included an affidavit ensuring quality, safety and efficacy; analysis protocol from another country; and a free sale certificate. The procedure that originally lasted 15 days was reduced to 7 days (Table 1) [10].

The Supreme Decree 001–2009-SA was issued to rule Law 29316, particularly the new requirements for the registration of pharmaceuticals, stating in part:

> "The Trade Promotion Agreement ...... establishes in its Chapter 16 provisions regarding the respect and safeguarding of Intellectual Property Rights, which must be incorporated into Peruvian legislation in this matter; ...... its amendment in Law 29316, which establishes standards related to the protection of test data or other undisclosed data on pharmaceutical products, which must be regulated;
>
> That, it is necessary to modify the system of registration of pharmaceutical products so that the health authority can demand certain information relevant to the evaluation and determination of the safety and efficacy of said products ......
>
> This Supreme Decree shall enter into force on the date of entry into force of the Trade Promotion Agreement signed between Peru and the United States" [11].

The National Drug Policy (NDP) was approved on December 24, 2004 [12]. However, the NDP did not define a timeline for implementation and it was not initiated until the enactment of Law 29459 in 2009. The objectives of Law 29459 were to adapt the national drug regulation to the requirements of the FTA, to implement new drug registration requirements, and to reach the objectives of the NDP of universal access and rational use of medicines.

The Law of Pharmaceutical Products, Medical Devices and Sanitary Products 29459 of February 2009 and its supreme decree 016–2011-SA stipulated all regulations, new requirements and changes for such products (Table 1) and

Table 1 A comparison between the registration laws before and after the Free Trade Agreement presenting the main changes related to medicines

Articles	Law 26842 of 1997 and D.S. 010–97-SA [10]	Law 29459 of 2009 [14] and D.S. 016–2011-SA [13, 14]

Type of pharmaceutical product	- Brand medicines
	- Generic medicines
	- Diet products and sweeteners
	- Homeopathic products
	- Diagnostic agents
	- Biologic products
	- Radiopharmaceutical agents
		- Medicines
		  * Pharmaceutical specialties
		  * Diagnostic agents
		  * Radiopharmaceutical agents
		  * Medicinal gases
		- Herbal medicines
		- Diet products and sweeteners
		- Biologic products
		- Compounding preparations

Requirements for registration and re-registration	- Affidavit assuring the quality, safety and efficacy of the product - Analysis protocol based on an authorized pharmacopeia of finished product - Free sale certificate and certificate[a] of consumption (if product is imported)	- Application form with character of affidavit - Specifications and analytical techniques of APIs, excipients, final product - Validation of analytical techniques of finished product - Flow chart and validation of process of manufacture - Stability studies - GMP certificate granted by Digemid or from a country with HRS - Free sale certificate or certificate of pharmaceutical product[a] (for import)
Timeframe application/ evaluation process	Automatic with presentation of requirements, no more than 7 days	Between 45 days to 1 year according to the product's category
Amount paid to get the registration license	10% of TU	59.74% of TU (category 1) 99.95% of TU (category 2) 99.65% of TU (category 3)
Term validity	5 years	5 years

[a]The Free Sale Certificate is an official document issued by the authority from the country of origin of the exported product that certified that the product is sold in the country of the manufacturer or exporter. The 'certificate of pharmaceutical product' from the International Commerce of WHO is a Free Sale Certificate
APIs Active pharmaceutical ingredients, *HRS* High regulatory surveillance, *TU* Taxation Unit

introduced the important terms of safety and efficacy within the regulatory authority and the Peruvian pharmaceutical sector. The Law stipulates the time allowed to review applications and grant marketing approvals according to the new categories of medicines:

– Category 1 (medicines in the essential medicines list): 45 to 60 days;
– Category 2 (medicines not in the essential medicines list but registered in countries of high regulatory surveillance (US, selected European countries, Japan, and Korea)): 45 to 90 days; and,
– Category 3 (other medicines): up to 12 months [13].

The fees for registration increased 10-fold and includes control activities and health surveillance. The technical requirements and the application documentation increased requiring presentation of therapeutic equivalence studies to demonstrate interchangeability, information on safety and efficacy (pre-clinical and clinical studies), a risk management plan for new medicines, Good Manufacturing Practice (GMP) certification, and analytical studies [14].

The technical information on safety and efficacy of the medicines must be submitted for registration and re-registration, but is not required for subsequent re-registrations unless it is required to address new safety and efficacy information. Registration and re-registration require studies of interchangeability; however, in vivo bioequivalent studies are only required for high risk medicines.

The Law also allowed from 3 to 10 years to comply with the requirements and studies for re-registration purposes. The GMP certificate must now be granted by DIGEMID, and quality control analyses are required for each lot that enters the market, except for biologics. Law 29,459 also includes chapters regarding universal access and rational use of medicines, promotion and research [14].

Health care and pharmaceutical systems in Peru

The Peruvian health care system is divided into public and private sectors. The public sector comprises the Ministry of Health (MoH), the National Institute of Social Security (NISS), the health services of the Armed Forces and the National Police, the regional health boards, and the local government. The public health sector is financed by subsidies (indirect contributions) and by social security (direct contributions). The government manages and finances health services and medicines through Integrated Health Insurance with a low cost or no cost to people below the poverty or extreme poverty levels respectively. NISS provides free health care and medicines exclusively for salaried workers and their family members in their own hospitals and clinics. The private sector sells services to NISS in their clinics and doctor offices. The military and police have their own health system and infrastructure. The private health care system is mainly represented by clinics and other private entities like companies providing health insurance plans.

The MoH provides health services for 60% of the population; NISS provides health services for 30% of the population entitled to social security; and the Armed Forces, National Police, and the private sector together provide services to the remaining 10% [15].

The public sector's procurement is both centralized for purchases and distribution of medicines at the national level, and decentralized for regional and local acquisitions. NISS performs centralized acquisitions of medicines and distributes them at a national level. Medicines are mostly distributed directly by the pharmaceutical manufacturers to hospitals and drugstore chains, also to large wholesalers, which mainly distribute brand imported medicines. Small wholesalers mainly distribute medicines to independent private community pharmacies. The retail sector has changed singularly; in the mid-1990s the market share of private pharmacies was around 86%, whereas in 2011 almost 60% of the market share was retained by drugstore chains [16].

The government's universal insurance coverage and purchase strategies provide price regulation for medicines for the public sector. Whereas, the constitution protects free market competition and bans price control measures in the private sector.

Study research questions
This study is intended to answer some of the research questions that arise as a result of the signing of the trade agreement and the subsequent implementation of the NDP.

- What is the impact of the NDP on the number of brand and generic anti-infectives registered in the country?
- What are the consequences of the NDP on the availability of anti-infectives at the retail pharmacy level?

Methods
Data sources
The evaluation was performed from January 2005 to April 2014 with the database provided by the Peruvian drug regulatory authority (DIGEMID).

The Anatomic Therapeutic Chemical (ATC) classification system at the WHO Collaborating Centre for Drug Statistics Methodology [17] was used to identify and categorize the anti-infectives from the DIGEMID database.

For the case study, data were collected from 10 retail pharmacies located in different socio-economic strata in the southern city of Arequipa, the second most industrialized

and commercial city of Peru. Lima, Peru's capital, was not chosen because the investigator wanted to determine the effect of the implementation far from the capital (in Peru, government policies are implemented first in the capital and then very slowly move to other parts of the country).

The metropolitan area of the province of Arequipa has 721 pharmacies and drugstores located among its 18 districts. Two pharmacies (1 privately owned by a university community health center, and 1 private with independent owner) were sampled from the low socioeconomic stratum representing 1.7% of the pharmacies in these districts. Two pharmacies (each from different pharmacy chains, one located inside a private clinic) were sampled in the districts of the high socio-economic stratum comprising a 1.4% sample. The other 6 pharmacies (3 privately owned, and 3 from different pharmacy chains) were representative of the middle socio-economic stratum comprising a 1.3% sample of the pharmacies in these districts. The socio-economic strata were determined using the poverty level per district from a study based on a population census of 2007 [18].

The districts with a poverty level of 26% or higher were considered in the low socio-economic stratum. The districts with a poverty level between 25 and 11% were considered within the middle socio-economic stratum and the districts with a poverty level of 10% or lower were categorized in the high socio-economic stratum [18]. The pharmacies were selected based on their location and type of pharmacy within the private sector. A convenience, non-random sample was selected from three different socio-economic strata representative of the city.

Data manipulation
The impact of the regulations on the pharmaceutical market was estimated by creating a registration history for each anti-infective in the period of 2005 to 2014, before and after the implementation of both the FTA and the NDP. The registration history included 8 statuses: 1 = New registration; 2 = Re-registered; 3 = Awaiting registration; 4 = Expired; 5 = Canceled; 6 = Not approved; 7 = Deserted or Disregarded; 8 = Suspended.

For the case study, pharmacies were visited only once. The data were collected from July 30 to August 15, 2014. The following information was recorded: brand name, international nonproprietary name of anti-infective, registration number, dose and manufacturer.

Data analysis
The frequency of anti-infectives registered for the first time was determined using the variable 'authorization date of first registration.' The number of anti-infectives re-registered in the study period was determined using the 'authorization and expiration date' of their registration considering that the license last 5 years. The anti-infectives for which companies

filed applications for registration at DIGEMID but did not obtain the authorization and registration number yet were considered as 'awaiting registration'. This situation started happening in 2008–2009 when the NDP was implemented, before the registration process lasted only 7 days. The number of anti-infectives awaiting registration was determined by the variable 'status of application' that was obtained from the DIGEMID database.

The DIGEMID website index was used to update the information from the database until August 2014 for statuses 3 to 8 (awaiting registration, expired, canceled, not approved, deserted or disregarded, and suspended registrations). The index is updated every month. The updated information was applied in the next part of the research, the case study.

Case study

A case study was performed to determine the availability of anti-infectives at retail pharmacies comparing these with the anti-infectives registered through DIGEMID. Data from the 10 retail pharmacies were matched with the anti-infectives DIGEMID database from January 2005 to August 2014, to record the registration history of each anti-infective. The proportion of generic and brand anti-infectives sold in each retail pharmacy was also calculated as well as their country of origin.

The registration expiration date and the ATC pharmacological-chemical class were determined for products with statuses 4 to 8.

Statistical analyses

Microsoft Office Excel 2013 was used to perform descriptive statistics. Sigma Plot 11.0 was used to perform chi-squared tests to assess differences in proportions. Mann-Whitney U test was performed when the chi-squared test determined statistically significant differences within the proportions. P-values < 0.05 were considered statistically significant.

Results

A total of 6112 anti-infectives with a unique health registration number were extracted from the DIGEMID database (January 2005 to April 2014) using the ATC classification system. There were 5007 antibacterials; 340 antimycotics; 143 antimycobacterials; and 622 antivirals.

Table 2 shows the 8 types of registration statuses used in this study. The number of anti-infectives with new registrations was quite consistent from 2005 to 2009 with 475 and 448 registrations respectively; however, the number of new registrations decreased from 2010 to 2013, with 91 and 80 respectively (Table 2). The number of anti-infectives that were re-registered declined from 236 in 2005 to 11 in 2013. There was a statistically significant difference ($p < 0.001$) between the type of registrations before and after the legislation. There also was a statistically

significant difference for new registrations ($p = 0.016$) and re-registrations ($p = 0.032$) before and after the implementation of the new legislation. The awaiting registrations started with 48 in 2009, increasing to 488 in 2013.

The number of registrations that expired from 2005 to 2013 went down and then up; in 2005 there were 466 expired registrations, in 2009 there were 212, and in 2013 there were 365. Furthermore, the canceled registrations increased from 10 in 2005 to 99 in 2008 and dropped again to 14 in 2013.

New registrations

The proportions of brand anti-infectives new registrations were greater than the ones for generics throughout the study period, and this difference was even greater from 2009 to 2013. However, the number of new registrations gradually decreased from 2005 through the first four months of 2014 (Table 3). There was a statistically significant difference ($p < 0.001$) in the number of brand and generics new registrations before and after the legislation. Bivariate analysis also found a statistically significant difference in the proportion of brand ($p = 0.016$) and in the proportion of generics new registrations ($p = 0.016$) before and after the legislation.

Re-registrations

The proportions for brand and generics were quite similar from 2005 to 2007. In 2008 brand anti-infectives reached 60.3% and generics reached 39.7% followed by small fluctuations through 2013, although, the number of re-registrations declined gradually from 2005 to 2013 for both brand and generics (Table 4). No significant differences ($p = 0.064$) were observed in terms of number of brand and generic anti-infectives re-registered before and after the implementation of the new legislation. However, there was a statistically significant difference ($p = 0.032$) for brand anti-infectives re-registered before and after the implementation of the new legislation and for generic anti-infectives only ($p = 0.016$). There were no anti-infectives re-registered through the first four months of 2014.

Awaiting registration

The proportions for brand anti-infectives were 75.0% ($n = 36$) in 2009, 58.2% ($n = 85$) in 2011 and 61.1% ($n = 116$) by April 2014. In contrast, the proportions for generics were 25.0% ($n = 12$) in 2009, 41.8% ($n = 61$) in 2011 and 38.9% ($n = 74$) by April 2014. The awaiting registrations numbers gradually increased from 2009 to 2013 for both types of medicines.

Case study

A total of 1105 anti-infectives were identified from ten community pharmacies in Arequipa, Peru.

Table 2 Registration statuses of anti-infectives (n) from January 2005 to April 2014

#	Registration status	2005	2006	2007	2008	2009	2010	2011	2012	2013	2014[a]
1	New registrations	475	528	510	623	448	91	60	140	80	35
2	Re-registrations	236	228	225	257	181	195	138	68	11	0
3	Awaiting registration	0	0	0	0	48	66	146	256	488	190
4	Expired	466	301	349	352	212	355	406	364	365	249
5	Canceled	10	13	43	99	60	47	44	23	14	15
6	Not approved	0	0	1	12	24	36	13	11	0	0
7	Deserted/Disregarded	0	0	0	0	5	10	7	11	2	0
8	Suspended	0	0	0	1	0	2	2	2	0	5

[a]Through April

There were 59.0% of generics in the low socio-economic stratum pharmacies and 16.0% in the high socio-economic stratum pharmacies (Fig. 1). There was a relationship ($p < 0.001$) between brand and generic anti-infectives and their socio-economic strata.

There were 69.0% brand anti-infectives of Peruvian origin in the low socioeconomic stratum and 68.0% and 48.0% in the middle and high socio-economic strata respectively. The non-Peruvian anti-infectives increased according to the socioeconomic stratum. In the case of generics (Fig. 2), the low socio-economic stratum pharmacies stocked 30.0% Peruvian anti-infectives and 70.0% non-Peruvian anti-infectives. However, the other two strata showed an opposite behavior: 73.0% and 74.0% Peruvian and 27.0% and 26.0% non-Peruvian anti-infectives.

The registration statuses of the anti-infectives found in the 10 retail pharmacies are shown in Table 5. The higher proportion of new registrations was observed in the pharmacies of the low socio-economic stratum; however, re-registrations were almost the same in the three strata as well as for those awaiting registration. Expired anti-infectives (status 4) were found in pharmacies in all three strata. The middle stratum pharmacies carried 2

anti-infectives with status 'not approved' and 2 with status 'deserted/disregarded.'

There were 82 anti-infectives with statuses 4 to 8 found in the 10 retail pharmacies by August 2014. After eliminating duplicates and triplicates, there were 57 unique anti-infectives (Table 6). Of the anti-infectives with status 4 (expired registration), 43 were brand and 9 were generic products; and from these, 33 were of Peruvian origin and 19 of non-Peruvian origin. Also, 18 of these anti-infectives had a registration expiration date of 2014; 14 had a registration expiration date of 2013; and 9 had a registration expiration date of 2011. Furthermore, this table shows the ATC classification for anti-infectives with statuses 4 to 8 found in the retail pharmacies. The majority were the combination of sulfonamides and trimethoprim followed by penicillin with extended spectrum and penicillin with beta-lactamase inhibitors as well as fluoroquinolones.

Discussion

The changes in the Peruvian drug legislation, as a consequence of the US-Peru FTA, have created uncertainty about their implications in the short and long term. Law 29459 caused considerable adjustments in the procedures for the registration of pharmaceutical products, medical

Table 3 Number and proportion of new registrations of brand and generic anti-infectives from January 2005 to April 2014

Years	Brand		Generic		Total
	n	%	n	%	N
2005	311	65.5	164	34.5	475
2006	335	63.4	193	36.6	528
2007	332	65.1	178	34.9	510
2008	451	72.4	172	27.6	623
2009	364	81.3	84	18.8	448
2010	70	76.9	21	23.1	91
2011	45	75.0	15	25.0	60
2012	103	73.6	37	26.4	140
2013	60	75.0	20	25.0	80
2014[a]	26	74.3	9	25.7	35

[a]Through April

Table 4 Number and proportion of brand and generic anti-infectives re-registered from 2005 to 2013

Years	Brand		Generic		Total
	n	%	n	%	N
2005	121	51.3	115	48.7	236
2006	116	50.9	112	49.1	228
2007	116	51.6	109	48.4	225
2008	155	60.3	102	39.7	257
2009	81	44.8	100	55.2	181
2010	114	58.5	81	41.5	195
2011	71	51.4	67	48.6	138
2012	32	47.1	36	52.9	68
2013	6	54.5	5	45.5	11

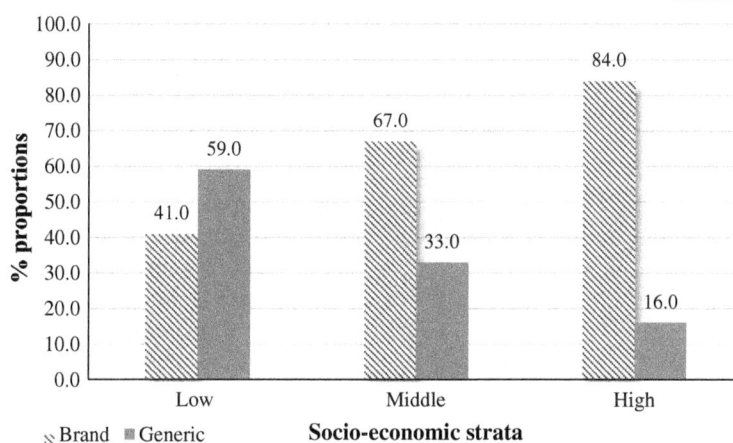

Fig. 1 Brand and generic anti-infectives available at 10 retail pharmacies cluster by socio-economic strata

devices and sanitary products. And the provision of data exclusivity may play a role in the long run.

Impact of the NDP (law 29459)

The new law's stricter requirements can explain the sudden decrease in the number of registrations. A study in March 2013, examined 11 procedures required by the MoH for the marketing of pharmaceuticals. The analysis of the perceptions of the companies found that the bureaucratic procedures were not consistent with the recent changes in the legal framework (Law 29459, and the DSs 014–2011-SA and 016–2011-SA); apparently increasing the time of DIGEMID's procedures may affect the launch of new pharmaceuticals in the Peruvian market [19]. Furthermore, data provided by wholesalers estimated that each procedure can cost up to $13,433 per medicine. This cost did not include the opportunity cost of the time elapsed between the initiation of the procedure to obtain the marketing approval and the effective

granting of the license. Although the registration fee and the cost associated with the new requirements can be considered modest by international standards, it might in fact become a market entry barrier for generic importers and domestic producers [16]. However, it can also contribute to the increase in the safety, efficacy and quality of registered medicines.

Since 2010, the government has requested GMP certificates in compliance with the new Peruvian standards. This requirement is also increasing the time needed to obtain marketing authorization. In 2011, Peru requested manufacturers, wholesalers, and importers of medicines to register and acquire the GMP from DIGEMID otherwise their medicines cannot be marketed in the country. DIGEMID has performed most of the inspections to production plants in China and India [20], countries with relatively low regulatory requirements.

The delay in approval of applications may also be related to logistical problems associated with the adaptation of

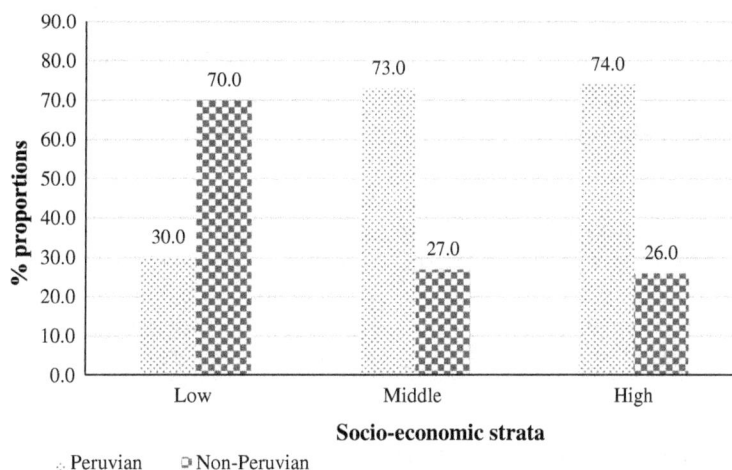

Fig. 2 Peruvian and non-Peruvian generic anti-infectives available at 10 pharmacies in Arequipa-Peru divided by socio-economic strata

Table 5 Registry statuses of anti-infectives by socio-economic strata from 10 retail pharmacies at Arequipa, Peru

#	Registration Status	Retail pharmacies by socio-economic strata					
		Low		Middle		High	
		n	%	n	%	n	%
1	New registrations	9	11.5	48	5.9	16	7.3
2	Re-registrations	22	28.2	228	28.2	53	24.3
3	Awaiting registration	42	53.8	471	58.2	134	61.5
4	Expired	4	5.1	56	6.9	14	6.4
5	Canceled	0	0	0	0	0	0
6	Not approved	0	0	2	0.2	0	0
7	Deserted/Disregarded	0	0	2	0.2	0	0
8	Suspended	1	1.3	2	0.2	1	0.5
	Total anti-infectives	78	99.9[a]	809	99.8[a]	218	100

[a]Percentage rounded error

DIGEMID reviewers to the new system that requires to evaluate pre-clinical and clinical studies. The previous system only required an affidavit proving safety, efficacy and quality.

The FTA required the Peruvian government to eliminate the 20% procurement subsidy for national companies. Now, national and foreigner companies can participate in public procurement under the same conditions. This will reduce the cost of medicines for the government but it could affect domestic pharmaceutical and/or wholesaler companies that would not be able to compete with a transnational company. This could be one of the reasons for the decline of Peruvian new registrations observed after 2009. Due to the pressures of the FTA, Peruvian companies could face intense competition but this can also reduce the presence of medicines without demonstrated safety, efficacy and quality.

Medicines in Peru are subjected to the following taxes: *Ad Valorem* import tax 9%, value-added tax (VAT) 16%, and local promotion tax 2%. However, medicines imported within the framework of the US-Peru FTA are exempted from the *Ad Valorem* import tax. Import duties applied to APIs and finished products are 6% and the VAT collected on finished products is 18% [21].

FTA provision on data exclusivity

Data exclusivity is a requirement demanded by the US FTA (called TRIPS plus). Until a five-year period elapses, data exclusivity prevents DIGEMID from utilizing confidential trial data submitted by the originator company to demonstrate the efficacy and safety of generic drugs [6]. Cortés Gamba et al. [22] compared Colombia with Venezuela and Argentina, the last two countries do not have data exclusivity regulations, and concluded that the entry of generics depended on market considerations and data exclusivity had minor effect on market competition.

On the other hand, two studies assessed the US-Jordan FTA and both concluded that the new data exclusivity regulation delayed generic entry and increased expenditures for medicines without generic competition [23, 24].

Data exclusivity has similar effect than a patent because it grants a temporary market monopoly and delays generic market competition. According to Seinfeld and La Serna [25], this practice would not affect generics competition because the generic companies typically wait between 3 to 5 years to see how the market for originators evolves before entering the market. However, data exclusivity can be especially important for medicines without patent protection or new formulations of existing medicines. In fact, in 2015, sponsor companies of 45 new chemical entities requested data exclusivity in Peru, of which 21 were enforced, 11 had already expired the exclusivity period, 11 were denied, and 2 were withdrawn [26]. As of October 2017, there were 27 new chemical entities including 6 antivirals with enforced data exclusivity and 5 new chemical entities including 2 antivirals waiting for first time marketing license that have requested data exclusivity [27].

Anti-infectives availability at the retail level

The modest Peruvian pharmaceutical market concentrates its production on generics and branded generics of good demand. This is confirmed by the results obtained from the 10 retail pharmacies in which almost the double of brand and generic anti-infectives were of Peruvian origin. The higher proportion of Peruvian brand anti-infectives in the low and middle socioeconomic strata is an indication that these anti-infectives are branded generics, not originators. The slightly higher proportion of non-Peruvian over Peruvian brand anti-infectives in the high socio-economic stratum pharmacies are an indication of the consumption of originator anti-infectives in this stratum. One of the pharmacies from this stratum is located in a clinic where most of the patients have private insurance; therefore, the pharmacy mostly sells originator products.

Peru commercializes 3 types of medicines: originators, branded generics and generics; however, DIGEMID only categorize two types of medicines: brand name (that include originators and branded generics) and generics. Branded generics are products with the same active ingredient(s) as an originator but are permitted to differ in shape, size, labeling, and excipients. Branded generics are typically marketed using a brand name [28]. A study determined that from 80% of brand name products registered at DIGEMID in 2013 only 24% were originators, the rest were branded generics [26].

In Peru, generics and branded generics are typically pharmaceutically equivalent but not bioequivalent to the originator. Furthermore, in some cases, they are only

Table 6 Characteristics of the 57 unique anti-infectives with statuses 4 to 8

Characteristics	Status 4 n	Status 6 n	Status 7 n	Status 8 n
Brand	43	1		1
Generic	9	1	1	1
Foreign	19		1	2
Peruvian	33	2		
Expiration date:				
2014	18			2
2013	14			
2012	5		1	
2011	9			
2010	3	1		
2008	1	1		
2007	2			
ATC – Anti-infective class:				
J01AA - Tetracycline	1	1		
J01CA - Penicillin extended spectrum[a]	9			1
J01 CE - Beta-lactamase sensitive penicillin	1		1	1
J01CF - Beta-lactamase resistant penicillin	1			
J01CR - Penicillin/beta-lactamase inhibitors	8			
J01DB - First generation cephalosporins[a]	3	1		
J01 DC - Second generation cephalosporins	1			
J01DD - Third generation cephalosporins	3			
J01EE - Combination sulfonamides/TMP[a]	11			
J01F - Macrolides, lincosamides	4			
J01G - Aminoglycoside antibacterial				1
J01MA - Fluoroquinolones[b]	8			
J01XD - Imidazole derivatives	1			
J02 AC - Triazole derivatives	1			

[a]Includes combinations with mucolytics/expectorants
[b]Includes combinations with phenazopyridine
TMP trimethoprim

pharmaceutical alternatives such as different salts, esters or complexes; or different dosage form or strengths but are prescribed or dispensed as interchangeable with the originator.

Peru's new regulation requires studies of bioequivalence; currently enforced for high risk medicines. This could imply better acceptance of generics if the government informs the public about the improved quality of these medicines. Although, this requirement could increase generics prices and limit their access, independently of patents or data exclusivity, as an indirect effect of the FTA.

A study of the Brazilian pharmaceutical policy and access to essential medicines concluded that the goal of availability of essential medicines in the public sector has not been reached yet. However, the authors also mentioned that because of the regulations about quality tests, bioequivalence/bioavailability (mandatory for most generics and branded generics), and medicine registration (2 years registration time) there was an increase in the number of generics in the market compared to the small proportion of such medicines in the Brazilian market at the beginning of the generic's policy implementation [29].

Indian and Chinese medicines are some of the cheapest in the Peruvian pharmaceutical market along with Latin American medicines. This explains the high percentage of generic anti-infectives of non-Peruvian origin in the low socio-economic stratum pharmacies. However, the middle and high socio-economic strata retail pharmacies kept a stock of Peruvian origin generics but from long time business manufacturers because they trust the quality of their products or because they are partners.

The sum of all 3 strata anti-infective stock reached 32.0% of generics and the rest were brand name. It is important to mention that 60.3% of generics are marketed in the public sector [30].

More than half of the anti-infectives in the 10 retail pharmacies were awaiting re-registration. Medicines applying for re-registration may continue in the market until the final decision is made. Anti-infectives awaiting registration can be anti-infectives that have not submitted GMP certificates, have failed plant inspections, or have not yet presented pre-clinical or clinical studies to prove safety and efficacy. Even more concerning, anti-infectives with expired registrations were found in all 3 pharmacy cohorts.

The anti-infectives mostly found were penicillins with extended spectrum, macrolides, cephalosporins, fluoroquinolones and combination of sulfonamides and trimethoprim (the government covers the treatments for HIV and tuberculosis in the public sector; this is why the majority of anti-infectives in the retail pharmacies were antibiotics). The public sector shows almost the same patterns, in a study conducted in four hospitals in four of Lima's provinces, the antibiotics used with high incidence were amoxicillin, ciprofloxacin, metronidazole and azithromycin [31]. Unfortunately, the use of these antibiotics for common pathologies increase the risk of bacterial resistance. Moreover, the situation in the private sector is quite different since the retail pharmacies do not ask for a prescription, although officially required, and many of the antibiotics are sold for minor infections or no bacterial infections at all; in 2010 60% of anti-infectives were sold without a prescription in the private sector and 10% in the public sector [32].

Limitations of the study

Only private settings were sampled for the case study; however, the study results have been compared and supported with public sector studies such as the Lima hospitals' study. Furthermore, although growth in overall consumption of medicines is explained mainly by the public health sector, the total cost of such consumption is more related to consumption by the retail private sector [16].

The study included a small, convenience sample of pharmacies and the results of the study cannot be generalized to the situation in Peru. However, when the data were compared to DIGEMID reports, which are performed at the national level, the results did not differ greatly.

The present study could not measure directly if the availability of anti-infectives decreased after the FTA and NDP at the retail level. Although, the low proportion of new registrations in stock could mean that the availability of anti-infectives has been affected. Further studies could assess the effect of the FTA on the prices of medicines. It maybe still early to assess the impact of data exclusivity on the access to generics; a previous study concluded that 10 years are reasonable to measure the effect on prices and access of such medicines [22].

Conclusions and Recommendations

This study found that the number of new registrations and re-registrations of anti-infectives dropped considerably after the implementation of the NDP in 2009. This drop is related to the longer time required for registration, the bioavailability and bioequivalence requirements, the GMP certificate requirement, and the first lot quality control defined by the NDP after the signing of the FTA.

The new regulation may affect the number of new registrations and the availability of affordable anti-infectives, and may also increase the safety, efficacy and quality of marketed medicines.

The following recommendation should be taken into consideration by the Peruvian government:

- FTAs may provide opportunities for changes in regulatory systems and improving the safety, efficacy and quality of medicines. Regulatory changes may occur without external changes, however, it may be difficult to reach a consensus with the pharmaceutical market stakeholders.
- Reducing the barriers to market competition, including IP regulation, should be one of the goals of the NDP. Negotiation of future FTAs should prioritize access to high quality affordable medicines.
- There is a need for implementing a comprehensive Generic Drug Policy, as part of the NDP, and inform the public how the new regulations will improve the safety, efficacy and quality of generics. It is important that prescribers and patients understand these changes and increase their trust on generics.
- Reinforce monitoring and surveillance of retail pharmacies to control the quality of drugs marketed in the country. Pharmacy surveillance must also assess the existence of the pharmacy license, the presence of the pharmacist, and the compliance with the prescription-only requirement for anti-infectives and other drugs.

Abbreviations

APIs: Active pharmaceutical ingredients; ATC: Anatomic Therapeutic Chemical; DIGEMID: (Dirección General de Medicamentos, Insumos y Drogas): Peruvian Drug Regulatory Authority; FTA: Free Trade Agreement; GMP: Good Manufacturing Practice; HIV: Human Immunodeficiency Virus; HRS: High Regulatory Surveillance; IP: Intellectual Property; MoH: Ministry of Health; NDP: National Drug Policy; NISS: National Institute of Social Security; TU: Taxation Unit; US: United States; VAT: Value-added Tax

Acknowledgements

The authors thank Dr. Cesar M. Amaro, former director of the Peruvian Drug Regulatory Agency (DIGEMID), for his unconditional help providing the database used in this study. We would also like to thank Dr. Enrique Seoane-Vazquez for his revision of the manuscript.

Authors' contributions

LA analysed and interpreted the data, sampled the data for the case study, and was a major contributor in writing the manuscript. The author read and approved the final manuscript. MM made substantial contributions to the conception and design of the work; and revised the work critically for important intellectual content. Both author read and approved the final version to be published.

Competing interests

The authors declare that they have no competing interests.

Author details

[1]Pharmaceutical Business and Administrative Sciences, MCPHS University, 179 Longwood Avenue, Boston, MA 02115, USA. [2]School of Pharmacy, MCPHS University, 179 Longwood Avenue, Boston, MA, USA.

References

1. Arnold P J, Reeves TC. Global trade and the future of national health care reform. Account Forum. 2006. https://doi.org/10.1016/j.accfor.2006.08.002.
2. Hayakawa K, Fukunari K. How much do free trade agreements reduce impediments to trade? Open Econ Rev.2014. https://doi.org/10.1007/s11079-014-9332-x.
3. Correa CM. Implications of bilateral free trade agreements on access to medicines. Bull World Health Organ. 2006;84(5):399–404.
4. Lopert R, Gleeson D. The high price of "free" trade: U.S. trade agreements and access to medicines. J L Med Ethics. 2013;41(1):199–223.
5. Stiglitz JE. Trade agreements and health in developing countries. Lancet. 2009;373(9661):363–5.
6. Office of the US Trade Representative. Peru trade promotion agreement. Executive office of the president U.S. Government. 2007. http://www.ustr.gov/trade-agreements/free-trade-agreements/peru-tpa. Accessed 16 Apr 2016.
7. Rangel BC. A new trade policy for America. In T. P. Stewart (Ed.). Opportunities and obligations: New perspectives on global and US trade policy. 2009. p. 295.
8. Roca S. Public health and intellectual property in the US-Peru TPA: Incredible but true: very few of the amendments introduced by US congressional democrats to the IP chapter of the US-Peru trade promotion agreement have been implemented by the Peruvian government. Bridges news. International Centre for Trade and Sustainable Development (ICTSD). 2009;13 Number 2. http://www.ictsd.org/bridges-news/bridges/news/21-public-health-and-intellectual-property-in-the-us-peru-tpa-incredible. Accessed 9 Feb 2015.
9. Law amending, incorporating and regulating miscellaneous provisions on the implementation of the trade promotion agreement signed between Peru and the United States. [Ley que modifica, incorpora y regula diversas disposiciones a fin de implementar el acuerdo de promoción comercial suscrito entre el Perú y los Estados Unidos]. No. 29316. Congreso de la República, Lima, Perú. 2009.
10. General Health Law. [Ley General de Salud]. No. 26842. Congreso de la República, Lima, Perú. 1997.
11. Regulation of article 50 of Law 26842, General Health Law. [Reglamento del artículo 50 de la Ley 26842, Ley General de Salud]. Supreme Decree 001-2009-SA. Congreso de la República, Lima, Perú. 2009.
12. Ministerio de Salud del Perú. Rapid evaluation -with indicators- of the national pharmaceutical situation. [Evaluación rápida – con indicadores - de la situación farmacéutica nacional]. MINSA, PAHO. 2005. No. 016.
13. Regulation of the registration, control and vigilance of pharmaceutical products, medical devices and sanitary products. [Reglamento para el registro, control y vigilancia de productos farmacéuticos, dispositivos médicos y productos sanitarios]. Supreme Decree 016-2011-SA. Congreso de la República, Lima, Perú. 2011.
14. Law of pharmaceutical products, medical devices and sanitary products. [Ley de productos farmacéuticos, dispositivos médicos y productos sanitarios]. No. 29459. Congreso de la República, Lima, Perú. 2009.
15. Arroyo J, Hartz J, Lau M. Human resources in health by 2011: Evidence for the decision making. [Recursos humanos en salud al 2011: Evidencias para la toma de decisiones]. Dirección General de Gestión del Desarrollo de Recursos Humanos. Lima: Ministerio de Salud. Serie Bibliográfica Recursos Humanos en Salud. 2011;14:116.
16. Coronado J, Espinoza J. Competition issues in the distribution of pharmaceuticals. Paris: Contribution from Peru. Proceedings of the Global Forum on Competition. Organization for Economic Co-Operation and Development. Directorate for financial and enterprise affairs competition committee; 2014. http://www.oecd.org/officialdocuments/publicdisplaydocumentpdf/?cote=DAF/COMP/GF/WD%282014%2922&docLanguage=En. Accessed 23 Feb 2015.
17. WHO Collaborating Centre for Drug Statistics Methodology Norwegian Institute of Public Health. ATC/DDD index. http://www.whocc.no/atc_ddd_index/ (2013). Accessed 15 Feb 2014.
18. Robles Chávez M, Ramírez Ramírez R. Province and district poverty map. the poverty monetary approach. [Mapa de pobreza distrital y provincial. El enfoque de la pobreza monetaria]. Survey Report. Lima- Perú: Instituto Nacional de Estadística e Informática (INEI). (Dirección Técnica de Demografía e Indicadores Sociales). 2009. https://www.mef.gob.pe/contenidos/pol_econ/documentos/Mapa_Pobreza_2007.pdf. Accessed 13 Nov 2014.
19. Dávila S, De la Cruz J, Salgado V, Serna L. Identification of provisions of the public administration that affect the private investment in the trade sector: Health, cosmetics and sanitary products. [Identificación de disposiciones de la administración pública que afectarían a la inversión privada en el sector comercio: Productos de salud, cosméticos e higiene]. Observatorio de Disposiciones de la Administración Pública que Afectarían a la Inversión Privada. Gerencia de Estudios Económicos. 2013. INDECOPI, 1.
20. Macdonald G. Peru's GMP requirements mean delayed approvals, says expert. In-Pharma Technologies, Dispatches from AAPS. 2012. https://www.in-pharmatechnologist.com/Article/2012/10/16/Peru-srequirement-for-Peruvian-GMP-certs-causing-delays. Accessed 23 Feb 2015.
21. Villar López RA. Republic of Peru, pharmaceutical country profile. In: Peruvian Minister of Health and Pan American Health Organization/World Health Organization (PAHO/WHO). 2012. http://apps.who.int/medicinedocs/documents/s19825en/s19825en.pdf. Accessed 15 Jan 2015.
22. Cortés Gamba ME, Rossi Buenaventura F, Vásquez Serrano MD. Ten years impact of data protection in medicines in Colombia. [Impacto de 10 años de protección de datos en medicamentos en Colombia]. Serie buscando remedio 2. IFARMA, Fundación Misión Salud. 2012. 978–958–57014-1-0.
23. Abbott RB, Bader R, Bajjali L, Abu ElSamen T, Obeidat T, Sboul H, et al. The price of medicines in Jordan: the cost of trade-based intellectual property. J Generic Med. 2013;9(2):75–85.
24. Malpani R. All costs, no benefits: how TRIPS-plus intellectual property rules in the US-Jordan FTA affect access to medicines. Oxfam International. 2007. https://policy-practice.oxfam.org.uk/publications/all-costs-no-benefits-how-trips-plus-intellectual-property-rules-in-the-us-jord-114080. Accessed 22 Jun 2017.
25. Seinfeld J, La Serna C. Why shouldn't data protection be an impediment to sign the US FTA? [Porque la protección de los datos de prueba en el mercado farmacéutico no debe ser un impedimento para firmar el TLC con los EEUU?]. Report (Documento de Discusión). Lima: Universidad del Pacifico; 2005.
26. Araujo L. Effect of the 2009 US-Peru free trade agreement on Peruvian new drug policies and the registration and quality of pharmaceutical products. In: Unpublished dissertation. Boston: MCPHS University, pharmacy school; 2015.
27. Dirección General de Medicamentos, Insumos y Drogas (DIGEMID). New medicines-new molecular entities with license and data protection u other safety and efficacy data not disclosed. [Medicamentos nuevos - nuevas entidades químicas con registro sanitario y protección de datos de prueba u otros datos sobre seguridad y eficacia no divulgados]. (Updated table Oct 2017). Ministerio de Salud, Lima, Perú 2018.
28. Kanavos P, Costa-Font J, Seeley E. Competition in off-patent drug markets: issues, regulation and evidence. Econ Policy. 2008;23:499–544.

29. Bertoldi AD, Helfer AP, Camargo AL, Tavares NU, Kanavos P. Is the Brazilian pharmaceutical policy ensuring population access to essential medicines? Glob Health. 2012;8:6.

30. Villarán R, Richter R. Pharmaceutical industry: Vitamin for the world economy. [Industria farmacéutica: Vitamina para la economía mundial]. Revista Trimestral de las Cámaras Alemanas en Perú y Bolivia "Made in Germany". 2012. http://www.camara-alemana.org.pe/publicaciones/migediciones/2012MIG-MARZO-MAYO.pdf. Accessed 23 Nov 2014.

31. Dirección Regional de Salud (DIRESA). Prescription and use of antimicrobials evaluation study in ambulatory care at hospitals of the regional health directory-Lima. [Estudio sobre la evaluación de la prescripción, uso de antimicrobianos en la consulta ambulatoria a nivel de los hospitales de la dirección regional de salud Lima]. Dirección Regional de Salud, Lima, Perú. 2012. http://www.digemid.minsa.gob.pe/UpLoad/UpLoaded/PDF/Publicaciones/URM/P22_2012-06-07_Estudio_Lima.pdf. Accessed 23 Jan 2015.

32. Crisante Nunez M. Situation of the medicines in Peru. [Situación de las medicinas en Perú]. [PowerPoint slides]. Minsa-Digemid, Lima-Peru. 2012. http://www2.congreso.gob.pe/sicr/cendocbib/con4_uibd.nsf/5A5BAF742D4D837C05257BE9006DF120/$FILE/Potencias_01-Situacion_medicamentos_Peru.pdf. Accessed 24 Nov 2014.

2

Evaluating availability and price of essential medicines in Boston area (Massachusetts, USA) using WHO/HAI methodology

Abhishek Sharma[1,2,3], Lindsey Rorden[1], Margaret Ewen[4] and Richard Laing[1*] ⓘD

Abstract

Background: Many patients even those with health insurance pay out-of-pocket for medicines. We investigated the availability and prices of essential medicines in the Boston area.

Methods: Using the WHO/HAI methodology, availability and undiscounted price data for both originator brand (OB) and lowest price generic (LPG) equivalent versions of 25 essential medicines (14 prescription; 11 over-the-counter (OTC)) were obtained from 17 private pharmacies. The inclusion and prices of 26 essential medicines in seven pharmacy discount programs were also studied. The medicine prices were compared with international reference prices (IRPs).

Results: In surveyed pharmacies, the OB medicines were less available as compared to the generics. The OB and LPG versions of OTC medicines were 21.33 and 11.53 times the IRP, respectively. The median prices of prescription medicines were higher, with OB and LPG versions at 158.14 and 38.03 times the IRP, respectively. In studied pharmacy discount programs, the price ratios of surveyed medicines varied from 4.4–13.9.

Conclusions: While noting the WHO target that consumers should pay no more than four times the IRPs, medicine prices were considerably higher in the Boston area. The prices for medicines included in the pharmacy discount programs were closest to WHO's target. Consumers should shop around, as medicine inclusion and prices vary across discount programs. In order for consumers to identify meaningful potential savings through comparison shopping, price transparency is needed.

Background

Lack of regular access to essential medicines remains a major public health concern globally. Essential medicines are identified by the World Health Organization (WHO) as those medicines which meet the global health needs of the majority population. The WHO Model Essential Medicines List is updated every two years in a transparent process [1]. While access has improved considerably since the introduction of the essential medicines concept in 1977, one-third of the world's population is still not treated with the needed medicines [2–5]. Millar et al highlighted the potential value of using the WHO Model Essential Medicines List to reduce costs and provide more equitable access to low-income patients in the United States (US) [2].

In low- and middle-income countries (LMICs), as many as 90 % of the population pay out-of-pocket (OOP) for their medicines [3, 6]. The US has also seen a shift towards high-deductible insurance plans, within the last decade. The majority (78 %) of plans, covering medical procedures and prescription medicines, now have a general deductible (the amount that must be paid OOP before an insurer will pay any expenses), half of which are over $1,000 [7]. Low medicine availability, high prices and poor affordability are key barriers to medicine access [5, 8–12]. In many high-income countries including the US, there are growing concerns about reduced medicine access for reasons including high medicine prices and copayments/deductibles, uninsured populations, lack of transparency in medicine price components, and health agencies' poor ability to negotiate procurement prices [13–17].

In 2001, a resolution (WHA 54.11) endorsed by the Member States of the World Health Assembly called for

* Correspondence: richardl@bu.edu
[1]Department of Global Health, Boston University School of Public Health, Boston, MA, USA
Full list of author information is available at the end of the article

a standardized methodology to monitor medicines prices to help improve access [18]. In response, the World Health Organization/Health Action International (WHO/HAI) Project on Medicine Prices and Availability was established. The primary aim of this project was to develop a standardized method to measure medicines' prices, availability, affordability and price components in a reproducible way so as to allow international comparisons over time. In 2003, after testing in nine countries, the standard WHO/HAI methodology was released, with a second edition published in 2008 [19]. To assess the surveyed medicines' consumer prices, WHO/HAI methodology employs international reference prices (IRPs) as an external benchmark. To measure prices, a median price ratio (MPR) is calculated by comparing the median consumer price of a given medicine with the respective IRP. International reference prices used in this survey were taken from the 2013 Management Sciences for Health (MSH) International Drug Price Indicator Guide [20]. The MSH reference prices, first published in 1986, are procurement prices obtained from both sellers and buyers and collected from government agencies, pharmaceutical suppliers, and international development organizations. The MSH prices are widely accepted as an appropriate reference standard [9]. These MSH procurement prices report the actual prices obtained by non-profit suppliers and government tenders (see Additional file 1: List of price sources for 2013 MSH Drug Price Indicator Guide), the robust nature of this data ensures international comparability. Governments should be procuring medicines on the international market at close to IRPs. But patient prices in the private sector have to take into account additional costs in the pharmaceutical supply chain (markups, tariffs, taxes and other costs). Because of these additional costs, WHO has set a target of four times the IRP for patient prices in the private sector. Recognizing medicine availability and prices as important components of access, the WHO medium term strategic plan 2008–2013 defines global and national targets for generic essential medicines, targeting 80 % availability in all sectors and median consumer prices to be no more than four times the IRP [21].

The WHO/HAI Project has been successful in developing a standard method for measuring price, availability, and affordability of essential medicines. As of 2014, more than 100 surveys had been conducted across the world, highlighting variations in medicine availability and prices by region, therapeutic category, and sector [9, 22]. The surveys provide transparency in price and availability reporting and inform medicines procurement globally.

In 2009, Cameron et al reported on medicine availability and prices in 36 developing and middle- income countries [9]. A key finding was that in the private sector the average MPR of originator brands (OB) by economic region

varied from 13.8 to 40.9. For generic medicines, the average MPR by economic region varied from 9.8 to 11. The price ratios were adjusted for purchasing power parity.

In 2012, the US accounted for 35 % of the global spending on medicines [23]. Americans face a high burden of medicine expenditure owing to a combination of unregulated prices and high OOP expenditures: an average per-capita OOP spending of USD 758 on medicines in 2012 [24]. In 2014, an estimated 22 % of the patients did not fill a prescription or skipped prescription doses because of the cost [25]. Patients who are uninsured, elderly, low income, or with high insurance copays are disproportionately unlikely to fill their prescriptions [17]. Therefore, concerns about medicine access, especially due to high prices, persist in the US.

There is a widespread perception that generic medicines, which now represent 86 % of US prescriptions [7], are available at competitive prices. While generics are cheaper than the OB, the nature of generic price competition in the United States sometimes leads to aberrations such as unexpected price hikes. For instance, the price of daily average dose of albendazole, an older broad spectrum anti-parasitic medicine, rose from USD 5.92 in 2010 to USD 11.96 in 2013, while it is less than USD 1 in many countries [5].

Consumer Reports regularly investigates the availability and prices of a limited number of generic medicines across various pharmacy options available to consumers in the US [24, 26–28]. They also compare the OB and generic medicines across chain and independent pharmacies, but do not compare consumer prices to the IRP.

In the relative absence of surveys of the actual prices paid by consumers for prescription medicines in the US, we believe our initial survey in the Boston area can indicate whether the WHO/HAI methodology would be applicable, and allow comparisons with the studies undertaken by Consumer Reports. Medicines included in this survey are used globally, treat common conditions, and appear on most US treatment guidelines. Many of the surveyed medicines were included in the 2009 study of medicine availability and prices in 36 developing and middle-income countries [9].

Our Boston study investigated prices and availability of OB and generic essential medicines across chain, independent, big-box retail stores, and in-store supermarket pharmacies. Prices were obtained for both generic and OB products, and were then compared with the MSH IRPs. To our knowledge, there are no peer-reviewed studies assessing the availability and prices of OB and generic medicines in the US using the WHO/HAI methodology.

Methods

A modified version of the WHO/HAI methodology was employed. A typical WHO/HAI survey collects data on availability and prices of a specified list of essential medicines plus supplementary medicines chosen by the investigator, and uses a standardized sampling frame including public-sector health facilities and registered private-sector retail pharmacies along with any other sector such as nongovernmental or mission hospitals. Since the US lacks public sector distribution of medicines, we analyzed the availability and prices of 25 essential medicines in a representative sample of private-sector retail pharmacies (chain and independent) and 26 essential medicines offered by private-sector pharmacy and pharmacy discount programs in the Boston area. Data on some additional medicines were collected to provide a more robust sample of discount schemes. The WHO/HAI methodology also assesses the affordability of medicines, expressed as the number of day's wages required by the lowest paid unskilled government worker to purchase a month's supply of medicines for chronic conditions and a weeks' supply for acute conditions. Accurately identifying the wage of a government worker in the Boston area is difficult hence affordability was not assessed.

Sampling
Survey facilities
A list of currently licensed retail pharmacies (chain and independent) in zip codes within the cities of Boston, Cambridge, and Brookline was obtained from the Massachusetts Health Care Safety and Quality website [29]. Systematic random sampling was employed to select 10 chain pharmacies from this list. Each was then matched to an independent pharmacy in close proximity, resulting in a total survey sample of 20 pharmacies. This study also included a sample of seven pharmacy discount programs offered by big-box retail stores as well as in-store or freestanding pharmacies, including Walmart/Sam's Club, Target, Hannaford, Walgreens, CVS, and Jewel-Osco. These programs offer a selection of medicines usually at prices of $4 per month or $10 for three months. These programs were selected using nonprobability, convenience sampling and the price data were collected, using public online sources, for the surveyed medicines in these programs. See Additional file 1: Survey facilities random sampling (methods) for further details.

Survey medicines
For the facility survey, 14 prescription medicines were selected from the WHO/HAI global core medicines list, and 11 commonly-used over-the-counter (OTC) medicines. The survey basket for the pharmacy discount programs consisted of 26 medicines identified from WHO/HAI global and regional (Latin America and the Caribbean) core medicine lists [3, 10]. All medicines were strength and dosage-form specific. Table 1 lists the survey medicines. There were 14 medicines common to both pharmacy facility and discount program surveys.

All surveyed medicines are commonly used and have an available IRP [9].

Data collection, entry, cleaning, and analysis
After prior notification, the data collectors (Master of Public Health (MPH) students undertaking practical fieldwork) visited the selected pharmacy facilities and identified themselves during October 2014. The data collectors obtained information, by physically inspecting the availability (in-stock) of the OB medicines and their generic equivalents on the day of survey. The data collectors also obtained information on the undiscounted retail prices of the OB and the lowest price generics (LPG) versions of the survey medicines using a standardized form developed by the WHO/HAI. These prices reflect the amount in US dollars that a patient without any health insurance or special medicine plan would pay to purchase a given medicine.

For the pharmacy discount programs, price data were obtained from public online sources during November 2014 (see Additional file 1: Pharmacy discount program analysis (methods)). The medicine unit prices collected from the facility survey were entered into the Excel-based WHO/HAI Medicine Prices Workbook, followed by double entry, automated and manual error-checking, and built-in automated analysis feature of the workbook [19]. The pharmacy discount program data were entered and analyzed using MS Excel. The facility survey workbooks have been submitted to HAI and will be posted on the HAI online price and availability database http://haiweb.org/what-we-do/price-availability-affordability/.

In the case of the facility survey, medicine availability is reported as the mean percentage of the retail pharmacies (overall and stratified by chain and independent) where a given medicine was found. To facilitate international comparisons, medicine-specific median price ratios (MPR) were calculated when prices were available from at least four facilities. The MPR refers to the ratio of a medicine's local median unit price (across pharmacies) as compared to the 2013 MSH international median unit reference price [19, 20].

To summarize the MPRs of OB and LPG medicines, we performed 'all medicines' and 'matched pair' MPR analyses, overall and by pharmacy-type. While the 'all medicines' analysis considers all the available MPRs for each survey medicine, the 'matched pair' analysis considers the available MPRs for only those survey medicines which existed in OB-LPG pairs. Using statistical software SAS version 9.3, we conducted hypothesis testing to see if availability and prices varied among pharmacies at alpha significance of 0.05 (marginal significance if p-value between 0.05–0.06) (See Additional file 1: Statistical analysis: facility medicine availability and prices (results)).

Table 1 List of medicines surveyed

Medicines	Strength	Dosage form/Unit	Pack size (recommended)[a]	Originator Brand
A. Over-the-counter medicines				
Acetaminophen/Paracetamol	325 mg	Tab/cap	100	Tylenol (McNeil)
Acetylsalicylic Acid	500 mg	Tab/cap	100	Asprin (Bayer)
Cimetidine	200 mg	Tab/cap	30	Tagamet (GSK)
Clotrimazole vaginal cream	1 %	Gram	24	Clotrimin (MSD)
Diphenhydramine HCl	25 mg	Tab/cap	100	Benadryl (McNeil)
Hydrocortisone topical cream	1 %	Gram	51	–
Ibuprofen	200 mg	Tab/cap	200	Advil (Pfizer)
Loratadine	10 mg	Tab/cap	30	Claritin (MSD)
Miconazole Nitrate topical cream	2 %	Gram	9	Monistat (McNeil)
Omeprazole	20 mg	Tab/cap	42	Prilosec (AstraZeneca)
Ranitidine	150 mg	Tab/cap	80	Zantac (Boehringer)
B. Prescription medicines				
Amitriptyline	25 mg	Tab/cap	100	Tryptizol (MSD)
Amoxicillin	500 mg	Tab/cap	21	Amoxil (GSK)
Atenolol	50 mg	Tab/cap	60	Tenormin (AstraZeneca)
Captopril	25 mg	Tab/cap	60	Capoten (BMS)
Ceftriaxone injection	1 g/vial	Vial	1	Rocephin (Roche)
Ciprofloxacin	500 mg	Tab/cap	10	Ciproxin (Bayer)
Co-trimoxazole suspension	8 + 40 mg/ml	Gram	100	Bactrim (Roche)
Diazepam	5 mg	Tab/cap	100	Valium (Roche)
Diclofenac	50 mg	Tab/cap	100	Voltarol (Novartis)
Glibenclamide	5 mg	Tab/cap	60	Daonil (Sanofi-Aventis)
Omeprazole	20 mg	Tab/cap	30	Losec (AstraZeneca)
Paracetamol (Acetaminophen)	24 mg/ml	Milliliter	60	Panadol (GSK)
Salbutamol inhaler	100 mcg/dose	Dose	200	Ventoline (GSK)
Simvastatin	20 mg	Tab/cap	30	Zocor (MSD)
C. Pharmacy discount program medicines				
Acute medicines				
Amoxicillin[b]	500 mg	Tab/cap	30	Amoxil (GSK)
Amoxicillin suspension	250 mg/5 ml	Milliliters	150 ml	Amoxil (GSK)
Azithromycin	500 mg	Tab/cap	3	Zithromax (Pfizer)
Ceftriaxone Injection[b]	1 g/vial	Vial	1	Rocephin (Roche)
Ciprofloxacin[b]	500 mg	Tab/cap	20	Ciproxin (Bayer)
Clotrimazole topical cream[b]	1 %	Gram	15 gram tube	Canesten (Bayer)
Diclofenac[b]	50 mg	Tab/cap	60	Voltarol (Novartis)
Furosemide	40 mg	Tab/cap	30	Lasix (Sanofi-Aventis)
Hydrochlorothiazide	25 mg	Tab/cap	30	Dichlotride (MSD)
Ibuprofen[b]	400 mg	Tab/cap	90	Brufen (Knoll)
Metronidazole	500 mg	Tab/cap	14	Flagyl (Sanofi-Aventis)
Omeprazole[b]	20 mg	Tab/cap	30	Prilosec (AstraZeneca)
Ranitidine[b]	150 mg	Tab/cap	60	Zantac (GSK)
Chronic medicines				
Amitriptyline[b]	25 mg	Tab/cap	90	Tryptizol (MSD)

Table 1 List of medicines surveyed *(Continued)*

Amlodipine	5 mg	Tab/cap	90	Norvasc (Pfizer)
Atenolol[b]	50 mg	Tab/cap	90	Tenormin (AstraZeneca)
Atorvastatin	10 mg	Tab/cap	90	Lipitor (Pfizer)
Captopril[b]	25 mg	Tab/cap	180	Capoten (BMS)
Clonazepam	2 mg	Tab/cap	90	Rivotril (Roche)
Diazepam[b]	5 mg	Tab/cap	90	Valium (Roche)
Enalapril	10 mg	Tab/cap	90	Renitec (MSD)
Fluoxetine	20 mg	Tab/cap	90	Prozac (Eli Lilly)
Glibenclamide[b]	5 mg	Tab/cap	90	Daonil (Sanofi-Aventis)
Metformin	850 mg	Tab/cap	180	Glucophage (BMS)
Phenytoin	50 mg	Tab/cap	90	Epanutin (Pfizer)
Simvastatin[b]	20 mg	Tab/cap	90	Zocor (MSD)

[a]For facility surveys (Table 1a-b), data collectors were instructed to obtain information for these medicine pack sizes (number of units). If not available, the information for the size immediately larger was collected
[b]Medicines common to both the pharmacy survey and pharmacy discount scheme surveys

For each of the pharmacy discount programs, medicine availability is reported as the percentage of the medicines included in pharmacy discount programs survey basket (See Table 1c) which were included in a given program. Furthermore, we calculated medicine-specific 'price ratio' using the following formula:

$$Price\ Ratio = \frac{Discount\ program\ unit\ price\ (USD)}{MSH\ median\ unit\ international\ reference\ price\ (USD)}$$

Results

The surveyed facilities varied in size, ranging from 720 to over 30,000 square feet. The space for pharmacy services including dispensing and products ranged in size from as much as 216 feet of shelf space for OTCs to no OTC shelving at all. Of the total 20 pharmacies sampled, data on OTC medicines were obtained from 17 pharmacies (10 chain; 7 independent). Only 14 pharmacies (8 chain; 6 independent) provided data on the prescription medicines. Pharmacy staff's busy schedules or unwillingness to cooperate appeared to be the main reasons for the sample drop-outs in the case of prescription

medicines. However, some independent pharmacies even refused to allow the collection of the OTC medicines information, which they referred to as "proprietary information".

Facility survey: availability of surveyed medicines

Table 2 summarizes the availability of OTC and prescription medicines, stratified by OB and generic equivalents, in chain and independent pharmacies. In general, the overall availability of OTC medicines was higher than the prescription medicines. The OB medicines were less available (prescription: 42.3 %; OTC: 73.8 %) as compared to the generic equivalents (prescription: 78.6 %; OTC: 85.6 %). However, this difference was statistically significant for prescription medicines only. The originator version of omeprazole was available in only 50 % of facilities; however the generic was available in 93 % of facilities. The OB version of OTC medicine clotrimazole, which was not available in any of the surveyed facilities, only had availability as generic in 58.8 % of facilities.

Table 2 Mean percentage availability of surveyed medicines in retail pharmacies

	Prescription medicines		Over-the-counter medicines	
	Originator Brand % (number of pharmacies)	Generic % (number of pharmacies)	Originator Brand % (number of pharmacies)	Generic % (number of pharmacies)
Chain	52.7 % ($n = 8$)	78.6 % ($n = 8$)	80.9 % ($n = 10$)	94.5 % ($n = 10$)
Independent	28.6 % ($n = 6$)	76.6 % ($n = 6$)	63.6 % ($n = 7$)	72.7 % ($n = 7$)
Overall	42.3 % ($n = 14$)	78.6 % ($n = 14$)	73.8 % ($n = 17$)	85.6 % ($n = 17$)

Overall mean availability of originator brand (OB) and generic equivalent (GE) versions of over-the counter (OTC) medicines is not statistically different (p-value = 0.24). However, the overall mean availability of OB and GE versions of prescription medicines is statistically different (p-value < 0.001). Availability of OB and GE versions of matched pairs was not statistically different (p-value > 0.05) from each other for neither OTC nor prescription medicines, in both chain and independent pharmacies. Mean availability of GE of OTC medicines was statistically different (p-value = 0.01) in chain and independent pharmacies. There was no statistically significant difference (p-value = 1.0) in mean availability of GE of prescription medicines among chain and independent pharmacies. The mean availability of OB version were statistically different among chain and independent pharmacies, in case of both OTC (p-value = 0.001) and prescription (p-value < 0.001) medicines

For prescription medicines, the availability of generic equivalents was similar (p-value = 1.00) among the chain (78.6 %) and independent pharmacies (76.6 %). However, the OB prescription medicines were relatively less available (p-value < 0.001) in independent pharmacies (28.6 %) as compared to the chain counterparts (52.7 %).

In the case of OTC medicines, both the OB and generic equivalent medicines were statistically (p-value = 0.01) more available in chain pharmacies (80.9 and 94.5 %, respectively) as compared to those in independent pharmacies (63.6 and 72.7 %, respectively). See Additional file 1: Tables S1–S4.

Facility survey: price of surveyed medicines
Over-the-counter medicines
Table 3 summarizes the MPRs of the surveyed OTC medicines. Overall, across all medicines in the analysis (Table 3a), the OB and LPG versions of surveyed OTC medicines were priced 21.33 (range: 11.41–41.24) and 11.53 (2.68–29.42) times the IRPs, respectively. Cimetidine had the highest MPR among both the OB (MPR: 41.24) and LPG medicines (MPR: 29.42). Loratadine and clotrimazole had the lowest MPRs among the OB and LPG medicines, which were 11.41 and 2.68 respectively.

The analysis of matched pairs (Table 3b) showed that overall the OB and LPG versions of the same products were priced 21.33 and 14.56 times the IRP respectively. The median price premium for OB versions was 46.5 % (range: 23.4–133.8 %) over the LPG price. In the case of both chain and independent pharmacies, the median MPRs of the OB were statistically higher (chain p-value = 0.008; independent p-value = 0.03) than that of the LPG medicines.

Across all medicines in the analysis, the unit price of OB medicines was 15.7 % higher in chain pharmacies than in independent pharmacies. The price of LPG medicines was 22.3 % higher in chain pharmacies than in independents. In the matched pairs analysis, the median MPRs of both OB and LPG versions of OTC medicines were higher in chain pharmacies as compared to independent pharmacies, however, the differences were not statistically significant (OB p-value = 0.81; LPG p-value = 0.20). Also see Additional file 1: Tables S5 and S7.

Prescription medicines
Across 'all medicines' (Table 4a), the OB and LPG versions of prescription medicines were 158.14 (range: 16.43–655.09) and 38.03 (12.52–155.46) times, respectively, the IRPs. Considering LPG versions, the median MPR in chain pharmacies (39.54) was higher than that in independent pharmacies (31.28), though this difference was not statistically significant (p-value = 0.31). In contrast, the median MPR for OB versions was higher in independent pharmacies (188.56) than in chain pharmacies (180.29), however no significant difference was found (p-value = 0.86). Notably, the MPR was calculated for only three prescription medicines pairs in independent pharmacies due to low availability.

In 'matched pair' analysis (Table 4b), the median MPRs of the OB and LPG versions of prescription medicines were statistically different from each other, both overall and within chain pharmacies. The median OB price premium was 299.1 % over the LPG price, ranging to as high as 1943.2 % in case of diazepam. Also see Additional file 1: Tables S6 and S8.

Table 3 Summary of median price ratios (MPR) of the surveyed over-the-counter medicines in retail pharmacies

3(a). All Medicines analysis

	Overall		Chain Pharmacies		Independent Pharmacies	
	Originator Brand (medicines = 9)	Lowest Price Generic (medicines = 11)	Originator Brand (medicines = 9)	Lowest Price Generic (medicines = 11)	Originator Brand (medicines = 9)	Lowest Price Generic (medicines = 9)
Median MPR	21.33	11.53	20.81	11.53	17.98	9.43
Minimum, Maximum MPR	11.41, 41.24	2.68, 29.42	11.41, 143.13	2.68, 112.08	11.69, 37.27	2.55, 31.58

3(b). Matched pair analysis

	Originator Brand	Lowest Price Generic	Originator Brand	Lowest Price Generic	Originator Brand	Lowest Price Generic
	OB-LPG pairs = 9		OB-LPG pairs = 9		OB-LPG pairs = 8	
Median MPR	21.33	14.56	20.81	15.81	17.81	9.50
Minimum, Maximum MPR	11.41, 41.24	5.40, 29.42	11.41, 143.13	5.79, 112.08	11.69, 35.15	3.55, 31.58

In 'all medicines' analysis, the overall median MPRs for the originator brand (OB) and lowest price generic (LPG) versions of the over-the-counter (OTC) medicines were marginally different (p-value = 0.056). In chain pharmacies, the median MPRs of the OB and LPG versions were not statistically different (p-value = 0.11). Whereas in the independent pharmacies, the median MPRs of the OB and LPG were statistically different (p-value = 0.004). Furthermore, the median MPRs of the OB version of OTC medicine in chain pharmacy were not statistically different (p-value = 0.96) from that in the independent pharmacy. Similarly, the median MPRs of the LPG versions were marginally different (p-value = 0.503) among the chain and independent pharmacies.
In 'matched pair' analysis, the overall median MPRs of the OB and LPG versions of OTC medicines were statistically different (p-value = 0.03). Within both chain and independent pharmacies, the median MPRs of the OB and LPG versions of OTC medicines were statistically different (chain p-value = 0.008; independent p-value = 0.03) from each other

Table 4 Summary of median price ratios (MPR) of the surveyed prescription medicines in retail pharmacies

4(a). All Medicines analysis

	Overall		Chain Pharmacies		Independent Pharmacies	
	Originator Brand (medicines = 10)	Lowest Price Generic (medicines = 13)	Originator Brand (medicines = 8)	Lowest Price Generic (medicines = 12)	Originator Brand (medicines = 3)	Lowest Price Generic (medicines = 10)
Median MPR	158.14	38.03	180.29	39.54	188.56	31.28
Minimum, Maximum MPR	16.43, 655.09	12.52, 155.46	29.29, 663.30	19.15, 168.73	29.52, 655.09	5.37, 122.38

4(b). Matched pair analysis

	Overall		Chain Pharmacies	
	Originator Brand	Lowest Price Generic	Originator Brand	Lowest Price Generic
	OB-LPG pairs = 10		OB-LPG pairs = 8	
Median MPR	158.14	35.15	180.29	39.54
Minimum, Maximum MPR	16.43, 655.09	12.52, 98.57	29.29, 663.30	28.73, 115.79

In 'all medicines' analysis, overall median MPRs of originator brand (OB) and lowest price generic (LPG) versions of the prescription medicines were statistically different (p-value = 0.04). In chain pharmacies, the median MPRs of OB and LPG versions were statistically different (p-value < 0.05). Significance could not be calculated among independent pharmacies due to low availability of originator products.

In 'matched pair' analysis, too few pairs of sampled prescription medicines were available in independent pharmacies to make meaningful comparisons within such facilities. The overall median MPRs of the OB and LPG versions of prescription medicines were statistically different (p-value = 0.03), both overall and in case of chain pharmacies

Pharmacy discount programs

Inclusion

Table 5 summarizes medicine inclusion and prices in pharmacy discount programs. Among the seven pharmacy discount programs surveyed, the overall inclusion percentage of studied medicines was variable, ranging from 42.3 % (Walmart/Sam's Club and Target $4/$10 program) to 100 % (Target prescription saver program). Overall, acute medicines were more frequently included than chronic medicines, with a mean inclusion of 71.4 % compared to 60.2 %, respectively. All pharmacy discount programs had higher acute medicine inclusion than chronic, except for the higher-priced Target prescription saver program, where 100 % of surveyed acute and chronic medicines were included.

Prices

Table 5 shows that among the surveyed pharmacy discount programs, the median of the MPR in which the discount program prices were compared to IRPs for the acute and chronic medicines were found to be 8.3 (range: 4.4–16.3) and 5.0 (4.1–13.7), respectively. Walmart/Sam's Club and target $4/10 discount programs had the lowest overall MPR of the programs at 4.4 (range: 3.3–18.8), whereas Target Prescription saver had the highest MPR of the programs at 13.9 (range: 2.9–81.3). Also see Additional file 1: Table S9.

Limitations of the study

Despite the strengths of the WHO/HAI methodology, there are some limitations of this study. First, we assessed the availability and prices for a specific list of medicines and did not account for other strengths, dosage forms or therapeutic alternatives. Due to the low availability of OB prescription products in independent pharmacies, we were unable to undertake meaningful 'matched pair' analysis of all prices. All pharmacists reported it would take them less than 24 hours to obtain specific prescription medicines that were not available in-store. In the case of the pharmacy discount programs, we assessed if a medicine was included in a given program but did not assess the physical availability for dispensing at the respective pharmacies. Also, our analysis is based on the data collected on the day of survey and may not indicate availability and prices over time. In addition, we did not account for any discounts or insurance, which vary by patient. Lastly, the results of the facility study may not represent medicine availability and prices in other US states, however we provide an initial reference point for future studies to be conducted in North America.

Discussion

To our best knowledge, this is the first WHO/HAI study to assess the availability and prices of essential medicines in private-sector retail pharmacies in the US. The availability of medicines is often suboptimal around the globe, for medicines to treat both chronic and acute conditions [9]. An analysis of findings from price and availability surveys conducted in 36 developing and middle-income countries in 2009 found the average availability of generics was 64 % in the private sector. Availability was very low in some countries (e.g. Chad 14 %, Philippines 34 %, Shangdong province, China 35 %) but good in others (e.g. Syria 98 %, Chennai, India

Table 5 Inclusion and price ratio of studied medicines in the pharmacy discount program

Type of Medicine	Walmart/Sam's Club		Target Prescription Saver		Target $4/$10		Hannaford		Walgreens		CVS		Jewel-Osco		Overall/Summary	
	Inclusion (%)[a]	Price Ratio [median (min, max)][b]	Inclusion (%)[a]	Price Ratio [median (min, max)][b]	Inclusion (%)[a]	Price Ratio [median (min, max)][b]	Inclusion (%)[a]	Price Ratio [median (min, max)][b]	Inclusion (%)[a]	Price Ratio [median (min, max)][b]	Inclusion (%)[a]	Price Ratio [median (min, max)][b]	Inclusion (%)[a]	Price Ratio [median (min, max)][b]	Mean Inclusion (%)[a]	Median of Price Ratios [min, max]
Acute n = 12[c]	50.0 %	4.4 (3.3, 18.8)	100.0 %	16.1 (3.3, 70.7)	50.0 %	4.8 (3.3, 18.8)	100.0 %	16.3 (3.3, 74.3)	66.7 %	8.3 (4.4, 25.3)	58.3 %	13.3 (3.3, 46.7)	75.0 %	5.4 (3.5, 18.7)	71.4 %	8.3 (4.4, 16.3)
Chronic n = 14[c]	35.7 %	5.4 (3.3, 16.8)	100.0 %	15.0 (2.9, 81.3)	35.7 %	6.7 (3.3, 15.2)	92.9 %	5.4 (3.3, 70.1)	57.1 %	8.2 (2.5, 16.8)	50.0 %	6.5 (3.3, 20.2)	50.0 %	4.7 (3.3, 16.8)	60.2 %	5.0 (4.1, 13.7)
Overall Inclusion and Price Ratios [Median (min, max)] n = 26	42.3 %	4.4 (3.3, 18.8)	100.0 %	13.9 (2.9, 81.3)	42.3 %	4.4 (3.3, 18.8)	96.2 %	13.3 (1.4, 74.3)	61.5 %	8.2 (2.5, 25.3)	53.8 %	8.2 (3.3, 46.7)	61.5 %	5.3 (3.3, 18.7)		

[a] Inclusion refers to the percentage of total surveyed medicines offered by a given pharmacy discount program

[b] Compares median of the calculated price ratios to the MSH median unit reference price

[c] n refers to the total number of medicines surveyed for acute and chronic medicines, respectively

92 %). Price premiums paid for OBs compared to generics ranged from 152 % in the private sector in upper-middle income countries to over 300 % in low-income countries [9].

In our study, while few patients pay full list prices, assessing the actual prices paid was not possible given that discounts are highly variable and cannot be standardized. While it is possible to assess individual level prices paid using prescription claims data, this data does not include the population of interest, such as patients without health insurance (~33 million i.e. 10.4 % of people in the US in 2014) [30] and/or those who pay OOP. Furthermore, as mentioned earlier, more people are opting for high deductible insurance plans; the number increased from 11.4 million in 2011 to 15.5 million in 2013. Notably 49 % of these people were age 40 and over, an age group with expectedly higher healthcare and prescription needs [31].

Results of our survey show that overall availability was similar to WHO's target of 80 %, except for OB prescription medicines, which had lower availability, especially in independent pharmacies. This may be due to several factors, including independent pharmacies' ability to procure OB prescription medicines quickly, low demand for such products, as well as the consumer and insurer trend towards purchasing generics whenever possible. Notably, availability was assessed in an environment with a highly developed supply chain, where pharmacies routinely request and can avail less commonly prescribed medications within several hours from other sources as needed. In such cases, availability is not an absolute barrier to access. However, it can become a barrier to access when considering that some patients may not return to retrieve their medicines due to the inconvenience of returning. Furthermore, availability estimates reflect the market, reflecting difference in availability of OB medicines among chain and independent pharmacies. Mail-order pharmacies were not included in this study, however, they will impact the overall availability of medicines for patients. Our results were consistent with the Consumer Reports findings which showed substantial price variations across pharmacies, and that savings were realized when patients purchased certain generic medicines at big box-stores such as Walmart and Target and pharmacy discount programs, paying a discounted retail price [26–28].

While noting the WHO target that consumers should pay no more than four times the IRPs, we observed that medicine prices were high in the Boston area compared to IRPs. The OB and generic versions of OTC medicine prices in Boston area were as high as 21.33 and 14.56 times the MSH IRPs, respectively. The prices of prescription medicines were particularly high, with OB and generic versions at 158.14 (range 16.43–655.09) and

38.03 (12.52–155.46) times the IRP, respectively. These patient prices in Boston for the prescription medicines were very high when compared to the prices paid for the same 14 medicines in the private sector of some other high-income countries. A medicine price survey in Bahrain, undertaken in 2013 using the WHO/HAI methodology, showed that patients were paying 34.78 and 13.85 times IRPs for OBs and LPG respectively. In 2011 in Tatarstan Province in Russia, patients were paying 13.05 and 4.12 times IRPs for OB and LPG respectively. In 2010 in a high-income Caribbean country, patients were paying 61.44 and 17.33 times IRPs for OB and LPG respectively [22]. While the data was not adjusted for purchasing power parity, it is clear that patient prices in Boston were substantially higher than in these three countries.

Interestingly, the OTC medicines were cheaper in independent pharmacies than in chain pharmacies. Although the OB prescription medicines were higher priced in independent pharmacies, LPGs were higher priced in the chain pharmacies. A contributing factor may be the recent increased cost to register a generic medicine in the US [32].

While the prices obtained in this survey may seem high in relation to the IRPs, most patients receive insurance assistance or discounts from their health payer for prescription medicines (but not OTC medicines). For many of the prescription medicines surveyed, pharmacy discount programs are available. With the wide range in insurance assistance and discounts across health insurance plans and by product, consumers generally do not know what they will be expected to pay for a medicine when dispensed at the pharmacy using insurance. This lack of transparency can be disadvantageous for consumers. For uninsured patients, while it would be desirable to fill prescriptions through pharmacy discount programs, we don't know if they are directed to these programs. Consumer Reports suggests that this is not the case [26].

This survey has been conducted in an intensely medicalized and urban environment. It is not clear what the results would be in other settings. The Boston survey will be conducted annually using the same methods to evaluate trends in medicine availability and price over time. It would be of interest to have similar surveys repeated in other areas to compare results.

Prescribers in the US should encourage consumers to consider the pharmacy discount programs, which offer generic medicines at lower prices. Unlike the facilities, the prices of medicines in the pharmacy discount programs were much closer to WHO's target of four times the IRPs. Our analysis shows that the cheapest medicines, when not using insurance, are from the discount programs offered in big-box retail stores and in-store and free standing pharmacies. However, inclusion of a medicine in a given pharmacy discount program and the price offered varied across programs, providing a reason for consumers to shop around.

If the policy in the US is not to regulate medicine prices, but rather rely on retail price competition, then a transparent system is needed that allows consumers to easily check prescription medicine prices at different pharmacies in order to identify potential savings. These benefits will need to be balanced against the cost of membership fees and the challenges of travel to sites with discounted prices. Consumers must be empowered to choose facilities and payment options most beneficial to them, whether that's paying with insurance at a traditional pharmacy, or foregoing insurance co-payments and opting for discounted medicines through pharmacy discount programs or other options. However, such decisions cannot be made without transparent prices that allow for comparison. The current lack of transparency even extended to our survey where 6 pharmacies (4 independent and 2 chains) failed to provide full price information for the prescription medicines surveyed.

Conclusion

The responsibility for ensuring price transparency rests primarily with policy-makers. Comprehensive policies are needed that are legally binding. Consumers (as well as healthcare providers and others) must be able to easily access regularly updated medicine price information in order to make informed decisions about the treatments.

Competing interests
The authors declare that they have no competing interests.

Authors' contributions
RL conceived the study idea. AS, LR and ME, RL conducted the literature review and planned the survey. AS and LR conducted the data entry and analysis. AS performed the statistical tests and wrote the first draft of the manuscript. All authors participated in the interpretation of results, revised the manuscript to its final stages, and approved the final version of the manuscript. The views expressed in this article are of the authors and not necessarily of the institutions they represent.

Acknowledgements
We thank the Massachusetts Board of Pharmacy for assistance in providing the register of pharmacies in electronic format. We are grateful to all the Boston University MPH students including Stephen Kimatu (Northeastern University) who undertook data collection, all the pharmacists who provided the medicine price data, and the experts and reviewers who provided very useful comments.

Author details
[1]Department of Global Health, Boston University School of Public Health, Boston, MA, USA. [2]Center for Global Health and Development, Boston University School of Public Health, Boston, MA, USA. [3]Precision Health Economics, Boston, MA, USA. [4]Health Action International, Amsterdam, The Netherlands.

References
1. WHO Policy Perspectives on Medicines - The Selection of Essential Medicines. Geneva: World Health Organization; 2002. http://apps.who.int/medicinedocs/pdf/s2296e/s2296e.pdf. Accessed 13 Jan 2016.
2. Millar TP, Wong S, Odierna DH, Bero LA. Applying the essential medicines concept to US preferred drug lists. Am J Public Health. 2011;101(8):1444–8.
3. Equitable access to essential medicines: a framework for collective action. Geneva: World Health Organization; 2004. http://apps.who.int/iris/handle/10665/68571. Accessed 5 April 2015.
4. Bazargani YT, Ewen M, De Boer A, Leufkens HGM, Mantel-Teeuwisse AK. Essential medicines are more available than other medicines around the globe. PLoS One. 2014;9:1–7.
5. Alpern JD, Stauffer WM, Kesselheim AS. High-cost generic drugs — implications for patients. N Engl J Med. 2014;371:1859–62.
6. Lu Y, Hernandez P, Abegunde D, Edejer T. The World Medicines Situation 2011: Medicine Expenditures. Geneva: World Health Organization; 2011. http://apps.who.int/medicinedocs/documents/s18767en/s18767en.pdf. Accessed 28 Dec 2014.
7. Medicine use and shifting costs of healthcare. Parsippany: IMS Institute for Healthcare Informatics; 2014. http://www.imshealth.com/en/thought-leadership/ims-institute/reports/use-of-medicines-in-the-us-2013. Accessed 28 Dec 2014.
8. Steinbrook R. Closing the affordability gap for drugs in low-income countries. N Engl J Med. 2007;357:1996–9.
9. Cameron A, Ewen M, Ross-Degnan D, Ball D, Laing R. Medicine prices, availability, and affordability in 36 developing and middle-income countries: a secondary analysis. Lancet. 2009;373(9659):240–9.
10. Cameron A, Roubos I, Ewen M, Mantel-Teeuwisse AK, Leufkens HGM, Laing RO. Differences in the availability of medicines for chronic and acute conditions in the public and private sectors of developing countries. Bull World Health Organ. 2011;89:412–21.
11. Kapczynski A. Engineered in India-Patent Law 2.0. N Engl J Med. 2013;369:497–9.
12. Cameron A, Ewen M, Auton M. The World Medicines Situation 2011: Medicines prices, availability and affordability. Geneva: World Health Organization; 2011. http://www.who.int/medicines/areas/policy/world_medicines_situation/WMS_ch6_wPricing_v6.pdf. Accessed 26 Dec 2014.
13. Soumerai SB, Ross-Degnan D. Inadequate prescription-drug coverage for Medicare enrollees-a call to action. N Engl J Med. 1999;340:722–8.
14. Husereau D, Cameron CG. Value-Based Pricing of Pharmaceuticals in Canada: Opportunities to Expand the Role of Health Technology Assessment? Ottawa, Ontario: Canadian Health Services Research Foundation; 2011. http://www.cfhi-fcass.ca/Libraries/Commissioned_Research_Reports/Husereau-Dec2011-EN.sflb.ashx. Accessed 27 Dec 2014.
15. Schoen C, Osborn R, How SKH, Doty MM, Peugh J. In chronic condition: experiences of patients with complex health care needs, in eight countries, 2008. Health Aff. 2009;28(1):w1–16.
16. The new drug war: Hard pills to swallow. The Economist. http://www.economist.com/news/international/21592655-drug-firms-have-new-medicines-and-patients-are-desperate-them-arguments-over. Accessed 28 Dec 2014.
17. Steinman MA, Sands LP, Covinsky KE. Self-restriction of medications due to cost in seniors without prescription coverage: a national survey. J Gen Intern Med. 2001;16(12):793–9.
18. WHO medicines strategy. Geneva: World Health Organization; 2001. http://apps.who.int/medicinedocs/documents/s16336e/s16336e.pdf. Accessed 29 Dec 2014.
19. Measuring medicine prices, availability, affordability and price components 2nd Edition. Geneva: World Health Organization and Health Action International; 2008. http://www.who.int/medicines/areas/access/OMS_Medicine_prices.pdf. Accessed 5 Sept 2014.
20. International Drug Price Indicator Guide. Medford: Management Sciences for Health; 2013. http://erc.msh.org/mainpage.cfm?file=1.0.htm&module=DMP&language=English. Accessed 1 Oct 2014.
21. Medium-term strategic plan 2008–2013. Geneva: World Health Organization; 2008.

22. Medicine Prices, Availability, Affordability & Price Components. Amsterdam: Health Action International. http://haiweb.org/what-we-do/price-availability-affordability/price-availability-data/. Accessed 25 Jan 2015.

23. The Global Use of Medicines: Outlook through 2017. Parsippany: IMS Institute for Healthcare Informatics; 2013. http://www.imshealth.com/en/thought-leadership/ims-institute/reports/global-use-of-medicines-outlook-through-2017. Accessed 29 Dec 2014.

24. Same generic drug, many prices. Consumer Reports Magazine: May 2013. http://www.consumerreports.org/cro/magazine/2013/05/same-generic-drug-many-prices/index.htm. Accessed 10 Dec 2014.

25. Sarnak Do, Ryan J. How High-Need Patients Experience the Health Care System in Nine Countries. The Commonwealth Fund. 2016, pub. 1856, Vol 1. http://www.commonwealthfund.org/~/media/files/publications/issue-brief/2016/jan/1856_sarnak_high_need_patients_nine_countries_intl_brief_v3.pdf. Accessed 18 Mar 2016.

26. 8 ways to save big on your medication. Consumer Reports, 2014. http://www.consumerreports.org/cro/magazine/2014/12/8-ways-to-save-big-on-your-medication/index.htm. Accessed 10 Dec 2014.

27. Surprising ways to cut your drug costs. Consumer Reports, 2013. https://www.bostonglobe.com/business/2013/11/17/surprising-ways-cut-your-drug-costs/6SqjMFE1BuUQ3RBdV3lkBK/story.html. Accessed 6 Jan 2015.

28. Pharmacy Buying Guide. Consumer Reports, 2014. http://www.consumerreports.org/cro/pharmacies/buying-guide.htm. Accessed 6 Jan 2015.

29. Office of Health and Human Services. Massachusetts Health Care Safety & Quality License Verification Site. https://checkalicense.hhs.state.ma.us/MyLicenseVerification/. Accessed 28 Sept 2014.

30. Smith JC, Medalia C. U.S. Census Bureau. Health Insurance Coverage in the United States: 2014. Washington DC: U.S. Department of Commerce; 2015. http://www.census.gov/content/dam/Census/library/publications/2015/demo/p60-253.pdf. Accessed 1 Mar 2016.

31. January 2013 Census Shows 15.5 Million People Covered by Health Savings Account/High-Deductible Health Plans (HSA/HDHPs). Washington DC: America's Health Insurance Plans, Center for Policy and Research; 2013. https://www.ahip.org/HSA2013/. Accessed 1 Mar 2016.

32. Generic Drug User Fee Act Program Performance Goals and Procedures. 2012. http://www.fda.gov/downloads/ForIndustry/UserFees/GenericDrugUserFees/UCM282505.pdf. Accessed 13 Jan 2015.

3

HIV/AIDS related commodities supply chain management in public health facilities of Addis Ababa, Ethiopia

Eyerusalem Berhanemeskel, Gebremedhin Beedemariam and Teferi Gedif Fenta[*]

Abstract

Background: A wide range of pharmaceutical products are needed for diagnosis, treatment, and prevention of HIV/AIDS. However, interrupted supplies and stock-outs are the major challenges in the supply chain of ARV medicines and related commodities. The aim of this study was to assess the supply chain management of HIV/AIDS related commodities in public health facilities of Addis Ababa, Ethiopia.

Methods: A descriptive cross-sectional survey complemented by qualitative method was conducted in 24 public health facilities (4 hospitals and 20 health centers). A semi-structured questionnaire and observation check list were used to collect data on HIV/AIDS related service, reporting and ordering; receiving, transportation and storage condition of ARV medicines and test kits; and supportive supervision and logistics management information system. In addition, in-depth interview with flexible probing techniques was used to complement the quantitative data with emphasis to the storage condition of ARV medicines and test kits. Quantitative data was analyzed using SPSS version-20. Analysis of qualitative data involved rigorous reading of transcripts in order to identify key themes and data was analyzed using thematic approach.

Results: The study revealed that 16 health centers and one hospital had recorded and reported patient medication record. Six months prior to the study, 14 health centers and 2 hospitals had stopped VCT services for one time or more. Three hospitals and 18 health centers claimed to have been able to submit the requisition and report concerning ARV medicines to Pharmaceutical Fund and Supply Agency according to the specific reporting period. More than three-fourth of the health centers had one or more emergency order of ARV medicines on the day of visit, while all of hospitals had emergency order more than 3 times within 6 months prior to the study. All of the hospitals and nearly half of the health centers had an emergency order of test kits more than 3 times in the past 6 months. Overall, nearly 3/4th of the health facilities faced stock-out of one or more ARV medicines and test kits on the day of visit.

Conclusion: There was no adequate data on patient medication record and stock status of HIV/AIDS related commodities. Moreover there were frequent stock-outs of ARV medicines and HIV test kits, which was an indicator of the weak supply chain management. Hospitals and health centers, therefore, should devise a system to capture and make use of patient medication record and stock status information so as to ensure continuous supply of the commodities.

Keywords: HIV/AIDS, ARV medicines, HIV test kits, Supply chain management, Pharmaceutical logistic, Ethiopia

* Correspondence: tgedif@gmail.com
Departement of Pharmaceutics and Social Pharmacy, School of Pharmacy,
College of Health Sciences, Addis Ababa University, Ethiopia, P. O. Box: 1176,
Addis Ababa, Ethiopia

Background

The human immune virus (HIV) epidemic remains a major global public health challenge including in Ethiopia. According to the 2014 estimate, Ethiopia had 793,700 people living with HIV with 15, 700 new HIV infections and 35, 600 AIDS-related deaths. The national HIV prevalence was 1.14 % in 2014 and it is declining significantly varying by age, gender and geographical location [1].

In the early 1980s when the AIDS epidemic began, people living with HIV were not likely to live more than a few years [2]. However, with the development of safe and effective medicines, HIV positive people now have longer and healthier lives [2, 3]. Initially, resource limited countries could not afford to provide antiretroviral therapy (ART) for their populations, and the life expectancy of HIV positive people remained low [4]. However, efforts have been made to make it more affordable within low- and middle-income countries [3, 5].

Supply chain management of essential health commodities, including high-value medicines like Antiretroviral (ARV) medicines, involves a series of activities to guarantee the continuous flow of products from the manufacture to consumers [6]. The nature of ART and the specific characteristics of ARV medicines and how they are used pose particular challenges for managing the supply chain for ARV medicines [7].

Effective pharmaceutical supply management and inventory control avoid stock out, loss due to unnecessary expiry, theft and ensure that the desired pharmaceutical products are available at all times in adequate quantity [8]. But in many low and middle income countries (LMICs), the capacity of the pharmaceutical supply management system has always been challenging and weak. The ARV supply chain management has become increasingly difficult due to increasing number of people on ART, increasing number of sites providing ART and a greater diversity of different ARV regimen [9].

Moreover, there are certain common challenges associated with the quantification of ARV medicines and supplies mainly in LMICs. Data on ART services and ARV medicine supply are limited and when available, are often unreliable or insufficient to be used for quantifying ARV medicine requirements [7]. An accurate quantification based on reliable data is essential for all health commodities but more so for HIV/AIDS related commodities because uninterrupted access for patients must be ensured [9]. A pilot study done in Ethiopia, however, showed that out of the 48 hospitals and health centers, 10(21 %) of the institutions didn't have HIV medicines and out of 27 health posts, 9 (33 %) did not have rapid diagnostic tests [10]. This shortage of critical medicines and supplies in health facilities may compromise appropriate clinical management which ultimately increases mortality and development of resistance pathogens causing a detrimental public health impact [11].

One of the major reasons that medicines are wasted is that they may have expired without anyone noticing that the shelf life date was approaching. This type of lose, however, is not acceptable to pharmaceuticals such as ARV medicines, which are very expensive [8]. Besides, due to poor handling of the available medicines and other pharmaceutical products by the patients and professionals, there is also a great loss of resources.

In addition to this, the 2010 World Health Organization (WHO) guideline and the latest 2010 Ethiopian standard treatment guideline recommend that ART should be initiated when the CD4 count falls below 350/μl for WHO stage 3 disease and should be initiated irrespective of CD4 count for stage 4 disease. If CD4 count is not available it should be initiated irrespective of total lymphocyte count [4, 12]. So it may lead to a drastic increase of the number of patients who are eligible for ART and thus creating an enormous burden to national health care system and health facilities [13, 14].

Assessing the supply chain of ARV medicines and HIV test kits is indispensible to improve access and thus provide quality services. Little has been done in this regard. However a pilot study done by Daniel et al. (10) tried to assess the availability of HIV medicines but did not address the other components of the supply chain management. This study was therefore conducted with the aim of comprehensively assessing the supply chain management of HIV/AIDS related commodities in public health facilities of Addis Ababa, Ethiopia.

Methods

A descriptive cross-sectional survey employing both quantitative and qualitative data collection technique was conducted in the selected public health facilities. All public health facilities providing voluntary counseling and testing (VCT), prevention of mother to child transmission (PMTCT) and ART services were the source facilities of the study. All healthcare professionals working in ART clinic of the selected health facilities and all documents that were used to manage the supply chain of HIV/AIDS related commodities were used as sources of information.

The numbers of health facilities to be included in the study were calculated by using the Logistic Indicators Assessment Tool (LIAT) for ARV medicines and Test kits [14, 15]. At the time of survey, a total of 11 public hospitals and 37 health centers were providing ART and VCT services. Of these, 20 health centers; two from each of the ten sub-cities where one health center with the highest number of patients on ART treatment and the other with the lowest patients burden were selected for the study. Selection of study hospitals was also done based on their ownership and patient burden i.e. hospitals were administratively stratified into those administered by the Regional Health Bureau and the Federal Ministry of Health (FMoH) and then selection of the health facilities was made by extreme sampling. Accordingly four governmental hospitals, two from FMoH and two from Regional Health Bureau, were included in the study. Two of the selected hospitals, one from each administrative category, had the lowest patient load while two of the remaining hospitals again one from each had the highest burden of patients.

A semi-structured questionnaire and observation check list were used to collect the quantitative data. A modified version of the LIAT for ARV medicines and test kits was used as a data collection tool [15, 16]. A total of 14 ARV medicines and five HIV test kits were selected for this assessment. A six month data (May 2013 to October 2013) were taken from bin card and VCT daily register to see the pattern of VCT service and stock status in hospitals and health centers. VCT daily register, ARV medicines and patient information sheets (PIS), ARV medicines dispensing register, patient tracking charts, ARV medicines dispensing register for post exposure prophylaxis, ARV medicines dispensing register for emergency supply, medicine reporting and requisition format (RRF), Model 19 (receiving voucher), bin card, medicine and supply expiry date tracking charts and temperature recording charts were the major documents checked and reviewed to get the required information.

An in-depth interview with flexible probing techniques was designed to collect the qualitative data from the key informants. The head of pharmacy departments, ART store managers, ART dispensers, Laboratory heads, VCT staff and ART coordinator from the selected hospitals and health centers were purposively identified as key informants for the study.

After the data was manually checked for completeness and consistencies, it was entered and analyzed by using SPSS version 20. Descriptive statistics including mean, percentage and standard deviations was used to present the quantitative data. The qualitative data analysis involved an intensive reading through the interview in order to identify key themes. Audio-recorded interviews were transcribed verbatim and the raw data was categorized under pre-developed coded themes and sub themes. A thematic analysis was then used to analyze the data.

Ethical approval was obtained from the Ethics Review Board of the School of Pharmacy, Addis Ababa University, Addis Ababa Regional Health Bureau and from the respective health facilities. Besides, a verbal consent was obtained from all participants before starting the actual data collection. Confidentiality and anonymity of information was maintained throughout the data collection and analysis period by not linking personal identifiers in the data presentations.

Results
HIV/AIDS related services
A total of 24 health facilities were visited during this assessment; of which 4 were hospitals and 20 were health centers. All selected facilities were providing VCT, PMTCT and ART services. The selected health centers had an experience on VCT service provision for an average of 9.1 years (SD = 1.4 and range from 6 to 11 years) and ART service provision for a mean period of 6.9 years (SD = 0.8 and range from 5 to 8 years); while hospitals had longer experience of providing VCT and ART services, 10.3 years (SD = 1.5 and range from 9 to 12 years) and 9 years (SD = 1.6 and range from 7 to 11 years) respectively.

A majority (65 %) of the health centers and half of the hospitals were not providing VCT service on the day of visit. Moreover, the VCT service was interrupted at least once in 14(70 %) of the health centers and 2(50 %) of the hospitals within six months prior to the commencement of the survey. When facilities had shortage of HIV test kits, they conducted tests only for emergency cases or for PMTCT. In the past six months prior to the study, VCT service was not provided by the health centers for longer period which averaging 39.8 ± 32.8 (range from 0 to 98) days compared to hospitals, 6.8 ± 11 (range from 0 to 23) days. Mostly the interruption was associated with stock-outs of HIV (1 + 2) Antibody Colloidal Gold (KHB) but shortage of stat pack and blood lancet were also mentioned as additional factors.

Regarding the ART services, majority (80 %) of the health centers and all of the hospitals had lists of recommended ARV medicine regimens to be prescribed and dispensed. A majority 16(80 %) of the health centers and only one hospital knew and reported their patient medication record. The rest, 4 health centers and 1 hospital were using ART clinic data to report to higher level. Two hospitals claimed that they were reporting the data from the ART pharmacy without retaining the copy of the reported data.

The key informants' interview with the heads of pharmacy departments and the data clerks in two of the hospitals revealed that their Electronic Dispensing Tool (EDT) was not working appropriately and thus both the ART pharmacist and the data clerk were facing difficulties in using the patient database. In addition to this, they said that they wouldn't use any paper based format to register patient data because of high patient burden. In another hospital, the head of the pharmacy and the ART pharmacist mentioned that they were only able to enter patient information without analyzing the data for further reporting. In addition to this, they also mentioned that due to negligence of the professionals and other factors, the data in EDT was not reliable. Even though they have been using PIS, they didn't use it appropriately.

All of the health facilities had EDT to dispense medicines to the patient and all, except one, of them were applying the EDT in their daily work. A majority 19(95 %) of health centers and 3/4th of the hospitals used both EDT and PIS to record the amount of medicines dispensed to the patients and other patient information. But, Dispensing Register was available and used only in 14 health centers and none of the hospitals. A majority of them had been dispensing a dose that ranges from 15 days to 3 months, depending on patients' condition. Erratic supply of medicines in some health facilities, however, was reported by the ART pharmacists that forced them to dispense medicines for a week, 3 days and even for a day; especially for TDF/3TC based regimen. Sometimes, they mentioned that they even referred patients to other health facilities.

Eighteen health centers and 2 hospitals used separate register for post exposure prophylaxis and for emergency. Patient Tracking Chart was being used by only 10 health centers and 2 hospitals. Nevertheless, absentee patients tracked by this chart were not called to attend the health facility mainly due to lack of telephone in these health facilities.

Reporting and ordering ARV medicines and HIV test kits

Store manager in one of the 20 health centers was not available during the study time and hence 19 key informants from the health centers and 4 from hospitals were considered. All health facilities reported using RRF to report consumption and order ARV medicines from the Pharmaceutical Fund and Supply Agency (PFSA) Regional Hub.

In a majority (89.5 %) of the health facilities, RRF was prepared and reported by the store manager alone. Thus, the store managers were responsible for determining the quantity of medicines. In the rest of the facilities, both the store manager and the head pharmacist claimed to have been involved in quantification. A majority (94.7 %) of the health centers and 3/4th of hospitals' store managers claimed that they had submitted their last report according to the schedule. A majority of the store managers 15(78.9 %) in health centers and 3(75 %) in hospitals had training on integrated pharmaceutical logistic system (IPLS).

A majority of the facilities had emergency orders in the past 6 months prior to the study. Only 3(15.8 %) of the health centers didn't have emergency orders. On the other hand, all of the hospitals reported that they had

emergency orders for more than 3 times within 6 months prior to the study (Table 1).

The reporting and requisition of test kits was done in combination with the ARV medicines by the main store manager in all the studied health facilities except one hospital and two health centers. The hospital had a separate store for test kits, so the RRF was prepared by separate store manager. In the two health centers the RRF was prepared by the laboratory head that never had training for the purpose. All hospitals reported the use of standard method to determine the quantity of HIV test kits but only 9(47.3 %) of the health centers did use the same during the quantification process. Most health centers mentioned the practice of rough estimation since they were unable to calculate the exact quantity of test kits due to frequent supply interruption. Generally, the reporting and the requisition of HIV test kits were more organized in hospitals compared with health centers.

All health facilities, except one, had emergency order of test kits in the past six months prior to the study. All of the hospitals and nearly half (47.4 %) of the health centers had an emergency order for more than three times in the past six months. They all agreed that in the majority of the cases they received the test kits on emergency order (Table 1).

Receiving and transportation of ARV medicines and test kits

All of the hospitals reported that they were not always getting the required quantity of ARV medicines and only 1 of the health center was always able to get the

Table 1 Frequency of emergency orders for ARV drugs and HIV test kits in the health facilities, Addis Ababa, 2013

	Proportion by type of health facility	
	Health centers; n (%)	Hospitals; n (%)
Frequency of emergency orders encountered for ARV in the last 6 months		
No emergency order	3(15.8)	0 (0.00)
One emergency order	4(21.1)	0 (0.00)
Two emergency orders	2(10.5)	0 (0.00)
Three emergency orders	6(31.6)	0 (0.00)
More than three emergency order	4(21.1)	4(100)
Frequency of emergency orders encountered for HIV test kits in the last 6 months		
No emergency order	1(5.3)	0 (0.00)
One emergency order	3(15.8)	0 (0.00)
Two emergency orders	2(10.5)	0 (0.00)
Three emergency orders	2(10.5)	0 (0.00)
More than three emergency order	9(47.4)	4(100)
Do not know	2(10.5)	0 (0.00)

quantified amount (Table 2). Regarding the average time interval between ordering and receiving of the medicines, three-fourth of the hospitals and 13(68.4 %) of the health centers received the products ordered between two weeks to one month of their order point (Table 2). But review of the health facilities' last report had showed that, on average the lead time was 37.5 ± 17.1 days and 34.2 ± 18 days in hospitals and health centers, respectively.

During the last order time, the average number of ordered ARV product was found to be 6. The mean percentage difference between quantity ordered and received was high for 3TC300/TDF300 (69.6 % ±17 %, (55 %, 93 %)) and D4T12/3TC60 (69.4 % ± 33.3 %, (45.8 %, 93 %)) in hospitals while it was high for D4T6/3TC30/NVP 50 (110.9 % ± 193.8 %, (0 %, 400 %)) and 3TC300/TDF300 (51.7 % ± 33.8 %, (0 %, 99 %)) in health centers for last report period (Table 3).

Supportive supervision

All of the health centers and $3/4^{th}$ of the hospitals were supervised by professionals from the Regional Health Bureau or FMoH during the past 6 months prior to the study. The study also showed that only 2 of the hospitals and a quarter of the health centers had received supportive supervision more than 3 months ago. All of the respondents said that their last supervision included review of stock cards and bin cards, physical stock count, storage condition, review of health commodity information management system (HCMIS) and EDT, PIS and dispensing register book, VCT tally and VCT daily register. They also discussed and facilitated removal of expired products from the stores.

Storage condition of ARV medicines and test kits

The stores of 19 health centers and 4 hospitals were assessed during the study time. There were 2 health

Table 2 Frequency of receiving the ordered quantity of ARV drugs and Average lead time for ARVs in hospitals and health centers, Addis Ababa, 2013

	Health centers; n (%)	Hospitals; n (%)
How frequently did you receive the amount of ARV drugs you ordered?		
Always	1 (5.3)	0 (0.00)
Most of the time	12 (63.2)	1 (25.0)
Sometimes	6 (31.6)	3 (75.0)
Never	0 (0.00)	0 (0.00)
Average lead time between ordering and receiving ARV drugs		
Less than two weeks	3 (15.8)	1 (25.0)
2 weeks to 1 month	13 (68.4)	3 (75.0)
1 month to 2 months	2 (10.5)	0 (0.00)
More than 2 months	1 (5.3)	0 (0.00)

centers which didn't have a bin card for ARV medicines and not included in the calculation of percentage of bin card updated. There were also 2 hospitals, which had updated bin card with 1 month and 2 months transaction; which were included in the calculation of availability of bin card for ARV medicines and bin card updated. But these two hospitals had no complete transaction for the past 6 months. Store manager of one of the hospital had a complete bin card of 9 ARV medicines, so only the bin card of the 9 products were used in the past 6 month stock status. The store manager of the second hospital didn't record the past 14 months transaction neither on bin card nor on the HCMIS; and thus the hospital was excluded in the calculation of past six months stock status of ARV medicines. The stock status was then calculated with these limitations.

Overall, 14(73.7 %) of the health centers and 3(75 %) of the hospitals had stock out of one or more ARV medicines on the day of visit. All of the hospitals and health centers faced stock out of 1 or more ARV medicines in the past months prior to the study time. EFV600, NVP200, NVP240 and D4T6/3TC30/NVP50 were stocked out both at hospitals and health centers.

The average number of products which were out of stock on the day of visit was 1.6 and 2.0 in health centers and hospitals respectively and it went as high as 6 and 4 in health centers and hospitals respectively. Mean number of out of stock products in the past six months prior to the study was 5.1 and 6.5 in health centers and hospitals, respectively (Table 4). The most frequent out of stock item in the past 6 months prior to the study in the health facilities was TDF300/3TC300. The mean duration of stock out was longer for D4T6/3TC30 (55.8 ± 45 days, (0, 109)) and TDF300/3TC300 (45.9 ± 45.5 days, (0, 165)) in health centers while it was long for TDF300/3TC300 (42.5 ± 60.1 days, (0, 85)) and NVP200 (36.5 ± 19.1 days, (23, 50)) (Table 3).

Decreasing the ordered quantity of ARV medicines and test kits by the supplier was mentioned as a main reason for the stock outs of these pharmaceuticals. In addition to this, respondents claimed that the transfer of patients from D4T to TDF/3TC based regimen was a major contributing factor for shortage of TDF300/3TC300.

According to majority of the store managers, stock movement was controlled using both bin card and HCMIS. Except 2 (10.5 %) of health centers; all of the health facilities used bin card on the day of visit. Besides, all health facilities used maximum-minimum stock control system to manage the stock of ARV medicines and as a result they were supposed to have maximum stock of 4 months, minimum stock of 2 months and an emergency stock of 15 days.

During the time of visit, average percentage of updated bin cards were 85.7 % in health centers and 96.9 % in

Table 3 Stock-out status of ARVs within 6 months prior to the study and percentage difference between ordered and received quantities of ARVs in health centers and hospitals, Addis Ababa, 2013

ARV drugs	Stock-out days of ARVs within 6 months prior to the study		Percentage difference between ordered and received quantities of ARVS			
	Health centers	Hospitals	Health centers		Hospitals	
	Average number of days ± SD	Average number of days ± SD	Mean percentage difference ± SD	(Min, Max)	Mean percentage difference ± SD	(min, max)
EFV50	12 ± 21	0	0	0	a	a
EFV200	10.1 ± 28	0	9.5 ± 21.2	(0, 47.6)	0	0
EFV600	18.8 ± 25	0	47 ± 32.3	(0, 80.7)	2.9 ± 2.7	(0, 11.5)
3TC300/TDF300	45.9 ± 45.5	42.5 ± 60.1	51.7 ± 33.8	(0, 99)	69.6 ± 17	(55, 93.4)
NVP 200	16.6 ± 30.8	36.5 ± 19.1	0	0	0	0
ZDV300/3TC150	9.7 ± 13.9	34.5 ± 14.8	27.1 ± 43.1	(0, 143)	34 ± 29.5	(0, 52)
ZDV300/3TC150/NVP200	13 ± 19.9	20.5 ± 4.9	14.8 ± 33.6	(0, 93.6)	50 ± 0	(50,50)
3TC30/ZDV60/NVP50	15 ± 17	0	0	0	0	0
NVP 240 ml	33.7 ± 46.7	29 ± 41	5.9 ± 16.6	(0, 47.1)	0	0
D4T12/3TC60/NVP100	20.1 ± 25	27 ± 0.0	27.8 ± 83.5	(0, 290)	0	0
D4T6/3TC30/NVP50	16.8 ± 24.4	0	110.8 ± 193.8	(0, 400)	0	0
3TC30/ZDV60	14.8 ± 21.8	16.5 ± 14.8	25.4 ± 35.9	(0, 50.8)	45.7 ± 12.7	(36.7,54.7)
D4T 12/3TC60	15.6 ± 33.1	0	0	0	69.4 ± 33.3	(45.8,93)
D4T 6/3TC30	55.8 ± 45	0	a	a	0	0

[a]means the product was not ordered by the health facility in last requisition and reporting reviewed
D4T = Stavudine; EFV = Efavernez; NVP = Nevirapine; TDF = Tenofovir; 3TC = Lamivudine; ZDV = Zidovudine

hospitals. Percentage of bin card updated varied from facility to facility with a range of 22.2– 100 % in health centers and 87.5–100 % in hospitals. All bin cards were updated in 3(75 %) of the hospitals and 10(58.8 %) of health centers. While the remaining hospitals and health centers had one or more un-updated bin cards.

Regarding the selected HIV test kits, (KHB, stat-pack, Uni-gold, blood lancet and EDTA capillary tube), at the time of the assessment only 10(52.6 %) of health centers and 2(50 %) of hospitals had a bin card. Regarding the stock status of test kits, 10(52.6 %) of the health centers reported stock-out of 1 to 3 test kits and all hospitals had stock out of 1 or 2 test kits. In a majority of the health centers and hospitals, Uni-Gold was out of stock on the day of visit more than other kits (Fig. 1). Average percentage of test kits which were out of stock on the day of visit was 29.5 % and 35 % in health centers and hospitals, respectively.

Except one hospital, all of the facilities had one central store for ARV medicines and test kits. The qualitative data obtained from observation checklist showed that appropriate arrangement of products with visible expiry dates and identification labels, first expired first out (FEFO) organization of product and accessibility of products for counting; cleanliness of the store, and thermometer usage were the major challenges identified in majority of the health facilities. Lack of ventilation, inadequate light of the store room and inadequacy of storage space were observed in a majority of the health centers and few hospitals. The stores in a majority of the health centers were highly overfilled and products were kept in a direct floor without a pallet. In addition, there was sign of rodents and insects in the majority of health centers and few of the hospitals.

It was also observed that, utilization of expiry tracking chart was very minimal both in the health centers and

Table 4 Proportion of ARVs managed and stocked out in in the health facilities on the day of visit and within 6 months prior to the study, Addis Ababa, 2013

	On day of visit				The past 6 months			
	Health centers		Hospitals		Health centers		Hospitals	
	Mean ± SD	(Min, Max)	Mean ± SD	(Min, Max)	Mean ± SD	(Min, Max)	Mean ± SD	(Min, Max)
No. of ARVs managed	12.2 ± 2	(8,14)	13.2 ± 3.8	(8,16)	12.2 ± 2	(8,14)	13.2 ± 3.8	(8,16)
No. of ARVs stocked out	1.6 ± 1.5	(0,6)	2 ± 1.6	(0,4)	5.1 ± 2.6	(1,11)	6.5 ± 2.1	(5,8)
% of ARVs stocked out	12.8 ± 11.3	(0,42.8)	17 ± 13.7	(0,30.8)	46.3 ± 23.3	(9.1,91.7)	56.3 ± 8.8	(50,62.5)

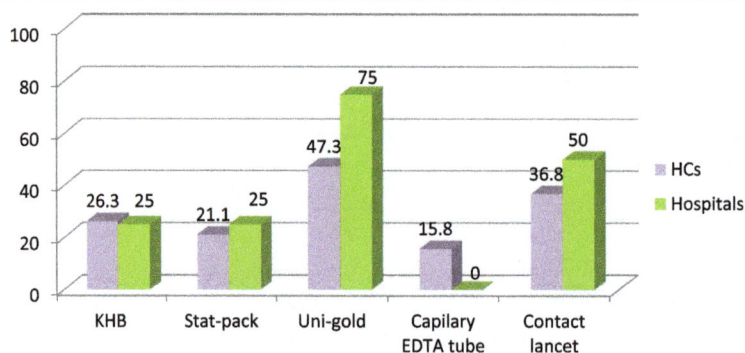

Fig. 1 Proportion of health facilities stocked out of HIV test kits on the day of visit in the, Addis Ababa, 2013

hospitals. Expired medicines and test kits were found on the shelves of some of the health centers and one hospital. On the contrary, majority of the health centers and hospitals were able to maintain the outer cartoon of the product in a good condition and they were able to separate the expired and damaged product from usable product either in the store room or in separate store. Moreover, the observation revealed that cartoons and products were protected from direct sunlight; stores were locked and the keys were maintained with the store manager, roofs were maintained in good condition to avoid sunlight and water penetration.

Logistic management information system

For majority of the health centers and hospitals, EDT was the main tool to record patient information even though there was risk of power interruption and risk of losing the patient data. EDT contains all the medicines currently dispensed at facilities unlike HCMIS. Since there is large number of HIV/AIDS patients, this computerized software eases the work of the health professionals and the data clerks at the dispensary. However, the professionals had reported drawbacks of the software; not easy to manipulate and get patient data by regimen type. So when the need arises, they relied on the data obtained from the clinic which had also some shortcomings.

Problem of data quality was also reported by majority of the health facilities. Only one health center was able to correctly report the ending balance as the stock on hand found in the central store room as well as in all other dispensing units, while the rest of the health facilities wrongly reported the ending balance as stock on hand kept in the store room only. Besides, deliberate manipulation of recording was reported by one store manager as there were cases where the supplier sent excess ARV medicines and thus the manager targeted to decrease the ordered ARV medicines. Hence, to prevent and minimize the fluctuations made by the supplier, the store manager of the health centers increased or decreased the balance to be reported accordingly.

Discussion

Although information about patients taking ARVs medicine by regimen data is crucial for the medicine supply chain management, it was only 16 (80 %) of the health centers and one hospital that were able to know the patient medication record data and reported appropriately. The main problem was related to inefficiency of the EDT and as a result some of the health facilities were using the ART clinic data as an alternative. Nevertheless, the report from the ART clinic lacked patient data on TDF/3TC/EFV and TDF/3TC/NVP; where these two medicines accounted near to quarter or more of the patients in the health facilities and other second line ARV medicines. Thus, this lack of adequate and accurate data might affect quantification and procurement planning for ARV medicines. Similarly, a study done by Allers et al. showed that, data on ART services and ARV medicine supply were limited and, when available, are often unreliable or insufficient to be used for quantifying ARV medicine requirements [7]. Another literature stressed the importance of information in medicine supply chain management to ensure that there are no interruptions in treatment and tests [5].

Adherence is an important issue in any antibiotic therapy but it is of a special concern when it comes to medicines like ARVs. HIV patients should be monitored and followed with much of concern. In this regard, the use of patient tracking chart is vital tool to monitor the adherence and thus recommended by the standard operating procedure for management of ART medicines in health facilities [8]. The present study, however, showed that only half of the health centers and hospitals had been using patient tracking chart. In those facilities which didn't use patient tracking chart, medicines were simply dispensed to patients who came to their dispensary but they didn't know how much of their patients were missed and treatment adherence is left to the patients. This practice could contribute to default of more patients, probably emergence of medicine resistance and loss of lives.

Our study also documented that in the studied health facilities, ART dispensers were dispensing doses that range from 15 days to 3 months depending on the patient's condition. Frequent stock-out of medicines and regimen change from D4T to TDF/3TC which is associated with shortage of TDF/3TC, however forced them to dispense medicines even for a single day. The percentage difference between quantities ordered and received was high for TDF/3TC both in health centers and hospitals. Such high percentage difference between ordered and received quantity was an indicative of interrupted supply chain. This kind of practice therefore might exhaust the patients and contribute for default. The present study result mirrors to a study in Mali, where forecasting became difficult due to shifting of patients to alternative first line and second line ART regimens [9].

Accurate quantification of HIV/AIDS related commodities is a complex process confined with multifaceted factors [17]. The present study revealed that even though both health centers and hospitals control their inventory using maximum-minimum stock inventory control system, frequent emergency order of ARV medicines was reported in the six months prior to the study. A majority of the health centers had one or more emergency orders while all of hospitals had emergence orders of ARV medicines more than three times. This might be associated with the relatively higher number of patients in hospitals than health centers.

This study also showed that only half of the hospitals and a quarter of the health centers had received recent supportive supervision more than 3 months ago. So, lack of planned and timely supportive supervision may also become a challenge in ensuring adequate supplies. A study done in Lesotho similarly revealed that there were challenges in the medicine supply management system, which were mainly due to the lack of supervisory site visits, leading to facilities over-stocking or under-stocking of certain items [18].

Failure to observe expiry dates of medicines might lead to the loss of a significant amount of resources, especially in resources limited countries. This type of loss is not acceptable to pharmaceuticals such as ARV medicines, which are very expensive [8]. Contrary to this fact, the present study showed that utilization of expiry tracking chart was minimal in health facilities and thus on the day of visit, expired medicines and test kits were found on the shelves of the health facilities. Similar to this finding, a study done in Lesotho showed that, ARV medicines were expired on the shelves in some facilities where inventory was poorly managed [18].

The present assessment also indicated that more than three fourth of the hospitals and health centers had stock-out of one or more ARV medicines on the day of visit and during the past 6 months preceding the survey date. TDF300/3TC300 was most frequent stock out item in the past 6 months both in hospitals and health centers. Mean number of stock out products in the past 6 month was 5.1 and 6.5 in health centers and hospitals, respectively. The percentage of products which were out of stock was 12.8 % and 17 % in health centers and hospitals, respectively. Regarding the test kits, all of the hospitals and 2 of the health centers reported stock out of one or more test kits on the day of visit. Different from this study, a study done in Oromia National Regional State showed that availability of first line ARV medicines was 100 % in health centers and 95 % in hospitals [19]. Another study done in Ethiopia also showed that stock outs for ARVs had been non-existent or minimal [14]. An assessment done in Sierra Leon similarly showed that there were stock-outs of EFV and second line medicines in ART providing facilities [7]. Concur to our finding, a study done in Uganda showed that, ARV shortages affected all ART providing facilities with considerable fluctuations. ARVs were available at 83 % and diagnostic kits at 70 % of the health facilities surveyed [20]. Similarly, Jonathan et al., showed that interrupted supplies and stock outs were the major challenges in the supply chain of ARV medicines in Africa [21].

Interruption of the supply of these medicines put individual patient at risk of disease progression and death, in medicine resistance development, hampers progress towards universal access, and diminishes the credibility of ART programs in the eyes of patients, community and healthcare providers and inadvertently putting the public health in danger [10]. So to prevent this kind of interruption, there has to be efficient supply chain. Effective medicine supply chain management and inventory control would help to avoid or at least minimize stock-outs, losses due to unnecessary expiry, theft and ensure that the desired pharmaceutical products are available at all times in adequate quantity [8].

Except 2 (10.5 %) of health centers; all health centers and hospitals used bin card for ARV medicines on the day of visit. Availability and practice of updating of the bin cards was relatively better in hospitals than health centers. Unlike ARV medicines, only 10(52.6 %) of health centers and 2(50 %) of hospitals had a bin card for the selected test kit on the day of visit. Consistent to this findings, a study done in Sierra Leone reported that the stock keeping practice in ART providing health facilities was not good where no bin cards were available for any of the ARV medicines or HIV test kits at any of the health facilities visited [22]. Contrary to the present findings, however, a 2009 evaluation done in Ethiopia indicated that the inventory control in all surveyed ART sites and use of bin cards and stock cards was found to be adequate [14].

To provide clients with high quality products and ensure efficient handling and use of products, each facility must have safe, protected and organized storage areas. The present assessment however, revealed that the storage facilities both in hospitals and health centers were far from adequate. The store premises and storage conditions were better in hospitals compared to health centers. Similarly, a study done in Sera Leon also stated that the storage condition observed in district and primary healthcare units was not generally in a good condition where expired medicines and kits were stored together with the usable commodities causing shortage of space in the health facilities [22]. An evaluation done in Ethiopia similarly showed that there were inadequate storage facilities, management, capacity, and temperature monitoring, especially for the cold chain [14].

The health facilities in Addis Ababa had both computerized and paper based LMIS. However, a majority of the health facilities had problems with the use of the automated LMIS. According to them, some features of the software were not easy to manipulate and fix the problem. As a result, relying on the computerized LMIS leave majority of the health facilities with incomplete and inaccurate data in both dispensary and store areas. A study suggested that computerized LMIS can greatly facilitate the work of supply chain managers and hence there is urgency to introduce user-friendly tools and software to support the management of logistics information system in the health facilities [23].

Conclusions

ART and VCT services started in Ethiopia over a decade ago. However, data on patient medication record and stock status of ARV medicines and Test kits is still inadequate. The present study demonstrated that a majority of the facilities in Addis Ababa didn't have patient tracking chart and consequently treatment adherence seemed to be left to the patients themselves. The reporting and receiving system of ART medicines were relatively more organized compared to HIV test kits in the studied health facilities. Though the stock status of ART medicines were controlled relatively in better way than HIV test kits, shortages of both commodities were common in both health centers and hospitals. Of all commodities; TDF/3TC, KHB and Uni-gold were the major out of stock items in the supply chain. For example, more than half of the health facilities were not providing VCT service on the day of our visit mainly due to lack of KHB. The storage condition of these commodities was not good but it was relatively better in hospitals than health centers. On the other hand, the stores and ART pharmacy sections of all health facilities had computerized LMIS. However, majority of the professionals who were supposed to run the system claimed that they were unable to manipulate and operate the software efficiently. Hence, introducing user-friendly tools and software is

essential to support the management of logistics information system in the health facilities.

Abbreviations

AA: Addis Ababa; AIDS: acquired immune deficiency syndrome; ART: antiretroviral therapy; ARVs: antiretroviral; D4T: stavudine; EDT: electronic dispensing tools; EDTA: ethylenediaminetetraacetica acid; EFV: efavernez; FEFO: first expired first out; FMOH: federal ministry of health; HCMIS: health commodities management information system; HIV: human immunodeficiency virus; IPLS: integrated pharmaceuticals logistic system; KHB: HIV (1 + 2) antibody colloidal gold; LIAT: logistic indicator assessment tools; LMICs: low and middle income countries; LMIS: logistic management information system; NVP: nevirapine; PFSA: pharmaceutical fund and supply agency; PIS: patient information sheet; PMTCT: prevention of mother to child transmission; RRF: report and requisition format; TDF: tenofovir; 3TC: lamivudine; VCT: voluntary counseling and testing; WHO: World Health Organization.

Competing interests

The authors of this manuscript declare that they have no competing interests.

Authors' contribution

EB conceived and designed the study, coordinated the data collection process, performed the data analysis and drafted the manuscript. GB participated in data analysis and corrected the manuscript. TGF participated in the design of the study, provided guidance in the overall process and corrected the manuscript. All authors read and approved the final manuscript.

Acknowledgement

The authors would like to acknowledge all study participants and individual who provided information. We are also grateful to Addis Ababa University School of Graduate Studies for sponsoring this research.

References

1. WHO. ETHIOPIA Update sheet on HIV - AIDS programme in 2014. 2015. http://www.afro.who.int/en/ethiopia/country-programmes/topics/4480-hivaids.html. Accessed 20 September 2015.
2. WHO. Fast facts about HIV treatment. 2009. http://www.who.int/mediacentre/factsheets/fs360/en/. Accessed 01 Jan 2012.
3. WHO. Global HIV/AIDS Response - Epidemic update and health sector progress towards Universal Access-2011 Progress Report. 2012. http://www.who.int/hiv/pub/progress_report2011/en/. Accessed 01 Jan 2012.
4. Walensky RP, Wood R, Ciaranello AL, Paltiel AD, Lorenzana SB, Anglaret X, et al. Scaling Up the 2010 World Health Organization HIV Treatment Guidelines in Resource-Limited Settings: A Model-Based Analysis. PLoS Med. 2010;7(12):e1000382.
5. AVERT. Universal Access to HIV/AIDS Treatment. 2010. http://www.avert.org/aids-hivtreatment.htm. Accessed 02 Dec 2012.
6. Chandani Y, Barbara F, Claudia A, David A, Marilyn N, and Alexandra Z. Supply Chain Management of Anitretroviral Drugs: Considerations for Initiating and Expanding National Supply Chains. Arlington, Va.: DELIVER, for the U.S. Agency for International Development. 2006. http://deliver.jsi.com/dlvr_content/resources/allpubs/guidelines/SCManaARVDrug.pdf . Accessed 23 March 2012.
7. Claudia A and Chandani Y. Guide for Quantifying ARV Drugs. Arlington, Va.: DELIVER, for the U.S. Agency for International Development. 2006. http://pdf.usaid.gov/pdf_docs/pnadg486.pdf. Accessed 13 March 2012.
8. RPM Plus. Standard Operating Procedures for Antiretroviral Drug at Health Facilities: Guidelines for Forms. Arlington: Management Sciences for Health; 2006.
9. Erik JS, Andreas J, Anne BS, Simon DM, Anthony DH, Francis A, et al. Antiretroviral drug supply challenges in the era of scaling up ART in Malawi. J Int AIDS Soc. 2011;14 Suppl 1:S4.
10. Daniel G, Tegegnework H, Demissie T, Reithinger R. Pilot assessment of supply chains for pharmaceuticals and medical commodities for malaria,

tuberculosis and HIV infection in Ethiopia. Trans Royal Soc Tropical Med Hyg. 2012;106(1):60–2.

11. Pasquet A, Messou E, Gabillard D, Minga A, Depoulosky A, Sylvie DB, et al. Impact of drug stock-outs on death and retention to care among HIV-infected patients on combination antiretroviral therapy in Abidjan, Côte d'Ivoire. PLoS One. 2010;5(10):e13414.

12. DACA. Standard Treatment Guidelines for General Hospital. Addis Ababa, Ethiopia: Drug Adminstration and Control Authority; 2nd edition. 2010.

13. Elke K, Yirga A, Katherine D, Peter G, Tesfaye A, Bud C. Implications of adopting new WHO guidelines for antiretroviral therapy initiation in Ethiopia. Bull World Health Organ. 2012;90:659–63.

14. USAID/ The Global Health Technical Assistant Project. RPM+/SPS and SCMS in Ethiopia: An Evaluation. DELIVER, for the U.S. Agency for International Development. 2009. http://pdf.usaid.gov/pdf_docs/Pdaco833.pdf. Accessed 29 Nov 2012.

15. USAID | DELIVER PROJECT, Task Order 1. Logistics Indicators Assessment Tool (LIAT): Antiretroviral Drugs. Arlington, Va.: USAID | DELIVER PROJECT, Task Order 1. 2009. http://deliver.jsi.com/dlvr_content/resources/.../LIAT_ARV.doc. Accessed 29 Nov 2012.

16. USAID | DELIVER PROJECT, Task Order 1. Logistics Indicators Assessment Tool (LIAT): Test Kits. Arlington, Va.: USAID | DELIVER PROJECT, Task Order 1. 2009. http://deliver.jsi.com/dlvr_content/.../LIAT_HIVTestKits.doc. Accessed 29 Nov 2012.

17. Family Health International. Strategies for an expanded and comprehensive response (ECR) to national HIV/AIDS Epidemic, Module 7: Managing the supply of drugs and commodities. 2008. https://www.k4health.org/sites/default/files/ECRenglish1.pdf. Accessed 15 Dec 2012.

18. Pharasi B. Assessment of the HIV/AIDS Medical Supplies and Laboratory Commodities Supply Chain in Lesotho. Arlington: Management Sciences for Health; 2009. http://apps.who.int/medicinedocs/documents/s16321e/s16321e.pdf. Accessed 29 Nov 2012.

19. Alemayehu L. Assessment of Supply Management Current Status for Antiretroviral Therapy (ART) in Oromia National Regional State, Ethiopia. Ethiopian Pharmaceutical Association, Book of Abstract. 2009. : http://epaethiopia.org/images/k2/38/32/abstract_2009.pdf. Accessed 19 Nov 2012.

20. Ricarda W, Peter W, Florian N, Florian S, Don de S. Scaling up antiretroviral therapy in Uganda: using supply chain management to appraise health systems strengthening. Global Health. 2011;7:25.

21. Jonathan D, Nana-Adjoa B, James R, Romuald JM. Medicines supply in Africa. BMJ. 2005;331(7519):709–10.

22. Allers C, Timothy O, Meba K, Sierra L. Supply Chain Assessment for ARV Drugs and HIV Test Kits. Arlington: USAID | DELIVER PROJECT Task Order 1; 2007. http://deliver.jsi.com/dlvr_content/resources/allpubs/countryreports/SL_SCAssARVHIVtest.pdf. Accessed 07 Feb 2013.

23. Wendy N, Yasmin C, Anubha B, Mimi W and Sarah A. Computerizing LMIS for managing HIV/AIDS commodities. : AIDS 2008 - XVII International AIDS Conference. 2008; Abstract no. MOPE0647. USAID/DELIVER Project.

4

Drugs for cardiovascular disease in India: perspectives of pharmaceutical executives and government officials on access and development

Charles Newman[1], Vamadevan S. Ajay[2], Ravi Srinivas[3], Sandeep Bhalla[4], Dorairaj Prabhakaran[2] and Amitava Banerjee[5,6,7*]

Abstract

Background: India shoulders the greatest global burden of cardiovascular diseases (CVDs), which are the leading cause of mortality worldwide. Drugs are the bedrock of treatment and prevention of CVD. India's pharmaceutical industry is the third largest, by volume, globally, but access to CVD drugs in India is poor. There is a lack of qualitative data from government and pharmaceutical sectors regarding CVD drug development and access in India.

Methods: By purposive sampling, we recruited either Indian government officials, or pharmaceutical company executives. We conducted a stakeholder analysis via semi-structured, face-to-face interviews in India. Topic guides allow for the exploration of key issues across multiple interviews, along with affording the interviewer the flexibility to examine matters arising from the discussions themselves. After transcription, interviews underwent inductive thematic analysis.

Results: Ten participants were interviewed (Government Officials: $n = 5$, and Pharmaceutical Executives: $n = 5$). Two themes emerged: i) 'Policy-derived Factors'; ii) 'Patient- derived Factors' with three findings. First, both government and pharmaceutical participants felt that the focus of Indian pharma is shifting to more complex, high-quality generics and to new drug development, but production of generic drugs rather than new molecular entities will remain a major activity. Second, current trial regulations in India may restrict India's potential role in the future development of CVD drugs. Third, it is likely that the Indian government will tighten its intellectual property regime in future, with potentially far-reaching implications on CVD drug development and access.

Conclusions: Our stakeholder analysis provides some support for present patent regulations, whilst suggesting areas for further research in order to inform future policy decisions regarding CVD drug development and availability. Whilst interviewees suggested government policy plays an important role in shaping the industry, a significant force for change was ascribed to patient-derived factors. This suggests a potential role for Indian initiatives that market the unique advantages of its patient population for drug research in influencing national and multinational pharmaceutical companies to undertake CVD drug development in India, rather than simply IP policy-directed factors.

Keywords: Cardiovascular, Stakeholder, Pharmaceutical

* Correspondence: ami.banerjee@ucl.ac.uk
[5]University of Birmingham Centre for Cardiovascular Sciences, Birmingham, UK
[6]Present address: Farr Institute of Health Informatics Research, University College London, 222 Euston Road, London NW1 2DA, UK
Full list of author information is available at the end of the article

Background

Cardiovascular Diseases (CVDs) are the principal cause of deaths globally [40, 46, 47, 52] and global spending on CVDs surpasses any other disease [3]. Low- and middle-income countries (LMICs) now shoulder the majority of the global CVD burden [40]; no country more so than India, where ischaemic heart disease (IHD) and stroke were the first and eighth largest causes of years of life lost to death and disability [14, 40]. The economic cost of CVD in India is estimated at $30 billion per annum [32] with future increases forecast [11, 21].

Drugs play an essential role in the prevention and treatment of CVD and its risk factors [3]. Access to drugs plays a significant part in reducing health inequality [12, 50, 51] and is influenced by both affordability and availability [37]. The Indian pharmaceutical industry is now the 3rd largest, by volume, in the world [31]. Furthermore, regardless of recent regulatory changes due to concerns largely about ethics, accountability and compensation [7], India remains one of the world's most attractive destinations for clinical trials [6]. However, marked inequalities in CVD drug access persist in India [43, 54] and improved access represents a key policy strategy.

Although prevalence studies from India suggested that CVD was more common in urban than rural regions [24], in more developed states of India such as Kerala, the rural–urban differences in cardiometabolic risk factors have largely disappeared and the risk factors are equal or slightly greater in rural subjects [38]. More than 70 % of India's population lives in rural areas and nearly 40 % of the population is below the poverty line [38], and CVD drugs are less likely to be taken in rural than urban settings [30]. Barriers to CVD drug availability in India include low utilization rates of evidence-based therapies [34], high out-of-pocket expenditure, long duration of therapy and high drug costs relative to income [37, 42]. The poorest are least likely to be able to afford cardiovascular (or any) medications and out of pocket expenditure on healthcare represents the highest proportion of household spending in this group [16, 25]. Over 80 % of CVD patients receive none of the recommended effective drug treatments [25] and low household wealth is the most important determinant. A major portion of overall out of pocket health spending (in excess of 45 %) is for medicines for chronic diseases and this proportion was as high as 64 and 58 % for cases of hypertension and diabetes, respectively [8, 19].

The Indian government spends just 1.2 % of the GDP on the health sector, which is among the lowest in the world [45]. Nearly 846 billion Indian rupees (INR) were spent out of pocket on health care expenses in 2004, amounting to 3.3 % of that year's gross domestic product (GDP). A major portion of overall out of pocket health spending (in excess of 45 %) was for medicines for NCDs and this proportion was as high as 64 and 58 % for cases of hypertension and diabetes, respectively [19]. As a result of increasing realization of health inequalities in terms of access to healthcare; out-of-pocket expenditure and poverty caused by healthcare expenditure; and an unsustainable national pharmaceutical policy, the Indian government sanctioned a $5.4-billion plan allowing government sector doctors to prescribe generic drugs to patients free of cost [20]. Generic medicines are typically 20 to 90 % cheaper than originator equivalents [17, 49].

Given the importance of CVD, drugs for its treatment and the scale of the Indian pharmaceutical sector, an evidence base is crucial to inform policymakers in India. Qualitative analyses of access to CVD drugs are very limited in low- and low-middle income countries, including India [29]. Government and pharmaceutical companies have been previously identified as the most powerful stakeholders in access to medicines [2]. Therefore we conducted a stakeholder analysis of government officials and pharmaceutical company executives regarding development of and access to CVD drugs in India.

Aims

Among government officials and pharmaceutical company executives, the aim was conduct a qualitative study to understand the perceptions of the Indian government and pharmaceutical industry about factors affecting the development of new CVD drugs and access to CVD medicines.

Methods
Inclusion criteria

Interviewees were eligible for inclusion if they worked at a policy-making level, either in a generation or advisory capacity, in either:

i) The Indian government with reference to CVD pharmaceuticals and/or healthcare (the Government Official sub-group).
ii) A national or multi-national pharmaceutical company, with a base in India, involved in the development of CVD medications (the Pharmaceutical Executive sub-group).

In addition, participants had to be able to communicate fluently in written and spoken English, and to provide informed, written consent.

Recruitment

Potential participants were contacted via e-mail, using existing contacts. Convenience sampling therefore formed a component of recruitment. However, strict adherence to the inclusion criteria ensured a purposive sampling method, thereby mitigating against the reported inadequacies of a solely convenience sampling approach [36, 41]. Once initial contact was made, informed consent was obtained using documents structured in line with WHO templates [53]. A conservative sample size of 12 participants was initially set [23].

Interviews

Semi-structured, face-to-face interviews were selected as the most appropriate method of data collection for three reasons. First, this technique allows interviewers to adapt their communication in response to a participant's behavioural or verbal cue, enabling taxing subjects to be addressed. Second, this method requires a smaller sample size than other qualitative methods [10], which was important given the expected difficulty in recruiting participants from government and pharmaceutical sectors. Third, group-orientated qualitative research methods were felt inappropriate for this study due to the potential for business-sensitive information to arise in the discussions.

Topic guides allow for the exploration of key issues across multiple interviews, along with affording the interviewer the flexibility to examine matters arising from the discussions themselves [5]. Moreover, semi-structuring limits 'dross rate', defined by Holloway and Wheeler [26] as information not relevant to the study. Therefore, a topic guide asking open-ended questions regarding three broad issues was constructed as a core component of the semi-structuring of interviews for this study (see Additional file 1). The three broad areas were: (i) role of India in the development of CVD medications both within India and throughout the world; (ii) influence of India in the availability and development of CVD medications in the world pharmaceutical market; and (iii) thoughts/beliefs on the pharmaceutical industry. The wide nature of the points covered in this guide allowed the interviewer the freedom to expand upon emerging themes as they arose during the interviews. Issues were approached from various time perspectives (past, present and future), as an intentional attempt to draw upon the full length of an interviewee's experience in their field. All interviews were undertaken in February and March 2015. Interviews were undertaken at a location of the interviewee's choice, in English. Each interview took place in an office environment in New Delhi, Bangalore or Mumbai. Only the interviewer and the participant were in each interview.

An audio recording was taken of all interviews. All interviews aimed to last no longer than 30 min. The interviewer would undertake all data analysis and was therefore tasked with transcribing each recording verbatim. In doing this, they became habituated to the data early on, a critical aspect of thematic analysis [9]. Audio software was used to slow the recording during transcription, in an attempt to reduce transcription error

rate. The interviewer then completed inductive thematic analysis, as per the distinct 6-stage guidance outlined by Braun and Clarke [9]. Following transcription, the interviewer read through the entire dataset twice to ensure a broad comprehension of the interviews was obtained. All semantic and relevant latent themes were then coded through line-by-line reading of the text, using *NVivo 10* qualitative data analysis software. Semantic grouping of the codes into candidate themes was then undertaken, forming an initial thematic map (see Fig. 1). These themes were then scrutinized for their legitimacy, as outlined by Braun and Clarke [9], and to ensure their internal homogeneity and external heterogeneity was present, as stipulated by Patton [44]. Subsequent adaptation of the first thematic map was required following this review process, resulting in the production of a final thematic map (Fig. 2).

Member checking aims to ensure results presented in qualitative analysis are both credible and reliable, avoiding data misrepresentation [10]. It was felt appropriate to complete this process, due to the potential for complex topics to have arisen during the interviews in this research. Therefore, after completing data analysis, the interviewer e-mailed participants a summary of the initial findings of their interview. Interviewees were asked to check this summary, ensuring that their anonymity had been preserved and nothing had been misinterpreted. No issues of data misrepresentation arose from this process.

Inclusion of a detailed summation of the full analytical process satisfies the assertion that "qualitative research is reliable if one can follow the 'decision trail' of the investigative process" [39]. The transparency resulting from the explicit account of the analytical process of this study should, therefore, increase the reliability of these findings, adding rigor to this research.

Results

Eleven interviewees were successfully recruited. Of those recruited, one participant was excluded as it became clear during the interview that they fell into neither one of the stakeholder sub-groups, and were in fact from an entirely clinical background. A final sample of 10 participants was therefore analysed, consisting of a Government Official sub-group ($n = 5$) and Pharmaceutical Executive sub-group ($n = 5$). The full participant recruitment pathway can be seen in Fig. 3. Participant demographic data are shown in Table 1. Actual interview times ranged from 28 to 46 min.

Responses to the issues outlined in the topic guide (Additional file 1) were broad. However, there were relatively few new viewpoints uncovered in the last interview in each participant sub-group. Two distinct themes emerged: i) Patient-derived Factors; ii) Policy-derived Factors. Both emergent themes and their key topics are

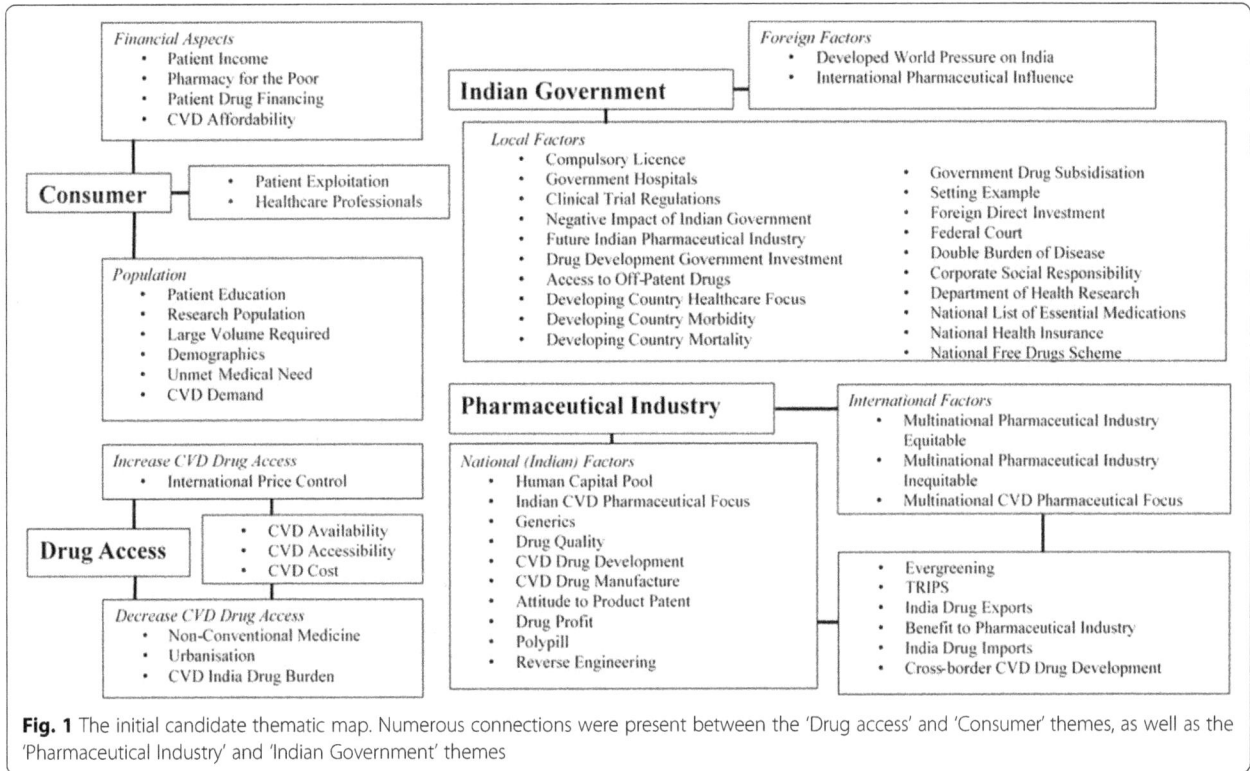

Fig. 1 The initial candidate thematic map. Numerous connections were present between the 'Drug access' and 'Consumer' themes, as well as the 'Pharmaceutical Industry' and 'Indian Government' themes

presented. Key issues are denoted as sub-headings under their respective theme.

Theme 1: patient-derived factors

The first distinct theme that emerged from the data contained factors that were either implicitly, or explicitly, linked to the Indian patient population.

1 (a) clinical trial regulations

One participant suggested that the recent tightening of clinical trial regulations in India was a positive factor affecting the role India plays in the development of CVD medicines:

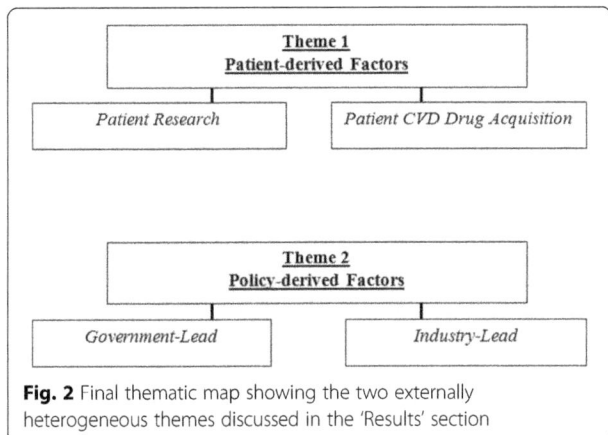

Fig. 2 Final thematic map showing the two externally heterogeneous themes discussed in the 'Results' section

P1 (Government Official sub-group): "The second thing that has happened which is quite good is tightening of [clinical trial] regulations... the patient population do not get exploited with loose clinical trial regulations."

The suggestion made by Participant 1 was not unanimously supported. Other participants, from both

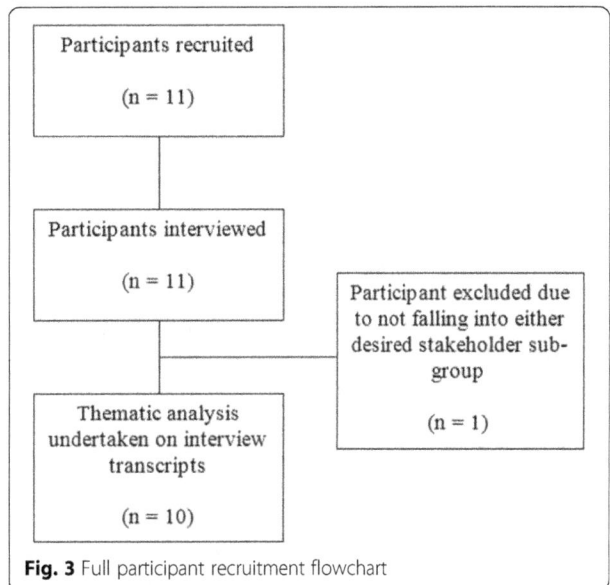

Fig. 3 Full participant recruitment flowchart

Table 1 Participant Demographic Table

Participant ID	Gender	Age (years)	Stakeholder sub-group	Time Working in Respective sub-group (years)
P1	Male	34	Government Official	6
P2	Male	50	Government Official	2.5
P3	Male	74	Government Official	49
P4	Male	53	Government Official	10
P5	Male	52	Government Official	16.5
P6	Female	53	Pharmaceutical Executive	20
P7	Male	46	Pharmaceutical Executive	19
P8	Male	40	Pharmaceutical Executive	13
P9	Male	50	Pharmaceutical Executive	20
P10	Male	52	Pharmaceutical Executive	15

Participant demographics and ID numbers

stakeholder sub-groups, suggested that present regulations applied too much pressure upon pharmaceutical companies, and were likely to deter drug research and development (R&D) in India:

> P3 (Government Official sub-group): "It's all negative [referring to the role the Indian government plays in relation to India's pharmaceutical industry]... there are three areas where we have problems with government... one is the clinical trial regulatory regime..."

> P6 (Pharmaceutical Executive sub-group): "The regulatory body, that sits in the government... in the last couple of years have come down with regulations related to pharmaceutical industry, which were very detrimental to the progress... on the clinical trial front... it's not possible to do studies with those regulations in mind..."

The differences in opinions highlight the complexity of the effects clinical trial regulations have had in India. Tight clinical trial regulations to promote ethical research may be motivated by concern for Indian patients, however, these rules may have a detrimental effect on the Indian pharmaceutical industry, according to participants in both stakeholder sub-groups.

1(b) benefits of undertaking drug development in India
Notwithstanding the conflicting opinion regarding drug regulations in India, participants highlighted numerous benefits to undertaking research in this nation. Firstly, the lack of exposure to previous pharmacological interventions mitigates against confounders present in other research settings, according to Participant 7:

> P7 (Pharmaceutical Executive sub-group): "I think what's good about India is that there... are a lot of drug naïve patients available... patients who have

never been treated with any drugs in the past... so... historically speaking they have a clean slate... and therefore... when you are looking for an effect of a particular drug it's much simpler because there are no... confounders..."

This positive factor was not mentioned at all by the Government Official sub-group, and introduced the idea that the Indian patient population may convey a clinical advantage over other nations, with reference to CVD drug development. Participant 7 reported that a further attraction for undertaking CVD medicine development in India stemmed from the large Indian population. They suggested the speed of research could be increased due to ease of patient recruitment:

> P7 (Pharmaceutical Executive sub-group): "Just by sheer population... it's possible to recruit patients fast... drug development and discovery... can be fast-forwarded... because of... this kind of [large] number of patients that we have."

This further example illustrates the importance patient-derived factors have in influencing pharmaceutical executive opinions regarding the best future focus for their business.

1(c) role of the media
Patient-derived factors are not all positive with reference to India's development of CVD medicines. One participant highlights how unethical research may have exploited patients in the past:

> P10 (Pharmaceutical Executive sub-group): "...and pharmaceutical industry... there are some bad players, and there have been some practices within the industry which were not the most ethical [towards patients] I would say,"

This interviewee went onto highlight the implicit role the media plays, through incomplete reporting, in tarring the wider reputation of the Indian pharmaceutical industry:

> P10 (Pharmaceutical Executive sub-group): "Having said that [referring to their previous comment regarding unethical research] I think... they [the pharmaceutical industry] want to do the right thing. Unfortunately, I think it is not publicised [to the patients] enough and... it becomes more of... a whipping law... in terms of any of the criticisms that come out..."

Therefore, whilst patient exploitation is not directly patient-derived, the subsequent detrimental influence of the media on patients is; through the resulting negative opinions of the drug industry. Media was not mentioned by the Government Official sub-group.

1(d) Patient Purchasing Power
Factors grounded in the patient population were commonly mentioned to affect availability of CVD medicines. Firstly, the ability of patients to purchase CVD medicines was highlighted as a significant barrier to CVD drug affordability, by both stakeholder sub-groups:

> P2 (Government Official sub-group): "Access is a function of economic strength of the people... if they... lack purchasing power, even if medicines are available in the villages... they won't be able to buy that [CVD medicine]."

> P7 (Pharmaceutical Executive sub-group): "I mean large population of India still lives in its villages... the poverty is just unbelievable... they don't have money to eat food, let alone have [CVD] medications."

The contextualisation of poverty in terms of geographic location by Participant 7 echoes, to some extent, the influence urbanisation has on access to CVD medicines according to another interviewee. Here, difficulties patients encounter in reaching government hospitals, and therefore accessing the CVD medicines and treatments available at these locations, is discussed:

> P6 (Pharmaceutical Executive sub-group): "I mean government hospitals are freely accessible... but even multi-speciality government hospital is very far from many of these rural areas, so many people will reach there only when they are in very bad shape..."

Patient purchasing power and finances are therefore somewhat linked to a person's physical location, in relation to the dispenser-point of the CVD drugs.

1(e) patient education
Another frequently mentioned factor which influences CVD drug access is educational level:

> P8 (Pharmaceutical Executive sub-group): "From the patient's perspective, cardiovascular disease is something which is a... chronic disease and it doesn't... kill people in a very short time. So I think that itself probably also means that patients are not paying too much of attention to the disease per se,"

> P5 (Government Official sub-group): "There is a question of [patient] education... better education... better lifestyle, those things ensure... you understand how you need to go for purchasing medicines."

Participants from both sub-groups hence spoke of the wider impact patient education has on their awareness to acquire CVD drugs.

1(f) Non-conventional medicine use
A participant in the Government Official sub-group also discussed the use of non-conventional medicine by patients, as a barrier to CVD drug access:

> P5 (Government Official sub-group): "Also it's [CVD drug access] a question of belief... some of the people... have the traditional way of thinking, so they do not go by the modern [CVD] medicines..."

Therefore, participants felt that patient education influences CVD drug access, not only through patient motivation to obtain medicine, but also by influencing the type of drugs being used. Patients may be harmed if alternative therapies being used are less clinically effective than conventional CVD drugs.

Theme 2: policy-derived factors
The second distinct theme that arose from this research regarded issues that were grounded in Indian drug policy.

2(a) Indian pharmaceutical industry focus and its effects
The predominant influence the Indian government has had in the past, according to both stakeholder sub-groups, is in directing the focus of the national pharmaceutical industry. Every participant stated the past, and to a certain extent present, role of the Indian pharmaceutical industry is in the production of off-patent, generic medicines:

> P2 (Government Official sub-group): "We [India] are the generics industry. We are not so much engaged in the new development of... [CVD] drugs."

P6 (Pharmaceutical Executive sub-group): "So I think if you look at Indian pharmaceutical industry, largely it's generics based."

Exploration of India's current pharmaceutical focus highlighted its role in the provision of low-cost, high quality medicines for the developing world and the West:

P3 (Government Official sub-group): "India could continue to be a major supplier of quality medicine to the third world countries, and also... in the West..."

P8 (Pharmaceutical Executive sub-group): "India has impacted the global pharmaceutical industry a lot by its generic drugs... provided to the global market, whether it is US, Europe, or it is Sub-Saharan countries...."

Furthermore, participants from both sub-groups touched upon the prospective focus of the Indian CVD pharmaceutical industry. Stakeholders stated the likely future for India will be to produce more complex, high-quality generics and to nurture stronger drug development:

P3 (Government Official sub-group): "...and within generic, Indian industry's also moving up the value chain. So, instead of plain generics, they're moving into a complex, or different chain of generics..."

B4 (Government Official sub-group): "The Indian pharmaceutical industry has largely been involved in manufacturing generics... but they do have some new fixed dose combinations and polypills which they developed recently,"

P2 (Government Official sub-group): "We [India] are the generics industry. We are not engaged in the new development of... [CVD] drugs, but our... aim is that [to become involved in the development of new CVD drugs]."

Despite the predicted transition of focus in the Indian industry, participants felt CVD generic medicines will remain a significant player in this market for the foreseeable future:

P10 (Pharmaceutical Executive sub-group): "...generics will still continue to be the primary driver of the [Indian pharmaceutical] market ..."

One participant suggested the Indian generic industry has cultivated an excessive amount of market competition, to the detriment of drug quality:

P10 (Pharmaceutical Executive sub-group): "The barriers to entry are so low to make new... generic medicine in India, you have got... 100 brands of atorvastatin now... do you think all 100 brands are going to behave the same way? Probably not... the quality control systems that we invest in, in this facility [referring to their own pharmaceutical company], are much more robust than... some mum and pap making tablets... in a garage..."

Participants also highlighted how generic CVD medicines increase access, as they are an economically viable option from a prescriber's perspective:

P9 (Pharmaceutical Executive sub-group): "Generics lower the cost of treatment, and hence give doctors the choice to prescribe a generic drug, when otherwise they may not have prescribed the innovator drug simply because of cost..."

In summary, according to participants, the Indian CVD pharmaceutical industry is currently centred on large-scale generic production. This role is likely to change in future to an increased focus on the production of high-quality generics and undertaking more drug R&D.

2(b) Indian human capital

Another significant impact government policy has had on the Indian CVD drug industry, according to this study's participants, has been the increased availability of scientific human capital:

P5 (Government Official sub-group): "Our Universities are also good in terms of producing quality professionals, and during the past 10 years a number of pharmacy colleges have been set up... we have good quality of professionals in the field of clinical trial and pharmaceutical technology and pharmaceutical R&D,"

P6 (Pharmaceutical Executive sub-group): "One thing which the [Indian] pharmaceutical industry has is lots of very highly skilled manpower..."

The pool of skilled academics available to undertake advanced drug research is therefore recognised by both stakeholder sub-groups. Furthermore, one participant implied this expert population is likely to grow, rather than decrease, over coming years due to return of trained Indian professionals to the country:

P8 (Pharmaceutical Executive sub-group): "You can find that a lot of them [Indian men and women] have gone abroad and specialized... in various [pharmaceutical] fields, even got work experience and are willing to come back [to India]..."

2(c) attitude to product patent

Indian drug policy is also linked to access to CVD medicines according this study's participants. The international pharmaceutical community would apparently prefer the Indian drug industry to have a more stringent product patent regime. However, a major barrier to this is product patent 'Evergreening', defined as a pharmaceutical company's extension of their monopoly on a drug beyond the usual term permitted by law [18]. Stakeholders form both sub-groups referred to this controversial attitude to patent law:

P4 (Government Official sub-group): "The multinational companies want a stronger patent regime in India... but the Indian companies don't want the multinational companies to Evergreen..."

P7 (Pharmaceutical Executive sub-group): "You see companies getting greedy... they have some small incremental innovation, and they want now again 20 more years after... the main... patent has... expired... If that can be prevented, then I think the basic intellectual property should belong to those who invest money in it..."

Despite international pressure for India to tighten its drug patent regime, one participant stated that India's present attitude to drug patents it not over-lenient, as it conforms to the Trade-Related Aspects of Intellectual Property Rights (TRIPS) agreement:

P3 (Government Official sub-group): "It's [India's product patent regime] not lax, we are conforming to the TRIPS agreement, whatever the standard TRIPS provided, we conform to that..."

Instead of being down to laxities in India's approach to intellectual property (IP), this participant suggested the international community were against India's present IP regime due to their success in producing high-quality generic medicines for the developed world:

P3 (Government Official sub-group): "Now 80 % of prescriptions in the US are of Indian generics, so the US generic companies are hurt... when you are successful... everyone is going to throw stone at you..."

Despite this defence of India's existing attitude to IP, it is likely that the Indian government will tighten regulations in the near future, according to Participant 4. This is due to the influence of other geo-political factors, like the US's provision of nuclear energy to India:

P4 (Government Official sub-group): "It's... rumoured that they [the Indian government] might have an agreement with the US in terms of... tightening the [drug] patent laws... to get other additional benefits... nuclear energy treaty was held hostage to many other things, so they [the Indian government] wanted to get that off the ground,"

India's compulsory licensing policy has allowed for past overruling of product patents in order to increase access to specific medicines. This initiative allows a government to develop patented drugs, without the patent-holder's permission [13]. However, one participant suggested this has detrimentally affected long-term access of novel CVD medicines in India, through mistrust between multinational companies and the Indian government:

P6 (Pharmaceutical Executive sub-group): "They [the Indian government] have asked the innovator... to give up their patent... you are making it [the CVD drug] available, but then... invalidating their [the innovator company's] patent in India... that will become a deterrent for new CVD drugs to come to India."

Therefore, there are perceived to be numerous external pressures on India attempting to direct the government's future attitude regarding IP. Altering attitude to IP may, through re-building trust with some multinationals, increase the amount of new CVD products being introduced into the Indian market, thereby potentially improving CVD drug access.

Discussion

Our study highlights three findings. First, both government and pharmaceutical participants felt that the focus of Indian pharma is shifting to more complex, high-quality generics and to new drug development, but production of generic drugs rather than new molecular entities will remain a major activity. Second, current trial regulations in India may restrict India's potential role in the future development of CVD drugs. Third, it is likely that the Indian government will tighten its intellectual property regime in future, with potentially far-reaching implications on CVD drug development and access.

The expiry of patents on $60 billion worth of drugs in 2010 suggests that India will remain a significant producer of generics [22]. The Indian pharmaceutical industry's increasing acquisition of resources to undertake independent R&D make it likely that drug development will gain in importance [27]. Whilst interviewees suggested government policy plays an important role in shaping the industry, a significant force for change was ascribed to patient-derived factors, contrary to current literature [27]. Therefore, there may be a potential role for Indian initiatives that market the unique advantages of its patient population for drug research in influencing national and multinational pharmaceutical companies to undertake CVD drug development in India, rather than simply IP policy-directed factors. It was suggested by one interviewee that rapid patient recruitment represented a major advantage of undertaking research in India. However, 2008 Federal Drug Administration (FDA) data suggest that at inspected clinical trial sites, China may be ahead of India in this regard, with India and China recruiting 8 and 13 participants per recruitment site respectively [33]. There is clearly a need for research into the factors which make India attractive to host CVD drug R&D before policy recommendations can be made, and comparative research with China will be beneficial to inform Indian policy [35].

Although current clinical trial regulations were implicated in restricting Indian CVD drug development, there are two arguments for their existence. First, deviations from ethical research practice have been documented in India previously [48] and therefore, more stringent regulations protect Indian patients from recurrence of such exploitation [35], reiterated by one participant in this study. Second, questions must be raised over the morality of undertaking research with a population that ultimately may not have access to the final product; such as in India where CVD drug availability is an issue. A fine line therefore exists, regarding clinical trial guidelines, between market facilitation and patient protection. However, it is clear that participants felt that the present balance is weighed against the CVD drug development industry. As with other heath policy domains, there is a role for an independent evidence-based appraisal of present clinical trial regulations in India [4] support the use of formal analytical institutes for the of health policy in LMICs, to ensure adequate patient protection, while allowing Indian pharmaceutical development.

Whilst one participant defended India's current stance, asserting that the government rigorously conform to TRIPS guidelines, other interviewees outlined the external pressure being placed on India to observe to tighter patent regulations. The European Union's Free Trade Agreement states Europe's intentions to seek regulations that go beyond the TRIPS agreement in developing countries [15]. Succumbing to such demands may afford India benefits to other sectors, such as energy, according to one stakeholder. Although IP regulations are praised in India for driving the development of a stronger R&D sector within the Indian pharmaceutical industry [27], there has been a lack of technology transfer since India's signing of the TRIPS agreement in 1992, along with a diminished focus on drug production as per the needs of the national population [1]. However, continued adherence to existing IP regulations may help reinforce trust between the Indian government and multinational drug industry, which is suspicious due to India's past compulsory licensing [28]. An improved relationship could persuade pharmaceutical companies to make novel CVD medicines readily available on the Indian market, something that they are presently reluctant to do according to this study. Further policy research should investigate the effects of tighter IP control and tighter clinical trial regulations on the scale of drug development in India.

Limitations
The small sample size of this study is a limitation. However, few novel topics emerged during the final interview of each stakeholder sub-group, suggesting theoretical saturation was being approached. Triangulation, the use of multiple researchers for data analysis [10], was not possible, and would have increased the validity of our findings. Our analysis considered two specific stakeholder subgroups in the Indian context for CVD drugs, and therefore, our findings cannot be generalized to other subgroups, countries or drug areas.

Conclusion
Among government and pharmaceutical stakeholders, our analysis suggested consensus around three barriers to new CVD drug development and access in India: (i) the prevailing culture, expertise and infrastructure of the drug industry favouring generic production; (ii) strict clinical trial regulations; and (iii) the current IP regime. The role of these different factors on CVD drug development and access in India should be the subject of further research.

Key messages

1. Both government and pharmaceutical participants felt that the focus of Indian pharma is shifting to more complex, high-quality generics and to new drug development, but production of generic drugs rather than new molecular entities will remain a major activity.
2. Current trial regulations in India may restrict India's potential role in the future development of CVD drugs.
3. It is likely that the Indian government will tighten its intellectual property regime in future, with potentially far-reaching implications on CVD drug development and access.

Approval
Ethical approval was awarded from the University of Birmingham BioMedical Science (BSc) Internal Ethics Review Committee (UK), and the Independent Ethics Committee of the Centre for Chronic Disease Control (India).

Competing interests

The authors declare that they have no competing interests.

Authors' contributions

AB had the idea for this study, and AB and CN developed the protocol. CN conducted the interviews under the supervision of VSA and RS. CN was responsible for transcription and CN and AB performed analyses. CN and AB drafted the manuscript. All authors read and approved the final manuscript.

Funding

The research has received funding from the European Research Council under the European Union's Seventh Framework Programme (FP/2007-2013)/ERC Grant Agreement no. 339239.

Author details

[1]University of Birmingham, Medical School, Birmingham, UK. [2]Centre for Chronic Disease Control, New Delhi, India. [3]Research and Information Systems for Developing Countries (RIS), New Delhi, India. [4]Public Health Foundation of India, New Delhi, India. [5]University of Birmingham Centre for Cardiovascular Sciences, Birmingham, UK. [6]Present address: Farr Institute of Health Informatics Research, University College London, 222 Euston Road, London NW1 2DA, UK. [7]School of Health, University of Central Lancashire, Preston, UK.

References

1. Abrol D. Post-TRIPS technological behaviour of the pharmaceutical industry in India. Sci Technol Soc. 2004;9(2):243–71.
2. Banerjee A. Whose responsibility is access to essential drugs for chronic diseases? Ethics Econ. 2006;4:2.
3. Banerjee A, Pogge T. The health impact fund: How might it work for novel anticoagulants in atrial fibrillation? Global Heart. 2014;9(2):255–61.
4. Bennett S, Corluka A, Doherty J, et al. Influencing policy change: the experience of health think tanks in Low- and middle-income countries. Health Policy Plan. 2011;27(3):194–203.
5. Bernard HR. Interviewing I: Unstructured and Semistructured. Research Methods in Anthropology. 5th ed. Plymouth: AltaMira Press; 2011. p. 158.
6. Bhatt A. India's next challenge: rebooting recruitment. Perspec Clin Res. 2014;5(3):93.
7. Bhosale N, Nigar S, Das S, Divate U, Divate P. Protection of human research participants: accreditation of programmes in the Indian context. Indian J Med Ethics. 2014;11:55–9.
8. Binnendijk E, Koren R, Dror DM. Can the rural poor in India afford to treat non-communicable diseases. Trop Med Int Health. 2012;17(11):1376–85.
9. Braun V, Clarke V. Using thematic analysis in psychology. Qual Res Psychol. 2006;3(2):77–101.
10. Braun V, Clarke V. Successful Qualitative Research. London: Sage; 2013.
11. Chaturvedi V, Bhargava B. Health care delivery for coronary heart disease in India - where Are We headed? Am Heart Hosp J. 2007;5(1):32–7.
12. Chen S and Ravallion M. 2008. The Developing World is Poorer than We Thought, But No Less Successful in the Fight Against Poverty. [Online]. World Bank Policy research Working Paper Series. Available from: http://ssrn.com/abstract=1259575 [Accessed 10 April 2015].
13. Chien CV. HIV/AIDS drugs for Sub-Saharan africa: How do brand and generic supply compare? PLoS ONE. 2007;2(3):e278.
14. Chow CK, Cardona M, Raju PK, et al. Cardiovascular disease and risk factors among 345 adults in rural India - the Andhra Pradesh rural health initiative. Int J Cardiol. 2007;116(2):180–5.
15. Correa C M. 2009. Negotiation of a Free Trade Agreement European Union-India: Will India Accept TRIPS-Plus Protection? [Online].Available from: http://www.oxfam.de/files/20090609_negotiationofafreetradeaggrementeuindia_218kb.pdf [Accessed 9 May 2015].
16. Daivadanam M. Pathways to catastrophic health expenditure for acute coronary syndrome in Kerala: 'Good health at low cost'? BMC Public Health. 2012;12:306.

17. Dunne S, Shannon B, Dunne C, Cullen W. A review of the differences and similarities between generic drugs and their originator counterparts, including economic benefits associated with usage of generic medicines, using Ireland as a case study. BMC Pharmacol Toxicol. 2013;14:1. doi:10.1186/2050-6511-14-1.
18. Dwivedi G, Hallihosur S, Rangan L. Evergreening: a deceptive device in patent rights. Technol Soc. 2010;32(4):324–30.
19. Engelgau MM, Karan A, Mahal A. The economic impact of Non-communicable diseases on households in India. Global Health. 2012;8:9.
20. Foy H. India to give free generic drugs to hundreds of millions. Reuters. 2012. http://www.reuters.com/article/us-india-drugs-idUSBRE8630PW20120705#TSACW5g2rmxxFMVj.97
21. Goyal EG, Yusuf S. The burden of cardiovascular disease in the Indian subcontinent. Indian J Med Res. 2006;124(3):235–44.
22. Greene W. The Emergence of India's Pharmaceutical Industry and Implications for the US Generic Drug Market. [Online]. Washington DC: US International Trade Commission; 2007. Available from: http://www.usitc.gov/publications/332/EC200705A.pdf. [Accessed 1 May 2015].
23. Guest G, Bunce A, Johnson L. How many interviews are enough? An experiment with data saturation and variability. Field Methods. 2006;18(1):59–82.
24. Gupta R, Guptha S, Sharma KK, Gupta A, Deedwania P. Regional variations in cardiovascular risk factors in India: India heart watch. World J Cardiol. 2012; 4(4):112–20.
25. Gupta R, Islam S, Mony P, Kutty VR, Mohan V, Kumar R, Thakur JS, Shankar VK, Mohan D, Vijayakumar K, Rahman O, Yusuf R, Iqbal R, Shahid M, Mohan I, Rangarajan S, Teo KK, Yusuf S. Socioeconomic factors and use of secondary preventive therapies for cardiovascular diseases in South Asia: The PURE study. Eur J Prev Cardiol. 2015;22(10):1261–71.
26. Holloway I, Wheeler S. Glossary. Qualitative Research in Nursing and Healthcare. 3rd ed. Wiley-Blackwell: Chichester; 2013. p. 338.
27. Kale D, Little S. From Imitation to Innovation: The Evolution of R&D Capabilities and Learning Process in the Indian Pharmaceutical Industry. Tech Anal Strat Manag. 2007;19(5):589–609.
28. Kapczynski A. Harmonization and its discontents: a case study of TRIPS implementation in India's pharmaceutical sector. California Law Review. 2009;97(6):1571–649.
29. Khatib R, Schwalm JD, Yusuf S, Haynes RB, McKee M, Khan M, Nieuwlaat R. Patient and healthcare provider barriers to hypertension awareness, treatment and follow up: a systematic review and meta-analysis of qualitative and quantitative studies. PLoS ONE. 2014;9(1):e84238.
30. Khatib R, McKee M, Shannon H, Chow C, Rangarajan S, Teo K, Wei L, Mony P, Mohan V, Gupta R, Kumar R, Vijayakumar K, Lear SA, Diaz R, Avezum A, Lopez-Jaramillo P, Lanas F, Yusoff K, Ismail N, Kazmi K, Rahman O, Rosengren A, Monsef N, Kelishadi R, Kruger A, Puoane T, Szuba A, Chifamba J, Temizhan A, Dagenais G, Gafni A, Yusuf S; PURE study investigators. Availability and affordability of cardiovascular disease medicines and their effect on use in high-income, middle-income, and low-income countries: an analysis of the PURE study data. Lancet. 2015 Oct 20.
31. Kiran R, Mishra S. Performance of the Indian pharmaceutical industry in post-TRIPS period: a firm level analysis. Int Rev Bus Res Papers. 2009;5(6):148–60.
32. Leeder S, Raymond S, Greenberg H, Liu H and Esson K. 2004. A Race Against Time: The Challenge of Cardiovascular Disease in Developing Countries. [Online]. New York: Columbia University Press. Available from: http://earth.columbia.edu/news/2004/images/raceagainsttime_FINAL_051104.pdf [Accessed 21 April 2015].
33. Levinson D. Challenges to FDA's Ability to Monitor and Inspect Foreign Clinical Trials. [Online]. India: Office of Inspector General; 2010. Available from: https://oig.hhs.gov/oei/reports/oei-01-08-00510.pdf [Accessed 3 May 2015].
34. Lonn E, Bosch J, Teo KK, et al. The polypill in the prevention of cardiovascular diseases: Key concepts, current status, challenges, and future directions. Circulation. 2010;122(20):2078–88.
35. Maiti R, Raghavendra M. Clinical trials in India. Pharmacol Res. 2007;56(1):1–10.
36. Marshall MN. Sampling for qualitative research. Fam Pract. 1996;13(6):522–5.
37. Mendis S, Fukino K, Cameron A, et al. The availability and affordability of selected essential medicines for chronic diseases in Six Low- and middle-income countries. Bull World Health Organ. 2007;85(4):279–88.
38. Menon J, Vijayakumar N, Joseph JK, David PC, Menon MN, Mukundan S, Dorphy PD, Banerjee A. Below the poverty line and non-communicable diseases in Kerala: The Epidemiology of Non-communicable Diseases in Rural Areas (ENDIRA) study. Int J Cardiol. 2015;187:519–24.

39. Morse JM, Barrett M, Mayan M, Olson K, Spiers J. Verification strategies for establishing reliability and validity in qualitative research. Int J Qual Methods. 2002;1(2):13–22.

40. GBD 2013 DALYs and HALE Collaborators, Murray CJ, Barber RM, Foreman KJ, Ozgoren AA, Abd-Allah F, Abera SF, Aboyans V, Abraham JP, Abubakar I, Abu-Raddad LJ, Abu-Rmeileh NM, Achoki T, Ackerman IN, Ademi Z, Adou AK, Adsuar JC, Afshin A, Agardh EE, Alam SS, Alasfoor D, Albittar MI, Alegretti MA, Alemu ZA, Alfonso-Cristancho R, Alhabib S, Ali R, Alla F, Allebeck P, Almazroa MA, Alsharif U, Alvarez E, Alvis-Guzman N, Amare AT, Ameh EA, Amini H, Ammar W, Anderson HR, Anderson BO, Antonio CA, Anwari P, Arnlöv J, Arsenijevic VS, Artaman A, Asghar RJ, Assadi R, Atkins LS, Avila MA, Awuah B, Bachman VF, Badawi A, Bahit MC, Balakrishnan K, Banerjee A, Barker-Collo SL, Barquera S, Barregard L, Barrero LH, Basu A, Basu S, Basulaiman MO, Beardsley J, Bedi N, Beghi E, Bekele T, Bell ML, Benjet C, Bennett DA, Bensenor IM, Benzian H, Bernabé E, Bertozzi-Villa A, Beyene TJ, Bhala N, Bhalla A, Bhutta ZA, Bienhoff K, Bikbov B, Biryukov S, Blore JD, Blosser CD, Blyth FM, Bohensky MA, Bolliger IW, Başara BB, Bornstein NM, Bose D, Boufous S, Bourne RR, Boyers LN, Brainin M, Brayne CE, Brazinova A, Breitborde NJ, Brenner H, Briggs AD, Brooks PM, Brown JC, Brugha TS, Buchbinder R, Buckle GC, Budke CM, Bulchis A, Bulloch AG, Campos-Nonato IR, Carabin H, Carapetis JR, Cárdenas R, Carpenter DO, Caso V, Castañeda-Orjuela CA, Castro RE, Catalá-López F, Cavalleri F, Çavlin A, Chadha VK, Chang JC, Charlson FJ, Chen H, Chen W, Chiang PP, Chimed-Ochir O, Chowdhury R, Christensen H, Christophi CA, Cirillo M, Coates MM, Coffeng LE, Coggeshall MS, Colistro V, Colquhoun SM, Cooke GS, Cooper C, Cooper LT, Coppola LM, Cortinovis M, Criqui MH, Crump JA, Cuevas-Nasu L, Danawi H, Dandona L, Dandona R, Dansereau E, Dargan PI, Davey G, Davis A, Davitoiu DV, Dayama A, De Leo D, Degenhardt L, Del Pozo-Cruz B, Dellavalle RP, Deribe K, Derrett S, Jarlais DC, Dessalegn M, Dharmaratne SD, Dherani MK, Diaz-Torné C, Dicker D, Ding EL, Dokova K, Dorsey ER, Driscoll TR, Duan L, Duber HC, Ebel BE, Edmond KM, Elshrek YM, Endres M, Ermakov SP, Erskine HE, Eshrati B, Esteghamati A, Estep K, Faraon EJ, Farzadfar F, Fay DF, Feigin VL, Felson DT, Fereshtehnejad SM, Fernandes JG, Ferrari AJ, Fitzmaurice C, Flaxman AD, Fleming TD, Foigt N, Forouzanfar MH, Fowkes FG, Paleo UF, Franklin RC, Fürst T, Gabbe B, Gaffikin L, Gankpé FG, Geleijnse JM, Gessner BD, Gething P, Gibney KB, Giroud M, Giussani G, Dantes HG, Gona P, González-Medina D, Gosselin RA, Gotay CC, Goto A, Gouda HN, Graetz N, Gugnani HC, Gupta R, Gupta R, Gutiérrez RA, Haagsma J, Hafezi-Nejad N, Hagan H, Halasa YA, Hamadeh RR, Hamavid H, Hammami M, Hancock J, Hankey GJ, Hansen GM, Hao Y, Harb HL, Haro JM, Havmoeller R, Hay SI, Hay RJ, Heredia-Pi IB, Heuton KR, Heydarpour P, Higashi H, Hijar M, Hoek HW, Hoffman HJ, Hosgood HD, Hossain M, Hotez PJ, Hoy DG, Hsairi M, Hu G, Huang C, Huang JJ, Husseini A, Huynh C, Iannarone ML, Iburg KM, Innos K, Inoue M, Islami F, Jacobsen KH, Jarvis DL, Jassal SK, Jee SH, Jeemon P, Jensen PN, Jha V, Jiang G, Jiang Y, Jonas JB, Juel K, Kan H, Karch A, Karema CK, Karimkhani C, Karthikeyan G, Kassebaum NJ, Kaul A, Kawakami N, Kazanjan K, Kemp AH, Kengne AP, Keren A, Khader YS, Khalifa SE, Khan EA, Khan G, Khang YH, Kieling C, Kim D, Kim S, Kim Y, Kinfu Y, Kinge JM, Kivipelto M, Knibbs LD, Knudsen AK, Kokubo Y, Kosen S, Krishnaswami S, Defo BK, Bicer BK, Kuipers EJ, Kulkarni C, Kulkarni VS, Kumar GA, Kyu HH, Lai T, Lalloo R, Lallukka T, Lam H, Lan Q, Lansingh VC, Larsson A, Lawrynowicz AE, Leasher JL, Leigh J, Leung R, Levitz CE, Li B, Li Y, Li Y, Lim SS, Lind M, Lipshultz SE, Liu S, Liu Y, Lloyd BK, Lofgren KT, Logroscino G, Looker KJ, Lortet-Tieulent J, Lotufo PA, Lozano R, Lucas RM, Lunevicius R, Lyons RA, Ma S, Macintyre MF, Mackay MT, Majdan M, Malekzadeh R, Marcenes W, Margolis DJ, Margono C, Marzan MB, Masci JR, Mashal MT, Matzopoulos R, Mayosi BM, Mazorodze TT, Mcgill NW, Mcgrath JJ, Mckee M, Mclain A, Meaney PA, Medina C, Mehndiratta MM, Mekonnen W, Melaku YA, Meltzer M, Memish ZA, Mensah GA, Meretoja A, Mhimbira FA, Micha R, Miller TR, Mills EJ, Mitchell PB, Mock CN, Ibrahim NM, Mohammad KA, Mokdad AH, Mola GL, Monasta L, Hernandez JC, Montico M, Montine TJ, Mooney MD, Moore AR, Moradi-Lakeh M, Moran AE, Mori R, Moschandreas J, Moturi WN, Moyer ML, Mozaffarian D, Msemburi WT, Mueller UO, Mukaigawara M, Mullany EC, Murdoch ME, Murray J, Murthy KS, Naghavi M, Naheed A, Naidoo KS, Naldi L, Nand D, Nangia V, Narayan KM, Nejjari C, Neupane SP, Newton CR, Ng M, Ngalesoni FN, Nguyen G, Nisar MI, Nolte S, Norheim OF, Norman RE, Norrving B, Nyakarahuka L, Oh IH, Ohkubo T, Ohno SL, Olusanya BO, Opio JN, Ortblad K, Ortiz A, Pain AW, Pandian JD, Panelo CI, Papachristou C, Park EK, Park JH, Patten SB, Patton GC, Paul VK, Pavlin BI, Pearce N, Pereira DM, Perez-Padilla R, Perez-Ruiz F, Perico N, Pervaiz A, Pesudovs K, Peterson CB, Petzold M, Phillips MR, Phillips BK, Phillips DE, Piel FB, Plass D, Poenaru D, Polinder S, Pope D, Popova S, Poulton RG, Pourmalek F, Prabhakaran D, Prasad NM, Pullan RL, Qato DM, Quistberg DA, Rafay A, Rahimi K, Rahman SU, Raju M, Rana SM, Razavi H, Reddy KS, Refaat A, Remuzzi G, Resnikoff S, Ribeiro AL, Richardson L, Richardus JH, Roberts DA, Rojas-Rueda D, Ronfani L, Roth GA, Rothenbacher D, Rothstein DH, Rowley JT, Roy N, Ruhago GM, Saeedi MY, Saha S, Sahraian MA, Sampson UK, Sanabria JR, Sandar L, Santos IS, Satpathy M, Sawhney M, Scarborough P, Schneider IJ, Schöttker B, Schumacher AE, Schwebel DC, Scott JG, Seedat S, Sepanlou SG, Serina PT, Servan-Mori EE, Shackelford KA, Shaheen A, Shahraz S, Levy TS, Shangguan S, She J, Sheikhbahaei S, Shi P, Shibuya K, Shinohara Y, Shiri R, Shishani K, Shiue I, Shrime MG, Sigfusdottir ID, Silberberg DH, Simard EP, Sindi S, Singh A, Singh JA, Singh L, Skirbekk V, Slepak EL, Sliwa K, Soneji S, Søreide K, Soshnikov S, Sposato LA, Sreeramareddy CT, Stanaway JD, Stathopoulou V, Stein DJ, Stein MB, Steiner C, Steiner TJ, Stevens A, Stewart A, Stovner LJ, Stroumpoulis K, Sunguya BF, Swaminathan S, Swaroop M, Sykes BL, Tabb KM, Takahashi K, Tandon N, Tanne D, Tanner M, Tavakkoli M, Taylor HR, Ao BJ, Tediosi F, Temesgen AM, Templin T, Ten Have M, Tenkorang EY, Terkawi AS, Thomson B, Thorne-Lyman AL, Thrift AG, Thurston GD, Tillmann T, Tonelli M, Topouzis F, Toyoshima H, Traebert J, Tran BX, Trillini M, Truelsen T, Tsilimbaris M, Tuzcu EM, Uchendu US, Ukwaja KN, Undurraga EA, Uzun SB, Van Brakel WH, Van De Vijver S, van Gool CH, Van Os J, Vasankari TJ, Venketasubramanian N, Violante FS, Vlassov VV, Vollset SE, Wagner GR, Wagner J, Waller SG, Wan X, Wang H, Wang J, Wang L, Warouw TS, Weichenthal S, Weiderpass E, Weintraub RG, Wenzhi W, Werdecker A, Westerman R, Whiteford HA, Wilkinson JD, Williams TN, Wolfe CD, Wolock TM, Woolf AD, Wulf S, Wurtz B, Xu G, Yan LL, Yano Y, Ye P, Yentür GK, Yip P, Yonemoto N, Yoon SJ, Younis MZ, Yu C, Zaki ME, Zhao Y, Zheng Y, Zonies D, Zou X, Salomon JA, Lopez AD, Vos T. Global, regional, and national disability-adjusted life years (DALYs) for 306 diseases and injuries and healthy life expectancy (HALE) for 188 countries, 1990–2013: quantifying the epidemiological transition. Lancet. 2015;386:2145–91.

41. Murray DM, Hannan PJ. Planning for the appropriate analysis in school-based drug-use prevention studies. J Consult Clin Psychol. 1990;58(4):458.

42. Osterberg L, Blaschke T. Adherence to medication. N Engl J Med. 2005; 353(5):487–97.

43. Patel V, Chatterji S, Chisholm D, et al. Chronic diseases and injuries in India. Lancet. 2011;377(9763):413–28.

44. Patton MQ. Qualitative analysis and interpretation. In: Laughton C, editor. Qualitative Research & Evaluation Methods. 3rd ed. London: Sage; 2002. p. 465.

45. Reddy KS, Patel V, Jha P, Paul VK, Kumar AK, Lancet India Group for Universal Healthcare, et al. Towards achievement of universal health care in India by 2020: a call to action. Lancet. 2011;377(9767):760–8.

46. Roth GA, Nguyen G, Forouzanfar MH, Mokdad AH, Naghavi M, Murray CJ. Estimates of global and regional premature cardiovascular mortality in 2025. Circulation. 2015;132(13):1270–82.

47. Roth GA, Forouzanfar MH, Moran AE, Barber R, Nguyen G, Feigin VL, Naghavi M, Mensah GA, Murray CJ. Demographic and epidemiologic drivers of global cardiovascular mortality. N Engl J Med. 2015;372(14):1333–41.

48. Sarojini N, Srinivasan S, Madhavi Y, Srinivasan S, Shenoi A. The HPV vaccine: science, ethics and regulation. Econ Pol Wkly. 2010;45(27):27–34.

49. Singal GL, Nanda A, Kotwani A. A comparative evaluation of price and quality of some branded versus branded-generic medicines of the same manufacturer in India. Indian J Pharmacol. 2011;43(2):131–6.

50. United Nations. 2000. United Nations Millennium Development Goals. [Online]. Available from: http://www.un.org/millenniumgoals/ [Accessed 15 April 2015].

51. von Schirnding Y. The world summit on sustainable development: reaffirming the centrality of health. Glob Health. 2005;1(1):8.

52. World Health Organization 2011. Noncommunicable Diseases Country Profiles 2011. [Online]. Available from: http://www.who.int/nmh/publications/ncd_profiles2011/en/ [Accessed 19 April 2015].

53. World Health Organization. Informed Consent Form Templates. [Online]. Available from: http://www.who.int/rpc/research_ethics/informed_consent/en/ [Accessed 23 April 2015].

54. Xavier D, Pais P, Devereaux P, et al. Treatment and outcomes of acute coronary syndromes in India (CREATE): a prospective analysis of registry data. Lancet. 2008;371(9622):1435–42.

5

Fighting falsified medicines with paperwork – a historic review of Danish legislation governing distribution of medicines

Rasmus Borup[1]*[iD], Susanne Kaae[1], Timo Minssen[2] and Janine Traulsen[1]

Abstract

Background: Many areas of pharmaceutical legislation in the European Union (EU) are harmonised in order to promote the internal market and protect public health. Ideally, harmonisation leads to less fragmented regulation and cross-border complexities. This study, however, focuses on an increasingly harmonised legislative area that is subject to increases in requirements and complexities: the distribution of medicines. This study compared Danish legislation governing the distribution of medicines before and after Denmark joined the EU in order to assess the impact of EU harmonisation, as well as to evaluate whether the drastic increases in requirements mandated by the Falsified Medicines Directive of 2011 correspond to a new approach to governing the pharmaceutical supply chain.

Methods: A review was conducted of 115 applicable Danish laws, executive orders and guidelines from 1913 to 2014. Legal requirements were organised according to the year they were published and the companies they affected. Greater changes in legislative requirements were developed through inductive content analysis.

Results: Early legislation positioned pharmacies as gatekeepers, requiring them to identify and stop medicines of substandard quality. Legislation to regulate the supply chain was slow to materialise. After Denmark joined the EU, the scope of legislation widened to include all actors in the supply chain, and the quantity of legislation increased dramatically. Simultaneously, requirements became more specific, thereby promoting a formalistic interpretation and focusing the attention of companies and authorities on predefined areas with little room to implement innovative solutions. Over time, documentation became the focus of legislation, requiring companies to provide documentary evidence for their compliance with legislation. The Falsified Medicines Directive continues these trends by increasing requirements for documentation and promoting a formalistic interpretation.

Conclusion: The legislative approach adopted since Denmark joined the EU gives companies and medicine inspectors little room to interpret legislation. The Falsified Medicines Directive does not depart from this approach. Legislation seems more focused on enforcing similar requirements than on benefiting public health. Legislation may benefit from allowing room for local interpretation of requirements.

Keywords: Harmonisation, Legislation, European Union, Falsified Medicines Directive, Enforcement

* Correspondence: Rasmus.Borup@sund.ku.dk
[1]Department of Pharmacy, University of Copenhagen, Universitetsparken 2, 2100 Copenhagen, Denmark
Full list of author information is available at the end of the article

Background

The European Union (EU) ensures that the quality, efficacy and safety of pharmaceuticals are regulated by similar legislation in all EU countries. Pharmaceutical legislation within the EU is harmonised to allow medicines to travel between EU countries with a minimum of barriers and to safeguard public health [1, 2]. As a result of harmonisation, EU member states have limited autonomy over the pharmaceutical legislation in their own country [3]. The EU claims that the harmonised rules contribute to a high level of safety for consumers [4]. However, others point out that breaking down trade barriers is in effect a deregulatory action likely to have negative effects on public health [5, 6].

Researchers who argue that harmonisation lowers requirements tend to focus on requirements relating to the development of medicines and to pay less attention to legislation governing manufacture and distribution [7–12]. Although research in the regulation of medicines' development is important, there may be something to be learned from looking at other areas of legislation, such as The Falsified Medicines Directive (the directive). Published by the EU in 2011, the directive aims to protect the public from falsified medicines. The directive imposes strong controls on the supply chain in order to keep falsified medicines out of European pharmacies. These measures have significant ramifications for supply chain actors [13–15], and some stakeholders, including manufacturers and medicine authorities, have argued that the directive raises the bar too high [16, 17]. As such, the directive does not seem to mirror the trend that harmonisation leads to deregulation.

In an effort to study the effects of EU harmonisation on the distribution of medicines, an area often ignored by researchers, this study analysed pharmaceutical legislation in Denmark before and after the country joined the European Community in 1973. Denmark is a small EU country with traditionally high regulatory standards, strong enforcement, a low level of corruption and a long history of pharmaceutical production.

Based on an historical review of legislation, this paper identifies characteristics in the developments in Danish legislation on the distribution of medicines, paying particular attention to changes after the Danish enrolment in the EU. In this context, this study examines whether the measures adopted in the directive introduced a new approach to governing the pharmaceutical supply chain.

Methods

This study used legislation governing the distribution of medicines as its empirical material. Although there are substantial and formal differences between laws, executive orders and guidelines, these differences will be ignored in this article. The most effective argument authorities have for enforcing rules in the pharmaceutical sector – regardless of whether these rules are written in a law, an executive order, or a guideline – is the threat of revoking a company's license to operate. This threat is only used when a company is overall non-compliant with the rules. However, rules written in laws, executive orders and guidelines all matter in the assessment of the compliance of a company, and they will therefore be referred to collectively as legislation and treated equally in this article.

It was decided to analyse past Danish legislation in order to answer the research question. As the first Danish Pharmacy Act was published in 1913, and due to the Danish tradition of manufacturing medicines locally at pharmacies, it was expected that distribution of medicines would be nearly non-existent in the early 1900s.

A documentary search of legislation from 1913 to the summer of 2014 was conducted to identify legislation governing the protection of medicines during distribution. Four different types of government publications were manually searched for relevant legislation at the Faculty of Law Library, Copenhagen: Proceedings from the former and current Parliament (*Rigsdagstidende* and *Folketingstidende*) as well as adopted laws (*Lovtidende*) and executive orders (*Ministerialtidende*). Legislation published after 1985 was available through the government website, www.retsinformation.dk. Danish legislation is indexed according to topic of legislation. The keywords used to identify legislation for this study were "pharmacy" (*apotek*), "medicines" (*medicin*), "pharmaceuticals" (*lægemidler*), and "health" (*sundhed*). Legislation was identified using the keywords and read by the first author before deciding whether to include it in the analysis. Documents were excluded if they did not relate to labelling, storage, distribution or manufacture of medicines. Documents were also excluded if they related only to specific types of medicines (narcotics, veterinary medicines, medical gasses), or, if reading determined that documents related only to manufacturing processes, pharmacy price setting or similar areas outside the scope of the study. When legislation referenced other documents (e.g. the pharmacopeia or EU guidelines), the referenced documents were located via the library or websites and included in the analysis. A total of 115 documents were identified as being relevant. Each document was then registered along with the year it was published (see Additional file 1).

Analysis

The documents underwent a three-step content analysis [18]. First, categories relating to handling of medicines during distribution and storage were inductively developed through thorough reading of the documents. Categories were developed to filter out legislative requirements related to reimbursement, ownerships of pharmacies, and other areas irrelevant to this study. A total of six different categories were developed: pre-purchase screening, detection (including complaints handling), stop and recall (including traceability), quality maintenance, preventing unauthorised handling, and management. See Table 1 for an explanation of each category. The categories were developed by the first author, presented to two Danish experts in legislation on distribution of medicines, and adjusted according to their feedback.

The first five categories of 'Quality Requirements' all relate to physical handling of medicines or preventing the distribution of substandard or falsified medicines. The category 'Management' encompasses requirements not related to the physical handling of medicines and not directly affecting the quality of the medicines, but rather the management of such activities. Although requirements in the category 'Management' do not directly affect the quality of medicines, this category was included in the analysis as it was clear even prior to the analysis that legislation often uses management tools to regulate the distribution of medicines.

Second, the documents were scrutinised by deductively identifying legislative requirements related to the categories and transferred to tables and organised according to the year published and the actors to which they applied. Third, tables were scrutinised by the first author and greater changes in requirements signalling a change in scope or adoption of new approaches were identified and validated via discussions with co-authors. Particular attention was given to the difference between the periods before and after Denmark joined the EU.

Results

The first Pharmacy Act was published in 1913, replacing the existing executive order from 1672. At this time, most medicines were manufactured locally at pharmacies from

Table 1 Categories of 'Quality Requirements'

Category of 'Quality Requirements'	Purpose of 'Quality Requirement'
Pre-purchase screening	To pre-qualify suppliers; evaluation of potential suppliers.
Detection (including complaints handling)	To evaluate the quality of received goods.
Stop and recall (including traceability)	To ensure that distributed products thought to be substandard or falsified are stopped or effectively and swiftly recalled.
Quality maintenance	To maintain the quality of the product while in the company's care.
Preventing unauthorized handling	To prevent products from moving into the illegal supply chain.
Management	To ensure that company activities are performed satisfactorily.

recipes published in the pharmacopeia. However, the industrial revolution was beginning to have an impact on the sale of medicines in Denmark. Pharmacies were able to buy both newly-developed (industrially-produced medicines) and traditional pharmacopeia-based medicines through foreign and domestic factories [19]. However, only pharmacopeia-based medicines were regulated in the beginning (see Fig. 1 for overview of developments).

Prior to the Danish enrolment in the European Community in 1973, three Pharmacy Acts were published approximately every 20 years. They focussed on pharmacy management and employee education as the most important tools to ensure high quality medicines, but provided very few details on how pharmacies should operate. Domestic factories and importers were also included in the scope of legislation, but they received similarly unspecific instructions. Common for all companies included in the legislation was the stipulation that they were subject to regular visits from health authority medicine inspectors. As pharmacies could only purchase pharmacopeia-based medicines from other pharmacies or domestic factories or importers, the supply chain was kept short and simple. Pharmacies were held responsible for the quality of any pharmacopeia-based medicine they sold, regardless of whether they manufactured or purchased the medicines [19–21].

Although the sales of newly-developed medicines had surpassed pharmacopeia-based medicines during the 1940s [22], legislation to regulate newly-developed medicines was slow to materialise. The measures taken to protect the quality of pharmacopeia-based medicines were not automatically applied to newly-developed medicines. For instance, companies manufacturing or distributing newly-developed medicines were not usually subject to legislation [21].

Denmark joined the EU (known as the European Community at the time) in 1973. The process of harmonising legislation with other member states fostered a new all-encompassing approach to regulating the manufacture and distribution of medicines. With the Medicines Act of 1975, legislation centred on the medicines instead of the pharmacy. The traditional distinction between pharmacopeia-based and newly-developed medicines ended. All companies physically handling medicines, whether through manufacture, storage, distribution or sale, were to be authorised and monitored through regular visits from medicine inspectors, resulting in an increase in the number of companies subject to legislation (see Table 2) [23].

The quantity of legislation rose remarkably after Denmark joined the EU (see Fig. 2). The rise in quantity correlated with increasing specificity of legislative requirements, initially in 1977 by establishing requirements for

Societal events   Legislative developments

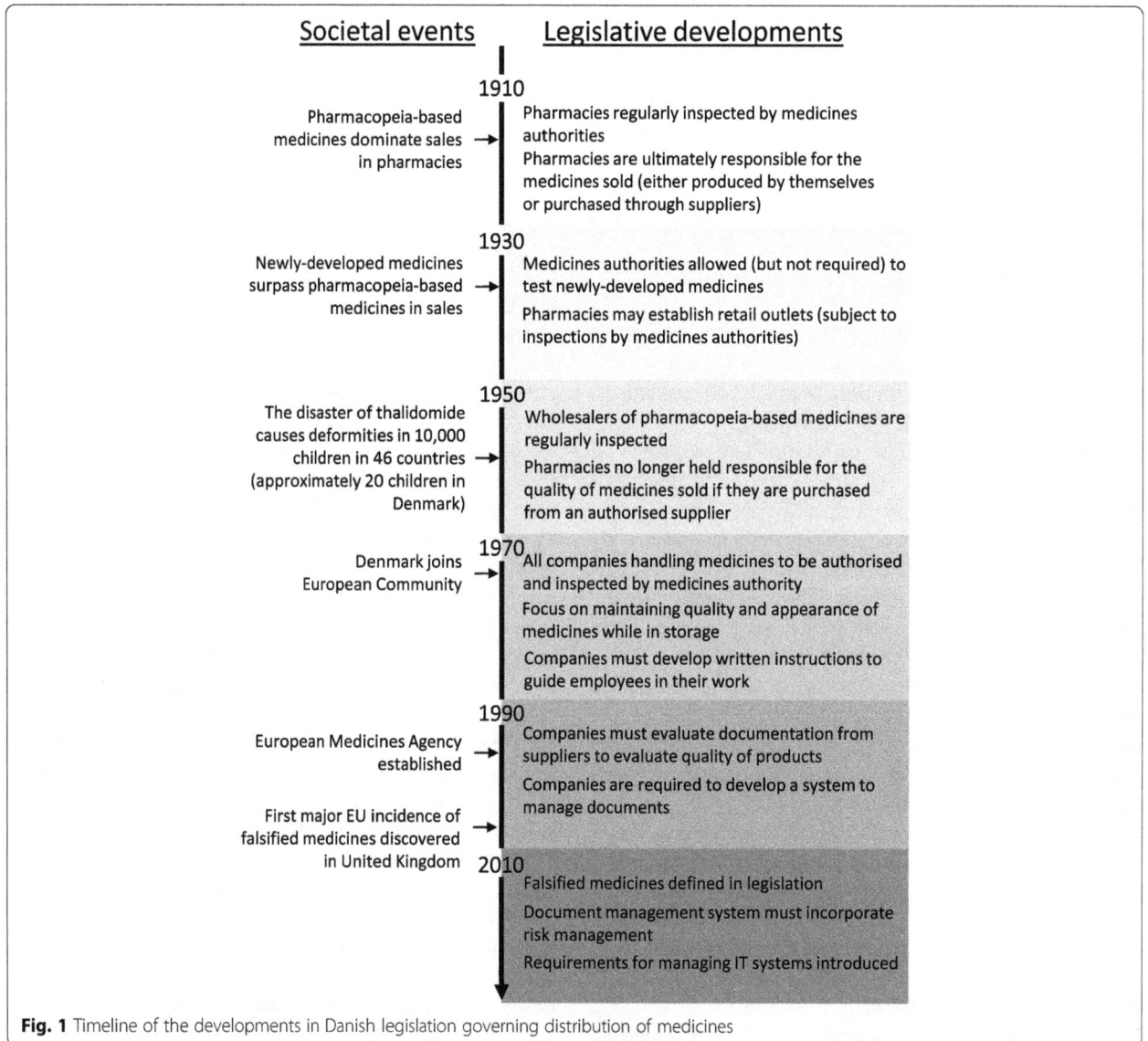

Fig. 1 Timeline of the developments in Danish legislation governing distribution of medicines

Table 2 The expansion of actors in the supply chain subject to legislation before Danish enrolment in the EU (left) and after enrolment (right)

Companies subject to Legislation in 1972 (prior to EU accession)	Companies subject to legislation in 2014 (after EU accession)
Pharmacies	Pharmacies
Manufacturers	Manufacturers
Retail outlets	Retail outlets
Wholesalers (for pharmacopeia-based medicines)	Wholesalers (for all medicines)
	Parallel importers
	Retail shops
	Internet shops
	Brokers
	Distributors of active pharmaceutical ingredients

the layout and cleaning of storage areas in order to maintain the quality of medicines. The same year, legislation began to require companies to produce written instructions and to record certain activities related to the handling of medicines. The focus on documentation and specificity of legislation continued, in 1997 resulting in the requirement to establish a document management system as well as written procedures describing document handling activities. The requirement for producing documentation today encompasses risk assessments of delivery routes, validation reports, auditing reports, training reports, qualification reports, corrective and preventive action reports, temperature evaluation reports, etc. As shown in Fig. 3, the number of different documents (procedures, records, descriptions, evaluation, etc.) required by legislation has risen dramatically since 1977.

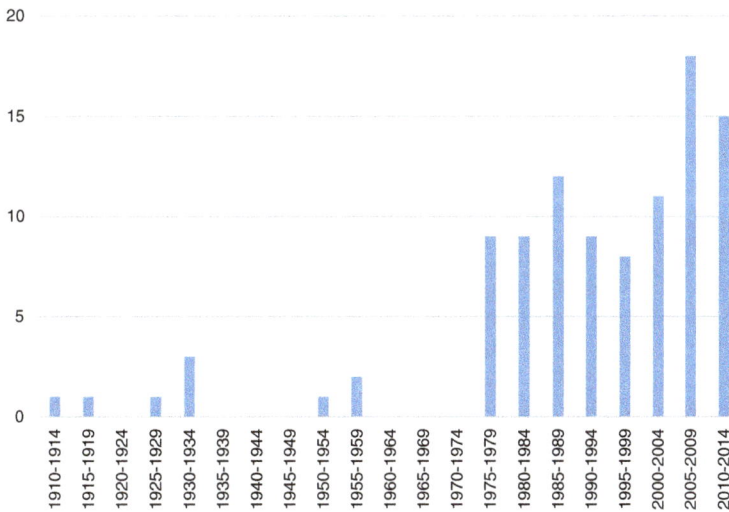

Fig. 2 The number of published pieces of legislation from 1910 to 2014 related to the distribution of medicines

The falsified medicines directive

The directive was partly implemented in Danish legislation in 2013, most notably introducing requirements for a new type of company, brokers, which have no physical contact with medicine, and expanding the regulated supply chain to include distributors of active pharmaceutical ingredients. The main component of the directive has yet to be implemented: by 2019, all pharmacies will be required to verify the authenticity of medicines before dispensing them by scanning a unique barcode printed on each package of medicine. The scanner will verify that the unique barcode is genuine by checking an EU-wide database accessible only to pharmaceutical manufacturers, wholesalers and pharmacies [24]. Data will be stored for later review by medicine authorities.

Although the specific focus on falsified medicines is recent, the requirement that pharmacies should only dispense medicines of good quality is by no means new. The directive may appear drastic to some stakeholders, but it continues the trends observed in Danish legislation since Denmark joined the EU, in particular by focusing on documentation and adding further specificity to requirements.

Discussion

Danish legislation was harmonised with EU member states in response to the Danish enrolment into the EU in 1973. Legislation has since continued to develop according to three main principles identified in this study: 1) Legislation has expanded to cover more types of actors, 2) legislative requirements have become increasingly specific, 3)

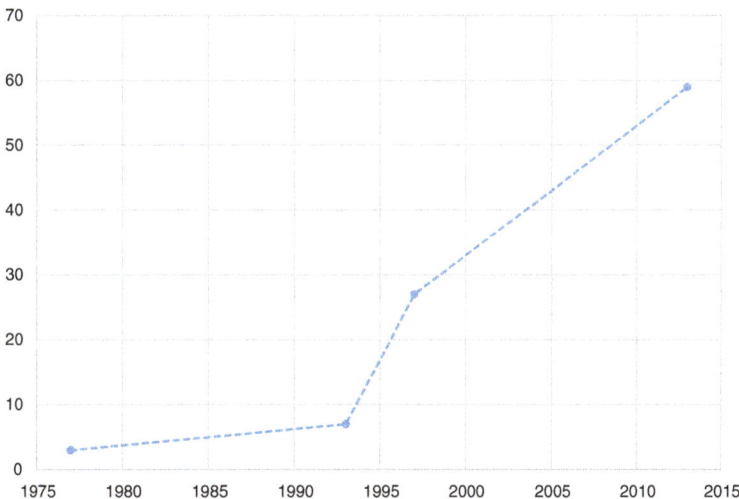

Fig. 3 The number of required documents for wholesalers

documentation has gained increasing importance. The consequences of these developments are discussed below.

More supply chain actors

The inclusion of different types of supply chain actors presents challenges, as requirements are rarely the same for all. Our data show that separate pieces of legislation are published to cover specific types of actors. Therefore, no one piece of legislation or one set of requirements applies to all actors in the supply chain. However, actors in the supply chain interact with each other, and legislation needs to regulate their interactions in a way that ensures the safety of medicines. For example, it is important to have a clear agreement on who is responsible for the quality of medicines during transport, the supplier or the purchaser. Similarly, it is important to make sure that a customer complaint made at a pharmacy is forwarded to the correct pharmaceutical company for further investigation. This study found that the legislation regulating the supply chain as a whole has become highly complex. Complexity inevitably makes compliance more demanding and is already forcing companies to hire experts in regulatory requirements [25]. As the Organisation for Economic Co-operation and Development suggested, resources might be put to better use by eliminating some of the legislative complexity [26].

Specific requirements

The increased specificity of legislation inevitably leads to a more formalistic interpretation of the rules, which can have both positive and negative consequences. On the one hand, specific requirements provide a clear checklist for authorities when assessing the compliance of companies during inspections, allowing them to focus on areas predefined as being the most important [27]. This also translates positively to companies, as they are more likely to know whether they are in compliance with requirements prior to inspections from authorities [28]. Specific requirements may also make compliance easier for some companies, as the important areas requiring attention and the level of attention required have already been identified and described in legislation [29].

On the other hand, some companies may want to focus on other areas or use strategies other than those prescribed by legislation. Companies may even want to change the way they handle medicines entirely. Such preferences are difficult to accommodate when legislation sets specific requirements [30]. Specific legislation therefore carries the risk that innovative and essentially better or less costly ways of performing tasks will not be implemented, an argument supported by previous studies on regulation of pharmaceuticals [31, 32].

Documenting instead of handling medicines

As shown in the analysis, recent requirements focus attention on documentation. By requiring companies to produce documentation of their compliance, medicine inspectors are able to discover events of non-compliance that happened in the past [33]. But as Power [34] describes, this type of compliance monitoring has a tendency to focus attention on the system of control rather than on the company's first order of business.

Companies are required to produce documents that describe most activities and to provide records to document the execution of these activities. Companies are required to establish elaborate management systems to manage the documents, as well as allocating employees to assess and maintain the systems. The resources that companies expend on complying with the requirements for document creation and maintenance are most likely considerable and could potentially be put to more productive use.

Harmonisation with enforcement in mind

This study found no signs of the deregulation typically reported when describing the effects of harmonising pharmaceutical legislation. On the contrary, requirements have increased following the Danish enrolment into the EU.

The more recent developments identified in this study promote a uniform enforcement of requirements: specific requirements promote the enforcement of similar standards in all member states, and the focus on documenting compliance deters non-compliance. Prior to joining the EU, Danish legislation was not focused on enforcement. Medicine inspectors would be unlikely to discover non-compliance, as requirements were broadly formulated and companies were not required to keep records of their activities. Enforcement therefore seems to have gained increasing importance in Denmark since joining the EU.

Although enforcement is obviously important, enforcement should not be the primary goal of legislation. Compliance monitoring should be performed using a minimum of resources, thereby allowing companies to focus on supplying medicines cheaply and timely while maintaining their quality. Further, legislation should allow room for companies and medicine inspectors to adopt the specific measures most suitable for promoting public health. Enforcing specific requirements with little view to the overall goal of legislation, protecting public health, may provide little value to patients.

This is exemplified in the directive that requires only prescription medicines to carry unique barcodes, thereby exempting non-prescription medicines. Although logically, voluntary use of unique barcodes on non-prescription medicines would only enhance the protection of public health, the European Commission, responsible for the legislation, has insisted on a formalistic interpretation of the directive and has refused to allow unique barcodes to be added to non-prescription medicines, even on a voluntary basis [35].

Hindering use of unique barcodes on medicines might ultimately lead to the consumption of falsified medicines by consumers. Such formalistic interpretation allows companies and EU member states little room to interpret legislation to fit local settings, even if such interpretation benefits public health [36].

The focus on enforcing similar requirements may be necessary for the EU to ensure the well-functioning of the internal market. However, it may be beneficial to adjust legislation and allow companies and medicine inspectors more discretion in implementing legislation. Recent pharmaceutical legislation may be too focused on enforcing harmonised requirements, rather than on making sure that requirements benefit public health. A similar view has been presented by Permanand [37].

The developments observed corresponds with Wards' description of New Public Management, where trust is "replaced by assessment at a distance" [38]. As Abraham has previously suggested that New Public Management has shaped pharmaceutical legislation [39], the developments observed in this study may benefit from being analysed in such a context.

Conclusions

This study did not find that Danish harmonisation with the EU caused deregulation. It did find, however, that the focus of harmonised legislation to enforce similar requirements for all might have unintended side effects. Rather than allowing companies and medicine inspectors to focus on protecting public health, harmonised legislation tends to focus attention on compliance with requirements that do not always fit the situation. This is exemplified by the Falsified Medicines Directive. There seems to be a risk that the overall goal of legislation, to protect public health, could become secondary to the efforts to ensure equal compliance among companies.

Keeping in mind that the protection of public health is an important goal of member states, we propose that legislation allows companies and medicine inspectors the possibility to interpret legislative requirements in order to make decisions that benefit public health.

Abbreviations
EU: European Union

Acknowledgements
The authors would like to thank our various Nordic colleagues who have commented on a previous draft of this article.

Funding
No external funding has been received for this study.

Authors' contributions
RB, SK, TM and JT conceived the idea. RB performed data collection and analysis. SK, TM and JT verified the analysis. RB wrote the manuscript and SK, TM and JT revised it. All authors read and approved the final manuscript.

Competing interests
The authors declare that they have no competing interests.

Author details
[1]Department of Pharmacy, University of Copenhagen, Universitetsparken 2, 2100 Copenhagen, Denmark. [2]Centre for Information and Innovation Law, University of Copenhagen, Studiestræde, 1455 Copenhagen, Denmark.

References
1. European Commission. The 'Blue Guide' on the implementation of EU product rules. 2015. Available from: http://ec.europa.eu/DocsRoom/documents/12661/attachments/1/translations/en/renditions/native.
2. European Union, Directive 2001/83/EC of the European Parliament and of the Council of 6 November 2001 on the Community code relating to medicinal products for human use. Official Journal of the European Union. 2001;L33:67.
3. Knill C, Tosun J. Public Policy: A New Introduction. London and New York: Palgrave MacMillan; 2012.
4. European Commission. Single Market for Goods. 2015. Available from: http://ec.europa.eu/growth/single-market/goods/index_en.htm.
5. Greer SL, et al. Health law and policy in the European Union. Lancet. 2013; 381(9872):1135–44.
6. Krapohl S. Thalidomide, BSE and the single market: an historical-institutionalist approach to regulatory regimes in the European Union. Eur J Polit Res. 2007;46(1):25–46.
7. Norris P. The impact of European harmonisation on Norwegian drug policy. Health Policy. 1998;43(1):65–81.
8. Vogel D. The globalization of pharmaceutical regulation. Governance. 1998; 11(1):1–22.
9. Abraham J, Lewis G. Harmonising and competing for medicines regulation: how healthy are the European Union's systems of drug approval? Soc Sci Med. 1999;48(11):1655–67.
10. Abraham J, Lewis G. Regulating medicines in Europe: Competition, expertise and public health. London and New York: Routledge; 2000.
11. Wiktorowicz ME. Emergent patterns in the regulation of pharmaceuticals: institutions and interests in the United States, Canada, Britain, and France. J Health Polit Policy Law. 2003;28(4):615–58.
12. Sauer F. European pharmaceutical harmonisation. Pharmaceutical Policy and Law. 2015;17:9–15.
13. Lisman J. The new EU legislation on falsified medicines: is it a step in the wrong direction? London: Scrip Regulatory Affairs; 2011. p. 7.
14. Gough P. Drug supply chain assurance issues for industry. London: Scrip Regulatory Affairs; 2013.
15. Willis C. What the EU has proposed for spotting fake medicines. Pharm J. 2014;292(7813). Online (URI: 20065511).
16. Schofield I. UK questions key facets of EU anti-counterfeiting plan. London: Scrip Regulatory Affairs; 2012.
17. Bruce F. EU generics industry complains of Efpia "misinformation" on counterfeiting. London: Scrip Regulatory Affairs; 2012.
18. Mayring P. Qualitative Content Analysis. Forum Qualitative Social Research. 2000;1(2). Art. 20. http://nbn-resolving.de/urn:nbn:de:0114-fqs0002204.
19. Danish Parliament. Law No 132 of 29 April 1913 about pharmacies. 1913.
20. Danish Parliament. Law No 107 of 31 March 1932 about pharmacies. 1932.
21. Danish Parliament. Law No. 209 of 11 June 1954 about phamacies. 1954.
22. Ministry of Interior. Report on the pharmacy sector etc. submitted by the Commission established by the Ministry of Interior on 22 January 1947

(Betænkning vedrørende Apotekervæsenet m.v. Afgivet af den af Indenrigsministeriet under 22. Januar 1947 nedsatte Kommission). 1952.

23. Danish Parliament. Law no 327 of June 26 1975 on medicines. 1975.

24. European Commission. Draft Commission Delegated Regulation supplementing Directive 2001/83/EC of the European Parliament and of the Council by laying down detailed rules for the safety features appearing on the outer packaging of medicinal products for human use. 2015; Available from: http://ec.europa.eu/growth/tools-databases/tbt/en/search/?tbtaction= search.detail&num=306&Country_ID=EU&dspLang=EN&BASDATEDEB=&bas datedeb=&basdatefin=&baspays=EU&basnotifnum=306&basnotifnum2=306 &bastypepays=EU&baskeywords.

25. Rahalkar H. Historical overview of pharmaceutical industry and drug regulatory affairs. Pharmaceut Reg Aff. 2012;11:002.

26. OECD. Better Regulation in Europe: Denmark, in Better Regulation in Europe. 2010.

27. Coglianese C, Nash J, Olmstead T. Performance-based regulation: Prospects and limitations in health, safety, and environmental protection. Administrative Law Review. 2003;55:705–29.

28. Burgemeestre B, Hulstijn J, and Tan Y-H. Rule-based versus Principle-based Regulatory Compliance. London: JURIX; 2009. p. 37-46.

29. Krähenbühl C. Gazing into the crystal ball: What will the EU-FMD safety features delegated act bring? European Industrial Pharmacy 2014; Available from: http://eipg.eu/wp-content/uploads/2014/12/eip23-dec14.pdf. Accessed 02 Oct 2016.

30. Black J. Forms and paradoxes of principles-based regulation. Capital Markets Law Journal. 2008;3(4):425–57.

31. Cacciatore GG. The overregulation of pharmacy practice. Pharmacotherapy. 1997;17(2):395–6.

32. Price II, WN, Making Do in Making Drugs: Innovation Policy and Pharmaceutical Manufacturing. Boston College Law Review. 2014;55(2). http://lawdigitalcommons.bc.edu/bclr/vol55/iss2/5.

33. Day L. What is documentation for? Am J Crit Care. 2009;18(1):77–80.

34. Power M. The audit explosion. London: Demos; 1994.

35. Bogaert PBC. The mysteries of the Falsified Medicines Directive- where is the logic on safety features? London: Script Regulatory Affairs; 2015. p. 1-3.

36. Kagan RA. Editor's introduction: understanding regulatory enforcement. Law Policy. 1989;11(2):89–119.

37. Permanand G, Mossialos E. Constitutional asymmetry and pharmaceutical policy-making in the European Union. J Eur Public Policy. 2005;12(4):687–709.

38. Ward SC. COMMENTARY: The machinations of managerialism: New public management and the diminishing power of professionals. J Cult Econ. 2011; 4(2):205–15.

39. Abraham J, Ballinger R. The Neoliberal Regulatory State, Industry Interests, and the Ideological Penetration of Scientific Knowledge: Deconstructing the Redefinition of Carcinogens in Pharmaceuticals. Sci Technol Hum Values. 2011;37(5):443–77.

6

Forces influencing generic drug development in the United States

Chia-Ying Lee[1*], Xiaohan Chen[1], Robert J. Romanelli[2] and Jodi B. Segal[1,3]

Abstract

Background: The United States (U.S.) Food and Drug Administration, as protectors of public health, encourages generic drug development and use so that patients can access affordable medications. The FDA, however, has limited mechanisms to encourage generic drug manufacturing.

Main results: Generic drug manufacturers make decisions regarding development of products based on expected profitability, influenced by market forces, features of the reference listed drug, and manufacturing capabilities, as well as regulatory restrictions. Barriers to the development of generic drugs include the challenge of demonstrating bioequivalence of some products, particularly those that are considered to be complex generics.

Conclusions: We present here a focused review describing the influences on generic manufacturers who are prioritizing drugs for generic development. We also review proposed strategies that regulators may use to incentivize generic drug development.

Keywords: Generic drug, Incentives, U.S. Food and Drug Administration

Background

The use of generic drugs products typically yields lower costs to insurers and patients than use of branded products. Efforts to increase generic drug utilization have proven helpful in reducing healthcare spending in the United States (U.S.) [1]. According to the most recent report from the Generic Pharmaceutical Association, generic drugs accounted for 88 % of all dispensed retail prescriptions in the U.S in 2014, while consuming only 28 % of total drug spending [2]. The use of generics, where available, is estimated to have saved the U.S. healthcare system $1.68 trillion between 2005 and 2014, with $254 billion saved in 2014 alone [2]. Patent expiration for a number of blockbuster drugs from 2010 to 2014, followed by the launch of generic equivalents, has played an important role in healthcare cost savings.

Despite evidence that generic drugs bring value to the healthcare system, these products are not uniformly valuable to their manufacturers. Manufacturers are appropriately deliberate about investing in the development of generic products. The United States (U.S.) Food and Drug Administration, as protectors of public health, encourages generic drug development and use so that patients can access affordable medications; however, the FDA has few mechanisms to incentivize generic manufacturing. Herein, we present a review aimed at exploring the forces that limit the development and production of generics in the U.S. and the ways in which the FDA could conceivably reduce barriers to the development of generic drugs. Our objective was to review the influences on manufacturers, which are the parties responsible for prioritizing drugs for generic development, as well as the strategies that regulators may use to incentivize generic drug development in the U.S.

Pathways to generic drug development

The Drug Price Competition and Patent Term Restoration Act of 1984, often referred to as the Hatch-Waxman Act, amended the Federal Food, Drug, and Cosmetic Act to create an abbreviated pathway for the approval of new drugs that are therapeutically equivalent to a branded drug [1].

* Correspondence: nicollelee@gmail.com
[1]Johns Hopkins University Bloomberg School of Public Health, Center for Drug Safety and Effectiveness, 624 N. Broadway, Room 644, Baltimore, MD 21205, USA
Full list of author information is available at the end of the article

Under this Act, a manufacturer needs only to demonstrate the bioequivalence of a generic product to a reference listed drug through an abbreviated new drug application (ANDA), rather than repeating the costly and time consuming safety and efficacy studies required of innovative, new chemical entities [3–5]. The FDA considers a generic drug to be bioequivalent to the reference listed drug if the rate and extent of absorption of the generic drug do not show a significant difference from the rate and extent of absorption of the listed drug when administered at the same molar dose of the therapeutic ingredient under similar experimental conditions in either a single dose or multiple doses [3]. Pharmaceutically equivalent drugs are products with the same active ingredients, dosage form, strength, and route of administration. Of these, those proven to be *bioequivalent* are consequently considered therapeutically equivalent or substitutable - with the expectation that they have the same safety and efficacy profile. Once the FDA approves the ANDA and the branded version is no longer protected by patent or market exclusivity, the generic product can be brought to market.

When identifying a new development target, generic manufacturers first seek an informed perspective on the competitive landscape about potential generic competitors before prioritizing resources and making a decision to proceed [6]. Strategies for generics development have evolved rapidly, responding to market dynamics [7]. Between 1984 and 2012, generic manufacturers focused largely on the production of "simple" to formulate small molecules, and won the market via mass production. The years between 2012 and 2017 have been called the "patent cliff", when many drugs considered to have been "blockbuster drugs' lost, or will soon lose, their patent protection. This opened important opportunities for generic manufacturers, who commonly apply one or more strategies. The first is the "portfolio-centric approach". Generic manufacturers include re-innovation design (i.e., the process of producing the next generation of generics with revised and refined features of successfully-launched products) in their portfolio ostensibly to provide personalized, cost-effective generic products that meet the demand of healthcare systems, policymakers, and patients [8]. One way is through what is called re-innovation or sometimes called the production of "super generics". The products have modifications beyond the originator generic; these often require a submission to FDA of a new drug application rather than an ANDA. An example is the generic drug, abraxane, which the manufacturer expected to gain market share over paclitaxel. The active ingredient, paclitaxel, is unchanged but abraxane has the molecule coated in albumin, allowing the company to claim fewer adverse reactions for the patient [9, 10]. The second is the "therapeutic area dominance". With this approach, generic manufacturers compete within a specialized area of generic

drugs such as cardiovascular, oncology, or rheumatology drugs [11]. For example, Relax Pharmaceuticals (an Indian generic manufacture) specializes in the manufacturing of generic antibiotics and gastrointestinal products. Finally, market experts have predicted that after 2017, when many branded drugs have lost their patent protection, generic manufacturers will shift resources to the production of complex generics such as drug/device combinations and sterile injectables, or may move into the marketplace for biosimilar products [5, 12].

Manufacturing considerations

When generic manufacturers are selecting products for development, the expectation of an adequate return on investment is the foremost consideration. This can be forecast, to some extent, by knowing the demand for the product and the requirements for production.

Market forces

Generic manufacturers understandably focus on drugs with a potential for high profit. Companies are often interested in developing a generic if the branded medication has a high average wholesale price, which is expected to translate into a profitable generic. Similarly, chronic diseases, with a larger population health burden, are also often targeted areas for generic manufacturers. For example, cardiovascular and central nervous system diseases are the two largest market segments, composing nearly 38 % of the global generic pharmaceutical market together [13, 14]. Generic manufacturers may also choose to avoid densely populated therapeutic classes, when deciding whether to join the competition.

Features of reference listed drug

The Hatch-Waxman Act defined single-dose pharmacokinetic studies as the method of establishing bioequivalence for *systemically* acting drug products. However, there are formulations or routes of administration where systemic blood levels cannot be used to determine bioequivalence, such as when the product is not intended to be systemically active. Therefore, drugs that are used topically in the eye; or dosage forms intended to act within the gastrointestinal tract lumen without absorption, do not have clear paths for demonstrating bioequivalence, which is a major deterrent to their production. The FDA has made significant progress in defining bioequivalence methodologies for many of these non-systemically active drug products; [15] however, a number of products remain without clearly defined methodology, including inhaled drug products and transdermal preparations. This impacts the production of generics for inhaled corticosteroids, such as for asthma treatment, and transdermal testosterone for hormone replacement, as examples. In the absence of product-specific guidance, drug developers may ask the

FDA development questions via the controlled correspondence process or request to meet with FDA scientists in pre-ANDA meetings. Sponsors also may develop their own analytical tools and study protocols through which they can demonstrate bioequivalence, and then work with the FDA for approval of their plan [2].

Manufacturing capabilities of complex drugs

Generic manufacturers also consider their technical ability to manufacture generic versions of branded products. They evaluate the complexity of the manufacturing that is needed to produce a generic equivalent, the cost of manufacturing, and their own research and development capabilities. For example, small molecule pharmaceutical products are simpler to create and therefore are more likely to be developed generically than complex large molecules. Dosage form also may play a role in generic drug development; solid oral forms (e.g., tablets, capsules) and parenteral solutions have a higher likelihood of being easily developed than more complex drug delivery systems (again, inhaled products, topical products). These differences are due to technological barriers and manufacturers' capabilities. For example, the drug delivery system development process is particularly complicated for inhaled products with manufacturers needing to work around the bans on ozone-depleting propellants and the multiple patents on hydrofluorocarbon-free devices. Generic manufacturers need sufficient research and development resources to manufacture these technically challenging generic products.

Innovative products have become increasingly complex and, necessarily, so have their generic equivalents [16]. Each complex generic is "complex" in its own way [17, 18] (Table 1). The development of complex generics requires substantial commitment from the manufacturer, which may lower the benefit to cost ratio for its production. The manufacturer may be asked to repeat clinical studies due to the challenges of demonstrating bioequivalence for these products or do additional physiochemical characterization testing [11]. Furthermore, for complex generics the pathway to drug approval may differ substantially from one product to another product; [13] the FDA's Office of Generic Drugs (OGD) manages each submission on a case-by-case basis. Complex generics are expected to eventually become a significant percentage of the generic market, but the approval challenges first must be overcome.

Table 1 Complex generics examples [11]

Complex Active Ingredients	Peptides, complex mixtures, natural source products
Complex Formulations	Liposomes and iron colloids
Complex Route of Delivery	Locally acting drugs
Complex Drug-Device Combinations	Metered dose inhaled products and transdermal systems

Materials challenges

Some generic products are challenging to develop because of inadequate source raw materials, although this is not unique to generics. The International Conference on Harmonization of Technical Requirements for Registration of Pharmaceuticals for Human Use guidelines are the main instructions for sourcing qualified raw materials for any drug manufacturing [19]. Drugs with carcinogenicity or toxicities may require suitable handling conditions in clinical practice and during development, which may be a deterrent to production, particularly if the return on investment cannot be assured [20, 21].

Regulatory considerations
180-day exclusivity period

The Hatch-Waxman Act gave additional protection to the inventors of innovative, new drugs by lengthening patent terms and by providing guaranteed periods of data exclusivity (5 years for a new chemical entity). The Act, in return, offers the first generic manufacturer to file an ANDA a 180-day period of market exclusivity. An effect of this regulation, however, is that the exclusivity period prevents other generic manufacturers from bringing their generic product to market during this time. This is typically not advantageous for consumers because it is not until roughly six generic products are available that the full cost savings of generics are typically realized; although the largest price decrease occurs with the entry of the second product [22].

Pay for delay

The 180-day exclusivity advantage provided to generic manufactures under the Hatch-Waxman Act encourages generic manufacturers to challenge the existing patents of brand manufacturers ("the Paragraph IV challenges"). It has, however, also encouraged generic drug manufacturers to settle and accept compensations from brand manufacturers for their delaying entry into the market [16]. This is counter to forces that encourage generic development and introduction to the market. Kesselheim describes studies measuring the impact of the Hatch-Waxman act; he notes that there are no well-controlled studies of the economic impact of Paragraph IV challenges and the effect of settlements on generic drug availability and public health outcomes [23].

These settlements have taken the form of a cash payment (so called "pay for delay") to reimburse some or all of a generic manufacturer's legal fees, or non-cash deals where the brand manufacturer agrees to purchase their product's active ingredients from the generic manufacturer or not to market their own generic version of the product (i.e., an authorized generic) for a period of time [21]. In one notable case of cash payments, Cephalon made reverse payments totaling $300 million dollars to four generic drug manufacturers to drop patent challenges and suspend marketing of generic versions of Cephalon's drug Provigil for six years. During that time, Cephalon earned an additional $4 billion dollars in sales for Provigil [24]. This was later found to be unlawful by the Federal Trade Commission (FTC) on the basis of these settlements being anticompetitive.

Pay for delay has posed a threat to the timely development of generic drugs and a substantial cost to the U.S. healthcare system. According to an FTC study, these deals cost consumers and taxpayers $3.5 billion in higher drug costs each year [25]. In 2013, there were more than 100 settlements reached between brand and generic manufacturers. In a suit filed by the FTC against the pharmaceutical company, Actavis, the U.S. Supreme Court ruled in 2013 that reverse payments are subject to U.S. antitrust laws [26]. Larger penalties to brand manufacturers, as well as generic manufacturers who accept such payments, may be needed to dissuade settlements that delay the availability of generic products. Hemphill and Lemley described a strategy called *earning exclusivity* that they proposed would improve the effect of the Hatch-Waxman Act on encouraging generic drug development [27]. They suggested that under the strategy of earning exclusivity, generic manufacturers would have to *earn* the 180-day exclusivity offered by FDA by successfully defeating the weak or bad patents on the branded products, without settlements. This would be done by demonstrating that the patent was invalid or by demonstrating that the generic product does not infringe upon the existing patent. Barr won an exclusive marketing rights challenge against Lilly for the production of a generic version of Prozac in 2000, which was 2 years before the patent was expected to expire [28].

Access to the branded reference products

Manufacturers, necessarily, must have access to the reference listed reference drug to perform the bioequivalence testing that the FDA requires of a generic product under an ANDA [29]. There have been instances, however, of brand manufacturers preventing generic manufacturers from accessing their product [23]. Some brand manufacturers have used the restrictions in their Risk Evaluation and Mitigation Strategies (REMS), and other restricted access programs, to prevent generic manufacturers from accessing brand drug samples for testing. These manufacturers have argued that they cannot provide generic manufacturers with samples of such REMS-covered products because doing so would be outside the FDA-sanctioned, restricted distribution pathway [30].

The Fair Access for Safe and Timely (FAST) Generics Act, first proposed in Congress in September 2014, was considered a solution to this REMS barrier [31]. The FAST Generics Act would create a pathway for generic manufacturers to secure a branded drug from its maker, wholesaler, or specialty distributor regardless of whether the product was subject to REMS, and impose stiff penalties for non-compliance. Ultimately, the branded drugs and their generic equivalents would then share a single REMS. At the time of writing, neither the House nor Senate has passed the FAST Generics Act [32].

Strategies for promoting generic drug utilization and development

In order to encourage generic drug development, two strategies have been frequently proposed by researchers and policymakers: implementing initiatives or reforms to increase generic utilization (thereby stimulating the generic economy by inducing demand) and offering aids or incentives for generic drug innovations [9, 33].

Godman and his colleagues proposed a 4 "E" methodology (Education, Engineering, Economics and Enforcement) for developing initiatives to increase generic drug utilization in Europe [8] (Table 2). Initiatives focusing on "Education" are usually programs that influence generic prescribing by disseminating educational materials. Initiatives that focus on organizational interventions ("Engineering") include agreements on price and volume of existing drugs or disease management programs. Financial incentives ("Economics") are for increasing generic drug utilization through the use of positive and negative incentives for physicians and patients. Finally, regulatory or law enforcement ("Enforcement") methods may include mandatory generic substitution laws to which pharmacists must adhere. Some of these initiatives can benefit generic utilization in the U.S., while others may face unique challenges in the U.S. marketplace.

Indeed, the U.S. healthcare system has mechanisms that promote generic usage. For example, most insurance companies incentivize patients to use generic drugs by requiring less cost-sharing for generic versus branded products. In addition, 14 states currently have mandatory generic substitution laws for pharmacists and the remainder, except Oklahoma, have laws permitting substitution by pharmacists [34]. However, it is unlikely that *federal* laws promoting generic substitution will be enacted due to the organization of the U.S. legal system, and "engineering"

Table 2 Strategies for increasing generics development and utilization: the four "E" method [8]

Education	Educational materials: treatment guidance and educational outreach visit
Engineering	Organizational interventions: agreements on price and volume of existing drugs
Economics	Financial incentives: positive and negative incentives for physicians
Enforcement	Regulatory or law enforcement: mandatory generic substitution laws

initiatives may be challenging given the fragmented nature of the U.S. healthcare system. Evidence is needed about the effects on generic development and utilization of those initiatives already in place, and future research should assess the potential impact of supplemental initiatives such as those involving education of patients and health care providers.

The above activities are promising but all hinge upon the production of new generic products. With more complicated branded products losing their patent protection, bioequivalence methodologies for complex drugs or dosage forms need to be developed. Guidance documents with updated standards or reference documents from the FDA may encourage generic manufacturers to proceed with the development of new products [8, 35]. Regular engagement with OGD may help drug manufacturers contain costs and decrease time-to-market delays. The OGD now has provisions to grant pre-ANDA meetings for complex generics [36].

Conclusions
We have described in this review select U.S. federal policies, and described the regulatory environment and market forces influencing generic developers. Generic drug developers choose candidate drugs based on the market forces, features of the reference listed drug, and manufacturing capabilities, as well as regulatory restrictions. With suitable policy and regulatory incentives to increase generic utilization or facilitate the generic drug development process, as described, generic manufacturers may be encouraged to develop new generic drugs that will help increase access to medications, improve population health, and contain healthcare spending.

Abbreviations
ANDA: Abbreviated new drug application; FAST: Fair Access for Safe and Timely; FDA: Food and Drug Administration; FTC: Federal Trade Commission; OGD: Office of Generic Drugs; REMS: Risk evaluation and mitigation strategy

Acknowledgements
We have no additional contributors to acknowledge in this manuscript.

Funding
Dr. Jodi Segal, Dr. Robert Romanelli, and Ms. Lee were funded by the Food and Drug Administration through grant U01FD005267. Ms. Chen was not funded for her work on this project.

Authors' contributions
CYL - Prepared a first draft of the manuscript. XC - Provided additional background research and drafted sections of the manuscript. RR - Provided critical suggestions and edited the final manuscript. JS - Conceived of the manuscript, drafted sections, and did the final editing. All authors read and approved the final manuscript.

Competing interests
The authors declare that they have no competing interests.

Author details
[1]Johns Hopkins University Bloomberg School of Public Health, Center for Drug Safety and Effectiveness, 624 N. Broadway, Room 644, Baltimore, MD 21205, USA. [2]Palo Alto Medical Foundation Research Institute, Palo Alto, CA, USA. [3]Division of General Internal Medicine, Johns Hopkins University School of Medicine, 624 N. Broadway, Room 644, Baltimore, MD 21205, USA.

References
1. U.S. Department of Health & Human Services, Office of the Assistant Secretary for Planning and Evaluation. ASPE issue brief. Expanding the use of generic drugs. 2010. Retrieved from https://aspe.hhs.gov/basic-report/expanding-use-generic-drugs.
2. Anonymous, Generic Pharmaceutical Association. Generic drug savings in the U.S.: Seventh annual edition: 2015. 2015. Retrieved from http://www.gphaonline.org/media/wysiwyg/PDF/GPhA_Savings_Report_2015.pdf.
3. U.S. Department of Health and Human Services Food and Drug Administration, Center for Drug Evaluation and Research (CDER). Guidance for industry: bioavailability and bioequivalence studies for orally administered drug products – general considerations. 2003. Retrieved from http://www.fda.gov/ohrms/dockets/ac/03/briefing/3995B1_07_GFI-BioAvail-BioEquiv.pdf.
4. U.S. Department of Health and Human Services Food and Drug Administration, Center for Drug Evaluation and Research (CDER). Guidance for industry: bioavailability and bioequivalence studies submitted in NDAs or INDs — general considerations. 2014. Retrieved from http://www.fda.gov/downloads/Drugs/GuidanceComplianceRegulatoryInformation/Guidances/UCM389370.pdf.
5. U.S. Department of Health and Human Services Food and Drug Administration, Center for Drug Evaluation and Research (CDER). Guidance for industry: bioequivalence studies with pharmacokinetic endpoints for drugs submitted under an ANDA. 2013. Retrieved from http://www.fda.gov/downloads/drugs/guidancecomplianceregulatoryinformation/guidances/ucm377465.pdf.
6. Ashburn TT, Thor KB. Drug repositioning: identifying and developing new uses for existing drugs. Nat Rev Drug Discov. 2004;3(8):673–83.
7. Barei F, Le Pen C, Simoens S. The generic pharmaceutical industry: moving beyond incremental innovation towards re-innovation. Generics Biosimilar J. 2013;2(1):13–9.
8. Ding M, Dong S, Eliashberg J, Gopalakrishnan A. Portfolio management in new drug development. In: Innovation and marketing in the pharmaceutical industry. New York: Springer; 2014. p. 83–118.
9. Ross MS. Innovation strategies for generic drug companies: moving into supergenerics. IDrugs. 2010;13(4):243–7.
10. Barei F, Le Pen C, Simoens S. The generic pharmaceutical industry: moving beyond incremental innovation towards re-innovation. Generics Biosimilars Initiat J. 2013;2(1):13–9.
11. Von Koeckritz K. Generic drug trends—What's next? Pharm Times. 2012; 78(4):78. Retrieved from http://www.pharmacytimes.com/publications/issue/2012/april2012/generic-drug-trends-whats-next--.
12. McKinsey & Company, Global Generics Interest Group. Generating value in generics: finding the next five years of growth. 2013. Retrieved from http://www.pharmatalents.es/assets/files/generating_value.pdf.
13. Godman B, Shrank W, Andersen M, et al. Comparing policies to enhance prescribing efficiency in Europe through increasing generic utilization: changes seen and global implications. Expert Rev Pharmacoecon Outcomes Res. 2010;10(6):707–22.
14. Chidambaram A. Global generic pharmaceutical market – Qualitative and quantitative analysis. 2013. Pharma Tech 2013 Conference. Retrieved from http://www.slideshare.net/AiswariyaChidambaram/pharma-tech-2013-aiswariya-chidambaram-fs.
15. U.S. Food and Drug Administration. Product-specific recommendations for generic drug development. 2016. Retrieved from http://www.fda.gov/Drugs/GuidanceComplianceRegulatoryInformation/Guidances/ucm075207.htm.
16. Srinivasan A. Complex generics: maximizing FDA approval potential. 2015. Retrieved from https://www.parexel.com/files/6714/3076/9385/ComplexGenerics_WPApril2015_final.pdf.
17. Sario N. Prescription drug market: the world is turning to generics. Market realist. 2015. Retrieved from http://marketrealist.com/2015/03/analyzing-prescription-market-branded-generic-drugs/.
18. Lionberger R. Complex Generic Drugs. GPhA Fall Technical Meeting, Bethesda, MD. 2013. Retrieved from http://www.fda.gov/downloads/aboutfda/centersoffices/officeofmedicalproductsandtobacco/cder/ucm374191.pdf.

19. Bowman D. A quick guide for sourcing biopharmaceutical raw materials. BioProcess international. 2015. Retrieved from http://www.bioprocessintl.com/upstream-processing/biochemicals-raw-materials/quick-guide-sourcing-biopharmaceutical-raw-materials/.

20. Shargel L, Kanfer I, editors. Generic drug product development: solid oral dosage forms. Active Pharmaceutical Ingredients. Chapter 2. New York: CRC Press; 2013. p. 19–21.

21. American Society of Health-System Pharmacists. ASHP guidelines on handling hazardous drugs. Am J Health Syst Pharm. 2006;63(1):1172–93.

22. Wiske CP, Ogbechie OA, Schulman KA. Options to promote generics markets in the Unites States. JAMA. 2015;314(20):2129–30.

23. Kesselheim AS. An empirical review of major legislation affecting drug development: past experiences, effects, and unintended consequences. Milbank Q. 2011;89(3):450–502.

24. Federal Trade Commission. Settlement of Cephalon pay for delay case ensures $1.2 billion in Ill-gotten gains relinquished; refunds will go to purchasers affected by anticompetitive tactics. 2015. Press release. Retrieved from https://www.ftc.gov/news-events/press-releases/2015/05/ftc-settlement-cephalon-pay-delay-case-ensures-12-billion-ill.

25. Federal Trade Commission. Agreements filed with the Federal Trade Commission under the Medicare Prescription Drug, Improvement, and Modernization Act of 2003. 2013. Retrieved from https://www.ftc.gov/sites/default/files/documents/reports/agreements-filed-federal-trade-commission-under-medicare-prescription-drug-improvement-and/130117mmareport.pdf.

26. Supreme Court of the United States. Federal Trade Commission v. Actavis, Inc. October term, 2012 No. 12–416. 2013. Retrieved from http://www.supremecourt.gov/opinions/12pdf/12-416_m5n0.pdf.

27. Hemphill CS, Lemley MA. Earning exclusivity: generic drug incentives and the Hatch-Waxman Act. Antitrust Law J. 2011;77(3):947–89.

28. Mclean B. Bitter Pill Prozac made Eli Lilly. Then along came a feisty generic maker called Barr Labs. Their battle gives new meaning to the term 'drug war. 2001. Accessed at http://archive.fortune.com/magazines/fortune/fortune_archive/2001/08/13/308077/index.htm.

29. Sarpatwari A, Kesselheim AS. Ensuring timely approval of generic drugs. Health Affairs Blog. 2015. Retrieved from http://healthaffairs.org/blog/2015/03/24/ensuring-timely-approval-of-generic-drugs/.

30. Brill A. Lost prescription drug savings from use of REMS programs to delay generic market entry. 2014. Matrix Global Advisors, Retrieved from http://www.gphaonline.org/media/cms/REMS_Studyfinal_July2014.pdf.

31. The 114th Congress. 1ST Session. H.R.2841. FAST Generics Act of 2015. 2015. Retrieved from https://www.congress.gov/114/bills/hr2841/BILLS-114hr2841ih.pdf.

32. Anonymous. Fast generics act reintroduced in congress. 2015. Retrieved from http://www.pharmacytimes.com/publications/issue/2015/september2015/fast-generics-act-reintroduced-in-congress.

33. Kaló Z, Holtorf AP, Alfonso-Cristancho R, Shen J, Ágh T, Inotai A, Brixner D. Need for multicriteria evaluation of generic drug policies. Value Health. 2015;18(2):346–51.

34. Survey of Pharmacy Law – 2015. Mount prospect. IL: National Association of Boards of Pharmacy; 2014.

35. Boehm G, Yao L, Han L, Zheng Q. Development of the generic drug industry in the US after the Hatch-Waxman Act of 1984. Acta Pharm Sin B. 2013;3(5):297–311.

36. U.S. Food and Drug Administration, Lionberger R. GDUFA regulatory science update. GPhA annual meeting. 2015. Retrieved from http://www.fda.gov/downloads/forindustry/userfees/genericdruguserfees/ucm434325.pdf.

7

Is there potential for the future provision of triage services in community pharmacy?

Louise E. Curley*, Janice Moody, Rukshar Gobarani, Trudi Aspden, Maree Jensen, Maureen McDonald, John Shaw and Janie Sheridan

Abstract

Background: Worldwide the demands on emergency and primary health care services are increasing. General practitioners and accident and emergency departments are often used unnecessarily for the treatment of minor ailments. Community pharmacy is often the first port of call for patients in the provision of advice on minor ailments, advising the patient on treatment or referring the patient to an appropriate health professional when necessary. The potential for community pharmacists to act as providers of triage services has started to be recognised, and community pharmacy triage services (CPTS) are emerging in a number of countries. This review aimed to explore whether key components of triage services can be identified in the literature surrounding community pharmacy, to explore the evidence for the feasibility of implementing CPTS and to evaluate the evidence for the appropriateness of such services.

Methods: Systematic searches were conducted in MEDLINE, EMBASE and International Pharmaceutical Abstracts (IPA) databases from 1980 to March 2016.

Results: Key elements of community pharmacy triage were identified in 37 studies, which were included in the review. When a guideline or protocol was used, accuracy in identifying the presenting condition was high, with concordance rates ranging from 70 % to 97.6 % between the pharmacist and a medical expert. However, when guidelines and protocols were not used, often questioning was deemed insufficient. Where other health professionals had reviewed decisions made by pharmacists and their staff, e.g. around advice and referral, the decisions were considered to be appropriate in the majority of cases. Authors of the included studies provided recommendations for improving these services, including use of guidelines/protocols, education and staff training, documentation, improving communication between health professional groups and consideration of privacy and confidentiality.

Conclusion: Whilst few studies had specifically trialled triage services, results from this review indicate that a CPTS is feasible and appropriate, and has the potential to reduce the burden on other healthcare services. Questions still remain on issues such as ensuring the consistency of the service, whether all pharmacies could provide this service and who will fund the service.

Keywords: Pharmacist, Community pharmacy services, Triage, Advice, Referral, Primary health care, Patient outcome assessment

* Correspondence: l.curley@auckland.ac.nz
School of Pharmacy, Faculty of Medical and Health Sciences, University of Auckland, Private Bag 92019, Auckland 1142, New Zealand

Background

The demands on primary health care services worldwide are growing [1], largely due to an ageing population which has subsequently led to increased strain on the primary health care workforce [2–5]. In order to overcome such challenges, primary health care systems have evolved to encompass new services and, in many countries, extended roles for community pharmacists [6, 7].

Triage has traditionally been described as the sorting and allocation of treatment to casualties, particularly in battlefield and disaster situations [8]. In this model, casualties are sorted based on a system of priority, designed to maximise the number of survivors [8]. The definition has been extended to refer to "The assessment of patients on arrival to decide how urgent their illness or injury is and how soon treatment is required" [9]. An example of the latter description includes the role of nurses in emergency rooms [8]. More recently, the term triage has been used increasingly to describe non-emergency situations in healthcare: one such example is Healthline in New Zealand, where members of the public can speak to a registered nurse who provides advice and directs patients to the most appropriate service [10].

Community pharmacy is recognised for its role as a common first port of call for patients in the provision of advice on minor ailments [11], and referral to an appropriate health professional when necessary [11]. Community pharmacies are available in most localities, often open at times when general practitioner (GP) services are not available, and no appointment is necessary to consult with a pharmacist [4, 5]. This raises the question of whether there is an opportunity to translate the concept of triage to a formalised service provided by community pharmacists.

It could be argued that elements of triage services in community pharmacy already exist. Worldwide, a number of medicines have been reclassified from prescription-only medicines to be available over-the-counter, as medicines available only from pharmacies [12]. Examples include chloramphenicol for the treatment of bacterial conjunctivitis [13] and trimethoprim for uncomplicated urinary tract infections [14] in New Zealand. This reclassification enables appropriately trained pharmacists to determine when to treat and when to refer the patient to their GP or other health professional, and thus includes an element of triage, although the skills and processes used to undertake this task are not currently referred to in this way.

Developing effective triage services in community pharmacy has the potential to reduce pressure on other health services, by reducing costs associated with unnecessary use of other more expensive healthcare services, such as visits to GPs and accident and emergency departments (EDs) at hospitals. In the year 2006 to 2007, it was reported in the United Kingdom (UK) that there were 57 million consultations with GPs involving a minor ailment, which had an estimated cost of £2 billion per annum [6]. In addition, a separate UK-based study found that of 353 observed GP consultations, 31 % were for minor ailments, of which 59 % could have been managed in a community pharmacy [15].

Research undertaken in Australia found that if the resources devoted to minor ailments were dealt with through community pharmacies, this redirection of resources could potentially free-up the equivalent of 500 to 1,000 full time GPs to treat more serious health problems [16]. In addition to GP visits, estimates have been made of the minor ailments managed in EDs and after-hours clinics, which could have been managed by a pharmacist [17–20], ranging from 5.3 % [17] to 8 % at EDs [19], and 28 % of adult attendances at afterhours primary care centres [20].

The potential for community pharmacists to act as providers of triage services has started to be recognised, and community pharmacy triage services are emerging in a number of countries. For example, the Swiss Pharmacists' Association has launched netCare in a select number of pharmacies [21]. netCare is a primary triage service using a structured decision-tree for 24 common conditions, where pharmacists can request a real-time video consultation with a doctor if necessary. In addition, minor ailment schemes have been implemented, for example, the Community Pharmacy Minor Ailments Scheme (MAS) [6, 21], which began in Scotland and is now available at some pharmacies across the UK. These minor ailment schemes have elements of triage within their structure and formalise the primary health care role of the community pharmacist for certain minor ailments, whereby designated patients can consult a pharmacist and, if necessary, obtain a pharmacist-prescribed medication from a limited formulary [21]. In Canada, two provinces (Nova Scotia and Saskatchewan) added minor ailments as an expanded aspect of practice in 2011. This new legislation broadened pharmacists' scope of practice, enabling them to prescribe certain medications for minor self-limiting and self-diagnosed ailments from a list of agents previously only able to be prescribed by a doctor [22].

The aim of this review is to explore the potential for community pharmacy provision of triage services. Specific objectives were:

- To explore whether key components of triage services can be identified in literature surrounding community pharmacy
- To explore the evidence for the feasibility of implementing community pharmacy triage services (CPTS)

- To evaluate the evidence of appropriateness of such services

Materials and methods

Working definition of triage

For the purposes of this paper, we used a definition of community pharmacy triage reported by Chapman et al. [23], In their report they described triage in this way "The provision of advice about how best to manage health issues – whether with a medical product or device or with non-drug measures, whether to seek assistance from a doctor or other health professional, and with what sense of urgency – is a primary health care service commonly provided by community pharmacies".

Definition of appropriateness

This review aimed to evaluate the evidence of appropriateness of CPTS. For the purposes of this study, appropriateness was considered in the light of clinical appropriateness and acceptability by other health professionals and patients.

Search strategy

We performed systematic searches in MEDLINE, EMBASE and International Pharmaceutical Abstracts (IPA) databases from 1980 to March 2016. The search strategy was designed to retrieve studies conducted on triage-like services in community pharmacy settings. Triage in community pharmacy is a relatively new and developing concept that does not have a clear definition; an initial search revealed that published literature on community pharmacy seldom uses the word triage; therefore, this review used several synonyms for the relevant activities that comprise our working definition of triage in community pharmacy to capture articles related to this concept.

Our search included both mapped and unmapped terms, which are illustrated in Fig. 1. In addition, the following text words and MeSH/EMTREE terms were used to identify additional relevant papers: (Mapped terms: pharmaceutical services OR pharmacies OR pharmacist OR community pharmacy services; unmapped terms: pharmac* OR community pharmac* OR retail pharmac* OR drugstore OR drug store) AND (Mapped terms: self medication OR self care OR non-prescription drugs OR behind the counter drugs OR referral and consultation OR gatekeeping OR triage OR primary healthcare OR patient centred care OR counselling; unmapped minor ailment).

Study selection

Inclusion criteria were formulated in relation to the research aims. First, papers were included only if they referred to community pharmacy settings and included a triage service (as defined above) in patients with a first presentation of a medical complaint. We excluded studies that were not written in English, did not have a full text article available, reviews, commentaries and letters to the editor. We also excluded studies that focused on services for monitoring chronic/long term conditions or were focussed on prescription services.

Data extraction and analysis

Two researchers (LC, JM) independently extracted study characteristics, using an extraction table. One researcher (LC) compared all extracted data and discussed discrepancies with other researchers (JShe, MM) when necessary. A summary of the data extracted from the studies is presented in Table 1. This includes the study design, aims, measurements taken, types of conditions, number of referrals and a summary of results. In addition, we recorded whether each study included the characteristics of community pharmacy triage, based on our working definition, in their study description: i.e. contact with the patient or caregiver, questions asked, urgency and level of care decided, advice given and decision made to treat or refer. Evidence of appropriateness in decision making, appropriateness of referral, adherence to referral advice, and the recommendations from the authors were extracted from the studies.

Results

Screening, selection and included studies

A diagrammatic depiction of the search strategy is included in Fig. 1. The searches in MEDLINE, EMBASE and IPA resulted in a total of 3597 titles. Studies were excluded if they were not related to community pharmacy triage or did not report outcomes related to patients. Duplicates were also excluded. The remaining studies ($n = 37$) reported aspects of triage in community pharmacy between 1980 and 2016 (Table 1). The studies were undertaken in the UK ($n = 16$), Europe ($n = 13$), Australia ($n = 6$), Canada ($n = 1$) and Singapore ($n = 1$).

Three main methodologies were used across the studies. Twenty-two of the studies in this review were cross-sectional observational studies with natural patients. Ten studies used a pseudo-patient methodology, which in our review was defined as studies where a trained person presented to a pharmacy asking for advice or a specific product as part of a predetermined case, and consultation was recorded and feedback given to the pharmacy. Lastly, questionnaires completed by healthcare providers and/or patients ($n = 5$) were also used where they described the aspects of a community pharmacy triage service.

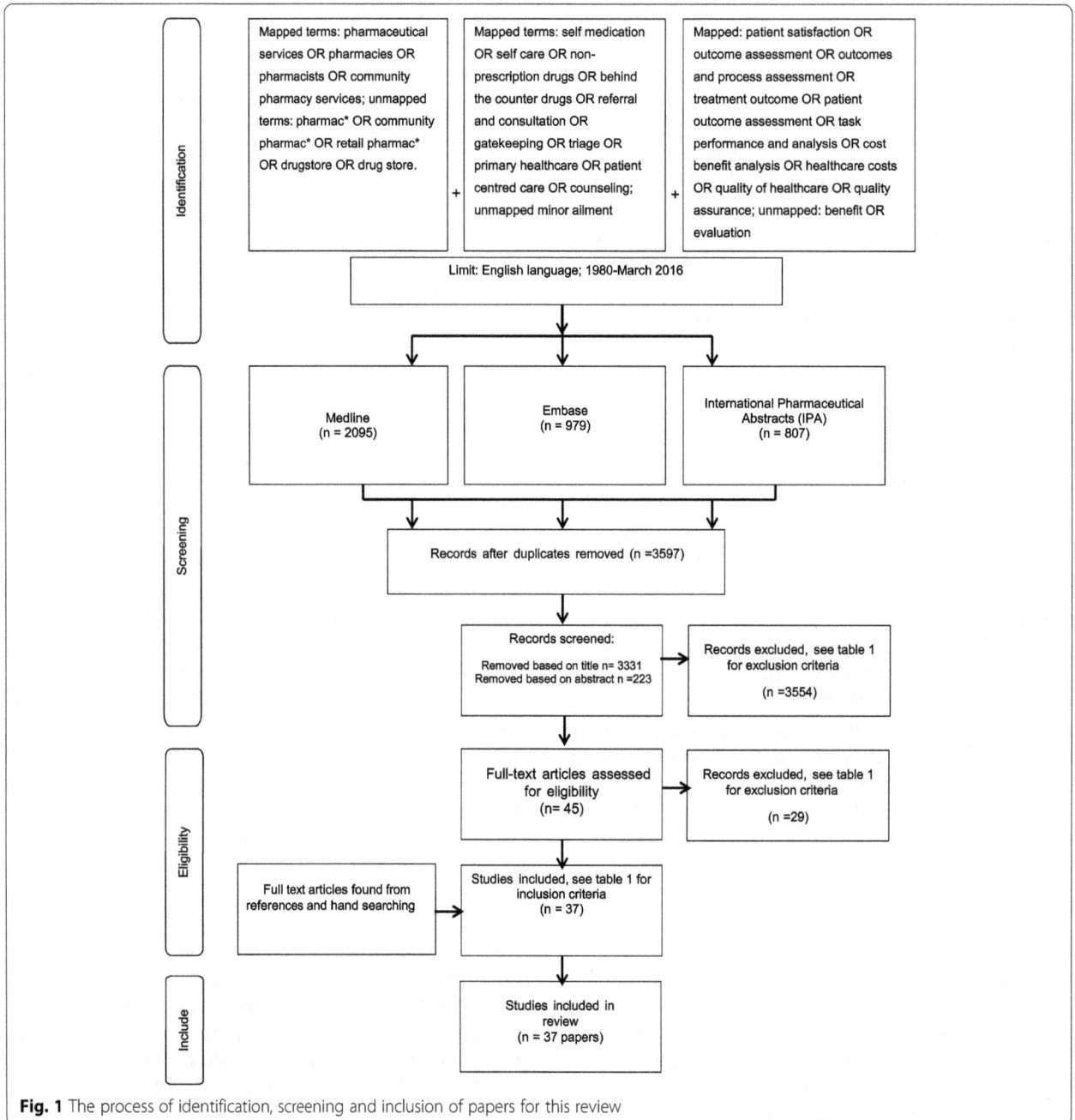

Fig. 1 The process of identification, screening and inclusion of papers for this review

Types of conditions

Thirteen studies included any minor ailment in community pharmacies across a given time period, whilst others presented results on specific conditions across a time period ($n = 24$). Observational studies of natural patients evaluated measures surrounding non-specific minor ailment presentations [11, 23–25]. Those that focused on specific condition presentations were: headache [26], back pain [26], head lice infestations [27], two studies focussing on erectile

dysfunction [28, 29] and four on gastrointestinal presentations [30–33]. All studies that used the pseudo-patient methodology focussed on specific conditions: allergic conjunctivitis [34], diarrhoea in an infant [35], abdominal pain [36], a gastrointestinal presentation [37], headache [36, 37], cough [38], insomnia [39], vaginal thrush [40] and three studies looked at ulcers/lesions in the mouth [41–43]. Four of the questionnaire-based studies investigated specific conditions: chloramphenicol use for bacterial conjunctivitis

Table 1 Overview of identified studies

Author (year) country [reference]	Key aims	Study design	Measurements	Participants	Proportion referred (%[n])	Summary of results	Contact between community pharmacy and the patient or caregiver/proxy	Questions are asked to determine the diagnosis	Urgency and level of care decided	Advice given	Decision made to treat or refer
Alkhatib et al. (2015) Australia [44]	To evaluate pharmacists' management of eye infections following the reclassification of ophthalmic chloramphenicol.	Cross-sectional postal survey to a randomized sample of community pharmacies.	Agreement or specific information by the pharmacist on: 1. Provision of ophthalmic chloramphenicol 2. Protocol and training 3. Pharmacist views 4. Demographics from recall	119 responses from pharmacist managers/ proprietors	Not recorded	Pharmacists' capability to treat acute bacterial conjunctivitis was improved and pharmacists felt that there was better utilisation of their professional skills. There was improved access to treatment options for patients. More education and training was signalled by some and use of protocol differed by age group. More sold OTC in larger pharmacies in metropolitan areas, no change in number of prescriptions for chloramphenicol. No evaluation of service.	✓	✓	✓	✓	✓
Baqir et al. (2011) UK [6]	To assess what action patients using MAS would have taken if the MAS had not been in place and to approximate the net cost impact.	A cost minimization analysis of submitted claims data. One item questionnaire for consumer.	Patients were asked what action they would have taken if the MAS was not in place. The calculated net cost impact of the MAS using standard health-care reference costs.	396 patient claims were recorded	Not recorded	Savings of NHS resources over 1 month equated to £6739.01. Estimation of which resources would be used if not in place identified GPs and EDs as the next port of call.	✓	✓	✓	✓	✓

Table 1 Overview of identified studies *(Continued)*

Berger et al. (2005) Germany [37]	To assess the quality of patient counselling in community pharmacy and evaluate a new method of feedback.	Observational study using pseudo-customer methodology	All aspects of the interview, recommendation and advice.	49 community pharmacies	90 % [27] of cases that warranted referral	More assessment was conducted when patient presented with symptoms than a product request. Some appropriate self-medication advice provided in 74 % of visits, usually not sufficient. One of the two cases the optimal decision was referral, whereas the other case medication and advice was sufficient. 90 % of cases that warranted referral were referred but only 30 % with necessary urgency.	✓	✓	✓	✓
Bilkhu et al. (2013) UK [34]	To determine and quantify questioning and management of a patient with presumed allergic conjunctivitis.	Observational study using pseudo-customer methodology	All aspects of the interview, recommendation and advice. The type of pharmacy staff who was involved in the consult	100 community pharmacies	14 % [13]	Average questions asked 3.5 ± 2.6. Differential diagnosis questioning and management of allergic conjunctivitis by community pharmacies in this study was lacking. Referral to optometrist comprised 2 % of the 100 pharmacies. 91 % advised on treatment.	✓	✓	✓	✓
Blenkinsopp et al. (1991) UK [50]	The aims of the study reported evaluation of pharmacist used referral cards	Questionnaires completed by both pharmacist and GP	1. Usefulness and acceptability of the notification card 2. The use of the card in the reporting of suspected adverse drug reactions from the community pharmacist to the GP 3. Acceptability and value of such a card	Six pharmacies, 15 general practices in two towns	Not recorded % [120]	71 % of patients who were referred to their GP by the pharmacist did so. Overall, 12 % of cards issued were for a suspected adverse drug reactions. Their was a positive perception of the cards by all parties - patients, doctors and pharmacists. Of the referrals GPs felt 88 % of cases were referred appropriately.	✓	✓	✓	✓

Table 1 Overview of identified studies (*Continued*)

Study	Aim	Study type	Description	Sample	Referral rate	Key findings					
Bojke et al. (2004) UK [7]	To investigate the effects of an intervention to provide easier access to pharmacists for patients with minor ailments.	Analysis of consultation numbers and types. Patient minor ailment type and influencing factors.	1. Effects of the intervention on the total number of consultations by GPs and on the mix of patients seen by the GP. 2. Factors affecting patients' choices between GP and pharmacist consultations for minor ailments	1521 consultations of which 575 patients took the pharmacy option to treat minor ailment	Not recorded	The total number of GP consultations was unaffected but the intervention led to the number of minor ailments consultations decreasing. The main reason behind patient choice in consulting the GP/ pharmacist was the type of minor ailment. Distance did not alter patient choice.	✓	✓	✓	✓	✓
Chui et al. (2005) Singapore [53]	To identify pharmacist's approach in providing advice and consumers' behaviour in self-treatment and their perception of the community pharmacist's role in advice.	Two structured questionnaires	The pharmacists and consumers were surveyed independently using two structured questionnaires.	44 pharmacists and 181 patients	15.5 % [28] said that pharmacists had referred them to a GP.	The majority of pharmacists gave advice on self-medication to at least 10 patients per day. The majority of patients (90.9 %) were at least somewhat satisfied with advice provided.	✓	✓	✓	✓	✓
Coelho et al. (2014) Portugal [24]	To determine the prevalence of self-medication and to evaluate the clinical impact of pharmaceutical counselling.	Cross-sectional observational study	All aspects of the interview were recorded including the recommendation advice and when referred	298 patients	9.1 % [27]	51.3 % presented asking for advice, 48.7 % asking for a specific product. 9.1 % referred to GP. Follow up - After 1 week of pharmaceutical intervention, 86.8 % had a positive impact, half of referred patients made GP visit, 80 % of counselled patients had improved symptoms.	✓	✓	✓	✓	✓
Chapman et al. (2010) Australia [23]	To understand the nature and impact of primary health care that is provided by community pharmacies	Cross-sectional observational study	Consultations between customers and staff in community pharmacies. Interview with each customer post consultation and a follow-up phone call.	24 community pharmacies; 280 customers (telephone contact made with 252)	4.2 % (5.6 %) [12 direct (16 conditional)], in addition 3 % (8.3 %) [4 (11 conditional)] from proxy consultations	Most elements of consultation only took place when a customer sought advice versus a product. Most did not take the advice of referral from the community pharmacy.	✓	✓	✓	✓	✓

Table 1 Overview of identified studies (*Continued*)

Study	Aim	Design	Outcome measure	Result	Findings						
Driesen et al. (2009) Belgium [35]	To assess management of acute diarrhoea in an 8-month-old baby using a simulated patient scenario in a community pharmacy	Observational study using pseudo-customer methodology	This outcome was assessed against the three WWHAM questions that were defined as the most essential topics to be able to evaluate the situation	101 community pharmacies	31 % [not recorded]	The majority of pharmacists asked too few questions to adequately analyse the situation. Advice was given but insufficient counselling on medicines. 31 % referral including conditional, good counselling on dehydration. Authors reported too few questions asked to adequately assess the scenario.	✓	✓	✓	✓	✓
Erni et al. (2016) Switzerland [48]	To evaluate the impact of this new service as well as the added value for the health care system.	Cross-sectional study	Ailment, procedure of the consultation, treatment, patient information and outcomes of the follow-up call on a standardized form submitted to the study centre.	Pharmacists from 162 pharmacies performed 4118 triages.	7 % [288] (17 % required second opinion of medical practitioner)	4118 triages were completed by 162 pharmacists In 17 % of the cases the option to have a backup consultation was utilised. In follow-up calls, 84 % of the patients who were seen only by pharmacists reported complete relief or symptom reduction. Significant or complete remission was seen in 84 % of the patients triaged by the pharmacist. 9 % required another medical consultation, 7 % of patients needed further pharmacy treatment.	✓	✓	✓	✓	✓
Evans et al. (2005) UK [41]	To find out whether community pharmacy was offering appropriate advice to patients seeking advice on management of a persistent ulcer on the tongue.	Observational study using pseudo-customer methodology	The interviewer then recorded the advice given and noted whether the source was a pharmacist or a pharmacy assistant	40 pharmacists and 40 pharmacy assistants	Pharmacist: 81 % [33] Pharmacy assistant: 35 % [14]	The most appropriate outcome would be referral. Most pharmacists gave the correct advice of referral. Pharmacy assistants gave inadequate advice in most cases.	✓	✓	✓	✓	✓

Table 1 Overview of identified studies (Continued)

Study	Aim	Design	Data measured	Sample	%	Key findings				
Hafejee et al. (2006) UK [45]	To elucidate the range of skin problems currently encountered and knowledge to deal with these	Questionnaire survey	Pharmacists' dermatology education, patient resources available, and the nature of the skin problems for which patients consulted them and the follow-up arrangements.	20 community pharmacists and 735 dermatological presentations	84 % if symptoms did not resolve [not recorded]	There is high number of presentations for dermatological advice, and the presentations are varied. There is a need for more focused dermatology topic teaching for pharmacists both at undergraduate and postgraduate levels. 84 % of pharmacists told patients to consult their GP if symptoms did not resolve.	✓	✓	✓	✓
Hassell et al. (1997) UK [11]	Patients qualitative views on pharmacy services and roles	Ethnographic-style research study	Staff and patient interviews and non-participant observations of medicine and health interactions	Ten pharmacies, over 1000 patients interviewed and 44 telephone interviews	6 % [not recorded]	Patients used pharmacy instead of GP due to: costs, convenience, and illness seen as minor, to see if pharmacist thought they should see GP. Pharmacists play a major role in keeping minor ailments out of the GPs, and act as a referral mechanism if necessary. Follow up on a sample of the patients seen to check relief of symptoms/resolution of problem, but outcome not recorded.	✓	✓	✓	✓
Hassell et al. (2001) UK [51]	To assess the extent to which patients would visit a community pharmacy instead of a GP for management.	Intervention study	Transfer rates and reductions in general practice consultations for the 12 conditions. Prescribing outcomes and re-consultation rates.	Eight community pharmacies, 1522 patients	3.6 % [21]	37.8 % of eligible patients accepted offer of transfer to community pharmacy for consult and treatment. 3.6 % referred back to GP, 5.7 % re-consultation within 14 days. Pharmacy treatment acceptable and feasible	✓	✓	✓	✓

Table 1 Overview of identified studies (Continued)

Study	Aim	Study type	Method	Sample	Result	Outcome					
Jiwa et al. (2010) Australia [46]	To characterize factors affect pharmacists providing a referral for patients with lower bowel symptoms to consult a general practitioner	Questionnaire	Vignettes were constructed around 6 clinical variables and pharmacists were asked to describe a referral pathway.	167 community pharmacists and 1503 vignettes	69 % [1040]	Cases presented to pharmacists as vignettes. Pharmacist triage was in agreement with expert panel in 70 % of cases. Diarrhoea over referred and weight loss and rectal bleeding under referred.		✓	✓		✓
Jiwa et al. (2012) Australia [49]	To develop a tool to assist community pharmacists to triage patients presenting with cough	Assessment tool development and pilot of tool	Leicester Cough Questionnaire; Pharmacy Cough Assessment Tool including referral and follow up	Four pharmacies and ninety-nine subjects	37 % [37] (however 18 more qualified for referral)	The tool identifies patients with cough who might benefit from medical advice and may feasibly be used as an initial screening tool in the community pharmacy setting. 7/37 participants who were referred to their GP could be confirmed to have done so. Two were prescribed antibiotics; one was referred for a chest X-ray and one to a specialist.	✓	✓	✓	✓	✓
Kippist et al. (2011) Australia [39]	To investigate how community pharmacists respond to complaints of acute insomnia from people who seek self-treatment and determine the factors affecting this response.	Observational study using pseudo-customer methodology	Supply/non supply of a sleep aid and scores for pharmacists for skills in eliciting information prior to supply of medication	100 community pharmacies	4 % [4] (24 % of cases overall made some type of referral incl to revisit if no resolution)	Many pharmacists are responding appropriately. The most appropriate outcome would be non-supply of medicine A product was supplied in 96 % of visits; conventional medicines in 65 % of cases, and herbal/ homeopathic medicines 31 %.	✓	✓	✓	✓	✓

Table 1 Overview of identified studies (*Continued*)

Reference	Aim	Method	Outcome measures	Sample	Referral	Findings					
Krishnan et al. (2000) Germany [33]	To determine whether patients with dyspepsia had improved outcomes in quality of life scores comparing an intervention sand a control pharmacy	Observational and questionnaire	Quality of life scores before and after self-medication. Quantitative and qualitative evaluation of pharmacist advice	36 pharmacies 198 patients	10.8 % [21] and 68.7 % conditional referrals	Overall counselling in trained pharmacies was better than non-trained pharmacies. In general patients were asked comprehensive questions and provided with advice. Longer consults were associated with more satisfied reports. However, some pharmacists did not provide sufficient warning for those who were at risk. Drug related problems were not addressed sufficiently.	✓	✓	✓	✓	✓
Mansell et al. (2015) Canada [22]	To determine whether patients prescribed such treatment by a pharmacist symptomatically improve within a set time frame.	Online questionnaire for patients	Demographics, condition, pathway to encounter, outcome including satisfaction and further consultation needed.	Ninety pharmacies and 125 participants.	Not recorded	Trust in pharmacists and convenience was the most common reasons for choosing a pharmacist. 27.2 % would have chosen a physician or ED otherwise. Satisfaction with the pharmacist and service was strong; only 5.6 % felt a physician would have been more thorough. The condition significantly/ completely improved in 80.8 %; 4 % experienced side effects.	✓	✓	✓		✓
Marklund et al. (2003) [32] Sweden	To assess whether pharmacists make appropriate choices with patients with dyspepsia.	Assessment of referral cards	Demographics, reason for referral, assessment of referral	132 patients	Not recorded [132]	Of all of the patients who were referred, the assessors agreed that 90 % of the patients should have been referred to their GP.	✓	✓	✓	✓	✓
Martin-Morales et al. (2013) Europe [Greece and Spain] [28]	To assess pharmacists' ability to detect erectile dysfunction and encourage patients to seek medical evaluation.	Cross-sectional observational study in two countries	Proportion of men with a SHIM score ≤ 21 and, of those, the proportion who visited a physician and credited the pharmacist for their visit.	451 patients	77 % [348]	First health care professional approached - 50 % pharmacist, 18 % GP. Follow up phone call to verify the quality of the patient education provided and whether they visited GP. Less than 1/3 referred to GP had visited	✓	✓	✓	✓	✓

Table 1 Overview of identified studies (Continued)

Study	Aim	Method	Outcomes measured	Sample	Referral	Results				
Maunder et al. (2005) UK [63]	To assess the advice given by pharmacists on oral health and the role of pharmacists in oral healthcare services	Questionnaire	Pharmacy characteristics, products available, knowledge of pharmacists and promotional activities	17 pharmacies	94.1 % of cases to see the dentist and, 23.5 % to see the GP [not recorded]	Most common presentations during data collection was for ulcers and toothache/pain. Advice was given to see a dentist/Dr. Albeit pharmacists had little knowledge of the dentists in the area or emergency arrangements. Pharmacists were interested in having protocols for management of oral health care.	✓	✓	✓	✓
Mehuys et al. (2009) Belgium [30]	The role of the pharmacist in triage related to upper gastrointestinal presentations	Questionnaire-based referral tool	1. Nature of GI symptoms that people intend to self-medicate 2. Prevalence of alarm symptoms 3. Adherence to referral advice 4. Self-reported efficacy	592 patient consultations	21 % [124]	Only 51.7 % of the customers, who were referred, adhered to that advice. Overall 48.7 % of people reported symptom relief and of those given OTC treatment 95.1 % reported relief of symptoms.	✓	✓	✓	✓
Parmentier et al. (2004) UK [52]	To evaluate a scheme offering pharmacy referrals for minor ailments in a refugee community.	Intervention study	The presenting minor ailment and corresponding medication as recorded by the pharmacist.	2 community pharmacies, 184 refugees	1.1 % [2]	200 vouchers were distributed to 184 refugees. Of all the referrals, there were two clients who were referred to the GP and two advised to see the GP if symptoms persisted.	✓	✓	✓	✓
Phillips et al. (2001) UK [27]	Use of community pharmacy versus general practice was acceptable as the first point of call for head lice.	Before and after training study and questionnaires to health professional and patient	Before and after training where pharmacists were asked to record head lice consults	571 patient consultations	Not recorded	Patients treated for head lice by pharmacist rather than GP. Estimated savings during study period of up to £52000.	✓	✓	✓	✓

Table 1 Overview of identified studies (Continued)

Study	Aim	Method	Outcome measure	Sample	Referral rate	Results				
Ralph et al. (2001) UK [47]	To assess the ability of pharmacists to appropriately manage a range of genital symptoms	Questionnaire on case-based scenarios	Pharmacist perceptions on their ability to manage a range of genital symptoms and their knowledge of genitourinary services	28 community pharmacies	4–100 % dependant on the condition, some with OTC products	Range of symptoms/conditions surveyed. Focus on pharmacist knowledge of genitourinary services nearby - low. Showed that many pharmacists know when to refer STDs, but more education on services to refer to needed.	✓	✓	✓	✓
Rutter et al. (2004) UK [36]	To determine whether an appropriate course of action was taken by UK community pharmacists for cases of headache and abdominal pain	Observational study using pseudo-customer methodology	All aspects of the interview, recommendation and advice	28 community pharmacies	53.6 % [15]	Referral was expected outcome - advised in 53.6 % of cases. Most questions asked were relevant (66 %) but inadequate histories taken.	✓	✓	✓	✓
Schneider et al. (2011) Australia [38]	Evaluation of pharmacist assessment and triage when appropriate for chronic cough.	Observational study using pseudo-customer methodology	Demographic details, assessment questions, and advice provided.	155 community pharmacies	38 % [59] (36 % of these provided OTC supply also)	Referral was ideal outcome based on symptoms; only 38 % of cases were referred. Adequate assessment increased likelihood of referral. Consultations conducted by pharmacists were more likely to lead to appropriate outcome.	✓	✓	✓	✓
Scully et al. (1989) UK [43]	To assess the advice offered by pharmacy staff with a potential oral carcinoma	Observational study using pseudo-customer methodology	Advice and recommendation.	57 community pharmacies	8.8 % [5]	Referral was the ideal outcome based on the symptoms; only 8.8 % of consultations were advised to see a doctor ($n=4$) or a dentist ($n=1$), after medication advice.	✓	✓	✓	✓
Symonds et al. (2011) Europe [UK, Germany, Czech Republic and Spain] [29]	To determine if community pharmacists could appropriately recommend suitability for supply of sildenafil 50 mg for the treatment of erectile dysfunction	Cross-sectional observational study of natural patients	Concordance rate between pharmacist and physician recommendations.	53 pharmacists, 13 physicians and 346 participants	Not recorded	Agreement between pharmacist, GP and specialist recommendations assessed. 90 % of cases specialist agreed pharmacist gave an acceptable recommendation.	✓	✓	✓	✓

Table 1 Overview of identified studies (*Continued*)

Varela-Centelles et al. (2012) Spain [42]	To assess whether pharmacies and herbalist's shops were offering appropriate advice for patients seeking guidance on a potentially malignant oral lesion	Observational study using pseudo-customer methodology	Individual interaction with the interviewee according to a previously prepared script and details were recorded	306 community pharmacies and 154 herbalist shops	27.5 % [84] referrals and 36.3 % [111] referrals in addition to OTC sale	The most appropriate outcome was referral. Community pharmacies referred more than herbalists. Pharmacy assistants were more likely to recommend OTC remedies (55.6 % vs. 13 %) and significantly less likely to refer than were pharmacists.	✓	✓	✓	✓	✓
Vella et al. (2009) Malta [26]	To design two protocols to help pharmacists care for consumers seeking treatment for headache and back pain and assess pharmacists' management of these conditions	Observational study using pseudo-customer methodology	Data for each case and divergence from protocol	10 pharmacies and 212 patient interventions	Not recorded	Compliance higher when pharmacists responded to symptoms than when product asked for by name - less advice given when product requested.	✓	✓	✓	✓	✓
Watson et al. (2015) UK [64]	To compare health-related and cost-related outcomes of consultations for symptoms suggestive of minor ailments in EDs, GPs and community pharmacies.	Cross-sectional study	1. Whether health-related and cost-related outcomes differ between settings. 2. Whether satisfaction with index consultation is associated with health-related outcomes. 3. What factors (triggers) influence patients' choice of care setting.	377 patients participated, recruited from EDs (81), general practices (162) and community pharmacies (134).	Not recorded	Symptom resolution was similar across all three settings: ED (37.3 %), GP (35.7 %) and pharmacy (44.3 %). Mean overall costs per consultation were significantly lower for pharmacy	✓	✓	✓	✓	✓

Table 1 Overview of identified studies (*Continued*)

Study	Aim	Methodology	Measured	Number	Response rate	Findings
Watson et al. (2016) UK	To assess what factors predicted whether the supply of a guideline compliance for the supply/non-supply of non-prescription medicines.	Observational study using pseudo-customer methodology	The questions asked during the consultation and the outcome of the consultation	351 patient visits (but some missing data)	No: recorded	WWHAM questioning was associated with appropriate outcome. After adjusting for WWHAM scoring the outcome was twice as likely to have an appropriate outcome than other consultations. The likelihood of an appropriate outcome increased if the consultation was conducted by the pharmacist
Westerlund et al. (2003) Sweden [31]	To measure the outcomes of a counselling model for dyspepsia	Observational study using pseudo-customer methodology	All aspects of the interview, recommendation and advice and a follow up interview by research staff	33 pharmacy staff and 319 patients	12 % [39]	A counselling model to discover and resolve problems related to symptoms and drug use appeared to have a favourable impact on outcomes. Patient outcome: Only 1/5 customers referred contacted GP. 2/3 reported feeling better following self- care advice.
Westerlund et al. (2007) Sweden [25]	To assess the quality of self-care from pharmacist using IT clinical guidelines	Cross-sectional study, where outcomes were reviewed by a doctor and follow-up with the patient occurred	Questions asked and information given Follow-up with the patient	10 pharmacists and 250 customers	Not recorded	Self-care counselling when supported by IT-based clinical guidelines is high. Independent assessment found a 97.6 % of the consultations were appropriate. Follow-up found that there was a favourable feedback from patients. Referrals were not included in this study

[44], dermatological conditions [45], lower bowel conditions [46] and genital conditions [47].

Evidence for decision making

Appropriate diagnosis Appropriate decision-making with regards to treatment or referral requires eliciting a patient's relevant history via questioning. The appropriateness in decision making was evaluated by two main methods, observing community pharmacy staff actions with the use of specific guidelines or protocols and observing community pharmacy staff actions without their use.

Ten of the studies used current or newly developed guidelines which covered asking appropriate questions and differentially diagnosing presenting conditions, and identifying requirements for referral [25, 26, 28–32, 44, 48, 49]. Other studies evaluated decision-making by recording the number of questions asked and comparing them with a pre-determined list of questions [33, 34, 36–40]; and/or the use of mnemonics such as WWHAM (Who is it for? What are the symptoms? How long? Action tried? Medications taking?) [24, 35, 40].

When a guideline or protocol was used, accuracy in identifying the presenting condition was high with concordance rates ranging from 70 % to 97.6 % [25, 28, 29, 32]. In comparison, in studies where no specific guidelines/protocols were used, the authors of those studies concluded that too few questions had been asked to obtain sufficient information to undertake a valid analysis [34–36]. For example, results from the study by Berger et al. [37] found that 95 % of community pharmacy staff asked at least one question to assess the diagnosis in patients presenting with a condition, but only 47 % in a case where a specific product request was requested.

Fifteen studies evaluated the appropriateness of the decision made to treat or refer. The studies that used pseudo-patients compared the interaction with the 'patient' to predetermined optimal outcomes [34–39, 41–43]. Bilkhu et al. [34] found that the differential diagnosis was lacking in community pharmacy, whereby questions were not asked to distinguish the different types of conjunctivitis. In addition, some studies found that too few questions were asked to adequately assess the presented situation [34–36]. Schneider and colleagues [38] and Watson and colleagues [40] found that the likelihood of adequate assessment increased with the number of questions asked.

In six of the natural patient studies, another health professional reviewed the outcome [25, 29, 32, 46, 47, 50]. Marklund et al. [32] had a GP assess all referrals related to dyspepsia that were recorded by pharmacists; the study found that in 90 % of cases the GP agreed that the patient needed to be referred to the GP for either a prescription, or a medical examination. Westerlund and colleagues [25], had an independent doctor assess the self-care advice given by the pharmacist and found that it was appropriate in 97.6 % of cases. In the study by Blenkinsopp and colleagues a notification card was used to improve the communication between GPs and pharmacists. If the pharmacist decided that a patient should be referred to the doctor, a notification card was completed. The card was given to the patient to take with them to their doctor and a copy was stored at the pharmacy for their records. The results showed that 88 % of the referrals were appropriate according to the GP [50]. In a separate study by Symonds et al. the medical specialist agreed with 90 % of the recommendations made by the pharmacist after a follow-up assessment [29].

In the questionnaire-based studies [46, 47], cases were given to the pharmacist who then had to make a decision on the necessity to refer. These decisions were then evaluated by a medical expert. Jiwa and colleagues [46] found a 70 % agreement between an expert panel and the pharmacist and Ralph et al. [47] reported that "many pharmacists were able to manage sexual health problems adequately".

Between 66 % and 95.1 % of patients reported symptom relief or resolution in studies using a guideline or protocol [25, 30, 31, 48]. In the study that did not use a guideline or protocol, 86.8 % reported symptom relief or resolution [24]. In the study by Krishnan et al. [33] patients who presented with dyspepsia were contacted at 7 days post consultation with the pharmacist. One group of pharmacies had a training intervention on guidelines for counselling of patients with dyspeptic disorders and another was a control group of pharmacies who did not have this training; patients who attended both control and intervention pharmacies reported an improvement in quality of life scores at day seven [33].

Referral rates, appropriateness of, and adherence to advice of referral

Referral rates All studies, except two ($n = 35$), discussed the referral of patients to other healthcare providers by pharmacists or other community pharmacy staff. In addition, 27 studies (see Table 1) documented either the number of patients referred or the proportion of patients referred.

There was a wide variation in the proportion of patients referred to other health services after a pharmacist or community pharmacy staff consultation. When considering the referral rate in the natural patient studies which included any minor ailment presentation, a range of 6 % [11] to 9.1 % [24] was reported. When considering the condition-specific studies this range is much wider, varying from 12 % [31] for a study on patients presenting with dyspepsia to a 77 % referral rate in erectile dysfunction cases [28].

Nine studies used pseudo-patients and documented referral [34–39, 41–43]; seven of the studies used one scenario, and the other two had two different case scenarios [36, 37]. The most appropriate, predetermined outcome in eight of the cases used in these studies was referral [36–39, 41–43] and the number of recorded patient referrals ranged between 8.8 % [43] and 90 % [37]. Three studies consisted of patient scenarios that were considered to be appropriately managed by a community pharmacy staff member; in one study no referrals were recommended [37], and the remaining two reported referral rates of 14 % [34] and 31 % [35].

In most of the studies where referrals occurred, patients were referred to a GP, but there were instances discussing referral to other health professionals, dentists in particular [41–43].

Adherence to referral advice Five studies included follow up with the patient, to evaluate what proportion had taken the advice of the pharmacist to visit another health professional. In four studies, [24, 28, 30, 31] 20 %–51 % of patients had taken the advice of the pharmacist. One study found 71 % patients acted on the advice of the pharmacist; in this case a referral card had been given to the patient [50].

Reverse referral interventions
Whilst some studies involved patients presenting at the pharmacy directly, others described a reverse intervention service. These services offered a patient, who was seeking an appointment with a GP or nurse for treatment for a minor ailment, the option of a consultation with the community pharmacist instead. In such instances the community pharmacist could refer the patient back to the GP when necessary [7, 51, 52]. Hassell and colleagues found that the referral rate back to the GP was only 3.6 % [51] in one of their studies and 6 % [11] in the other. One study investigated refugees approaching either the nurse, support worker or reception staff at the refugee hostel about a minor ailment. Instead of being given an appointment with a GP, they were offered a voucher which they could exchange at a community pharmacy for an appropriate over the counter medication free of charge, after a consultation with the pharmacist [52]. This study had a low number of referrals (1.1 %) back to the GP [52].

Recommendations from study authors
Twenty seven studies included in this review noted recommendations on community pharmacy, based on their findings. These are summarised below.

Additional pharmacy staff education or training Increased education, training or support for community

pharmacy staff was suggested in eight of the studies in [33, 34, 39, 41, 42, 44, 45, 47]. In most cases, the recommendations were specific to the medical condition being studied, for example, appropriate advice for sexual health [47] and insomnia [39], differential diagnosis of ocular conditions [34, 44] and identifying signs of potential oral cancers with appropriate referral advice [41, 42]. In addition, Hafajee et al. recognised that there are a large number of dermatological presentations in pharmacy, and suggested increased education at both undergraduate and postgraduate levels [45].

Use of guidelines and protocols Eleven of the studies suggested that guidelines or protocols be developed and used by community pharmacy [11, 22, 29–31, 34–36, 42, 46, 49]. For example, Hassell et al. [11] proposed that guidelines could be developed by pharmacists in conjunction with GPs, and a two way referral system could be established. Mehuys and colleagues [30] advocated for the use of structured questionnaires during consultations, with treatment options that ensured the recommendations made were evidence-based. Westerlund et al. [31] suggested that a model designed to diagnose and treat problems related to symptoms be used in the community pharmacy setting.

More emphasis on appropriate advice to customers was recommended by three studies [26, 35, 39]. Importantly, Vella et al., found that when customers asked for a specific product they were much less likely to be given advice on the use of that product [26]. Furthermore, the provision of patient resources and educational material was suggested [28, 29, 45].

Documentation and integration of care Three of the studies made recommendations surrounding documentation of customer consultations and/or increased communication with the healthcare professional to whom the patient was being referred [48, 50, 53]. One study noted that the use of a notification card given to the patient to take to the health professional to which they were referred, improved patients following through on referral advice by pharmacists. The authors also suggested that more information could be included on this card, for example any screening measurements that had been taken, for example blood pressure, and this was being trialled [50]. Erni and colleagues [48] also proposed that future services needed better integration into the health system to ensure "its efficacy, safety, cost effectiveness and acceptance by patients".

Documentation of patient consultations would also allow for follow-up treatment. It was suggested that there was a need for follow-up of some patients to ensure that appropriate care had been given and modification of treatment was made if necessary [28, 30].

Privacy and confidentiality Phillips and colleagues [27] recognised the sensitive nature of certain conditions, and that some patients did not want to have a consultation in the pharmacy due to concerns about privacy. Having pharmacies with private consultation rooms may be beneficial for avoiding embarrassment and for ensuring confidentiality.

Access to the pharmacist In the studies where it was considered that the most appropriate decisions were made [38, 42], pharmacists had conducted the consultation and thus the authors suggested that access to a pharmacist for consultations are a necessity.

Increased public awareness of pharmacist services Chui et al. [53] recognised that education of the public about the services that pharmacists provide is important; in addition Hafejee and colleagues [45] noted that one inexpensive method to increase patients' knowledge of the roles pharmacists can play in managing their skin problems was by the use of leaflets.

Discussion

This review addressed the feasibility of, and evidence for a CPTS and attempted to identify the key characteristics of such a service that are described in the literature. This review has found that elements of a CPTS currently exist in community pharmacies; however, the components of this service may need revising as we move forward. The recommendations of the various authors identified key areas which would need to be addressed to ensure that the service is safe and effective in terms of the appropriateness of differential diagnoses and decisions to treat or refer.

Pharmacists were found to make appropriate differential diagnosis decisions in a number of studies. However, several studies that did not use guidelines/protocols noted that pharmacists or their staff did not ask sufficient questions to obtain enough information to allow them to accurately assess the patient's condition. It is important for any consultation, whether the decision is to recommend treatment or to refer, to include adequate investigation using an appropriate number of pertinent questions. When guidelines/protocols were used this increased the appropriateness of the outcome [25, 28, 29, 32]; protocols can prompt appropriate questioning [54]. However, to optimise their use this must be coupled with training and education; Alkhatib and colleagues [44] showed that despite the high compliance with protocol use in their study, 21.8 % of pharmacists felt they required additional training. Computerised decision support systems have been trialled in community pharmacy [25], and nurse-based triage [55] with some success. If this type of protocol system were to be utilised,

logistics of use would have to be further tested in a community pharmacy environment. Regardless of whether the guidelines/protocols are computer-based on not, guidelines must be reviewed on a regular basis to ensure that the recommendations are evidence-based [56].

Cost analysis was conducted in two studies based in the UK, which estimated the cost savings when patients sought advice from the community pharmacy in comparison to GPs or EDs [6, 27]. Both of these studies concluded that there would be a significant cost benefit of schemes such as the MAS.

Overall, when the appropriateness of pharmacist referral decisions was evaluated by another health care expert, a high level of concordance was found. However, to our knowledge, there have been no studies that have looked at the appropriateness of treatment provided by pharmacists for patients using community pharmacy triage-like services; studies assessing the perspectives and health outcomes for patients are also scant. Whilst OTC medications can be effective in symptom control and resolution, and many minor ailments are likely to resolve without treatment, treatment with OTC medications has the potential to mask conditions or contribute towards diagnostic delay at a GP/ED. Varela et al. [42] reported that when a pseudo-patient presented with symptoms reflective of oral cancer, few patients were appropriately referred. Similarly, Scully and colleagues [43] found that fewer than 10 % of pharmacy staff recommended referral when a patient presented with a history suggestive of oral carcinoma. In both cases, if a patient was prescribed an OTC medication, this could delay presentation at the doctor for accurate diagnosis.

In order to reduce the risk of inappropriate diagnosis and inappropriate treatment, training and the use of guidelines and protocols have been advocated [25, 28, 29, 32], to ensure that a comprehensive and relevant patient history is taken, and to guide differential diagnosis. Hassell et al. [11] proposed that guidelines could be developed by pharmacists in conjunction with GPs, and Mehuys et al. [30] highlighted the need for evidence-based recommendations within such guidelines. Erni and colleagues [48] described the netCare triage service where 24 decision trees were developed. What is not yet known is whether the implementation of these guidelines would necessarily result in compliance. Alkhatib et al. [44] found that 55.5 % of pharmacists self-reported "always" using the specified protocol for the provision of ophthalmic chloramphenicol and a further 29.4 % used the protocol "usually". Nonetheless, 6.7 % "never" used the protocol.

Varela-Centelles et al. reported that pharmacist interactions with patients led to a higher proportion of appropriate decisions being made [42] than when consultations were with pharmacy support staff. In a study by Sheridan

Is there potential for the future provision of triage services in community...

77

et al., pharmacy assistants saw themselves as being the first point of contact within the pharmacy [57], and the same study also found that pharmacists perceived pharmacy assistants as "gatekeepers" to the pharmacist. For a CPTS, it is therefore important to ensure that pharmacy support staff have adequate training, and they know when to refer to the pharmacist. The use of protocols can guide this process. However, this then raises the question of whether a future CPTS should be restricted to accredited pharmacies where staff have undertaken specific training and the pharmacies meet certain criteria.

There have been contrasting perspectives from healthcare professionals with respect to the community pharmacy's role in the triage of minor ailments. Morris and colleagues surveyed GPs' opinions on the treatment of minor ailments by GPs and potentially pharmacists [1]. Whilst there were favourable responses toward pharmacists in this role from some, others expressed concerns about the quality of pharmacists' advice they did not know and only 50.9 % of GPs would recommend their patients seek advice from a pharmacist [1].

Patients have also been reported to have mixed perceptions about the role of pharmacists in healthcare. A study by Gidman et al. [58] described opinions of the public toward the role of the pharmacists and pharmacy services, including their role in the management of minor ailments. Some patients viewed the role of the pharmacist as a dispenser of medicines prescribed by the doctor and raised concerns about the incomplete nature of the services provided by community pharmacies and their lack of communication with GPs. On the other hand, others viewed pharmacists' knowledge of OTC products to be greater than that of the GP and expressed their trust in the pharmacist as being able to competently deal with minor self-limiting conditions [58]. Erni and colleagues [48] proposed that future triage services need better integration into the health system. This notion was also highlighted by Blenkinsopp et al. [50] and Marklund et al. [32] where referral cards were used between pharmacists and GPs.

Integrated computer-based healthcare services which link pharmacy and GP data, for example, are attainable. Whilst the studies in this review did not discuss whether IT integration was available, examples do exist. In New Zealand, "Testsafe" is a medical information sharing service for certain areas of the country, which gives healthcare providers access to diagnostic test results, reports and medicines information for their patients, in addition what medications have been dispensed by community pharmacists [59]. Such a system could be used for pharmacists to report on CPTS interactions.

This review did not focus on the funding of CPTS in pharmacies; however, it is evident that cost is an important factor in considering the service's feasibility. First of all, there is the issue of whether patients will pay for such a service. If a patient payment is required, one needs to consider whether they will use the service, in situations where GP and ED visits are free of charge, as in the UK. Conversely, in New Zealand, for example, unless you are under the age of 13, there is a cost associated with visiting a GP and thus a CPTS which is free of charge may be more attractive to patients. If no patient charge is to be made, this leaves the issue of who would fund the service.

One purpose of a recognised CPTS is to reduce the burden on other health providers such as GPs and EDs. Hassell et al. [51] found that diverting those seeking treatment for minor ailments from GPs to community pharmacies resulted in a 37.8 % reduction in GP consultations for 12 self-limiting conditions, although the overall GP workload did not decrease.

New and emerging services pertaining to the provision of advice and treatment for minor ailments, for example the MAS, are being utilised in some countries [6, 22, 52]. When questioned, patients who have used services such as the MAS, reported that if these pharmacy services were not available, they would have visited a GP or emergency services [6]. In addition, reverse referral interventions appear promising in reducing the workload of the GP for minor ailment consultations as they have resulted in few referrals back to the GP [7, 11].

An ideal CPTS needs to be one that is accessible [24] and that the public is aware of [28, 53], with sufficient resources, including competent staff that are available to appropriately question, diagnose and then either resolve or refer patients to the appropriate healthcare provider when necessary. Furthermore, communication and an interprofessional collaborative relationship between pharmacists and other healthcare professionals are integral to the success of a CPTS. Whilst a previous model developed referral cards to be taken by the patient to the referred provider [50], integrated computer-based systems may also be useful [25, 31]. Furthermore, having mutual support between GPs and pharmacists could allow for the potential of a two-way referral system [11]. In the netCare model, access to a dedicated GP to request a second opinion was available to pharmacists, which was used in only 17 % of cases [48]. This back-up consultation access may be valuable. Finally, documentation of the triage interaction is an important aspect of a potential service, and would allow for follow-up consultations to be arranged and medical notes available for re-assessment, and also allow the potential for auditing of services for quality.

It is important to differentiate community pharmacy triage from ED triage. In ED, the triage of patients involves the presenting condition being assessed for urgency and a decision on how soon treatment is required

[60], and hence ED triage encompasses the management of the full range of presentations from minor to life threatening [60]. However, in community pharmacy, an additional factor needs to be acknowledged – that there are many situations in which pharmacists are not able to treat, even if they are considered relatively minor and non-urgent. Thus triage in community pharmacy is not the same as triage in ED. The importance of a clear definition of CPTS is therefore essential.

Whilst the definition used in this review (from Chapman et al. [23]) describes elements of this service, the variability in current triage services suggests that this may not be sufficient to adequately define a CPTS. Community pharmacy triage may be best described as structured service which responds to contact initiated by the patient or caregiver for advice or a specific product request. This is then followed up with appropriate questioning with the decision to treat or refer to another health practitioner. Ideally, this should then be documented in the patient's notes held in the pharmacy and available to the GP in the patient's electronic health record, in an integrated health system. For the presentations that do not require referral to another health care provider, treatment and advice should be recommended based on evidence-based information.

We must also bear in mind that countries worldwide differ in their provision of prescription and non-prescription medicines. There are differences in regulations about where certain medications can be legally sold and by whom. For example, in the United States [33] all non-prescription medications do not have to be sold in a pharmacy setting. This is in stark contrast to many countries in Europe where all medicines have to be sold in a pharmacy [33].

Furthermore, we chose to define "appropriateness" in the light of clinical acceptability by other health professionals and patients. However, there is lack of clarity around how or whether appropriateness could also be expanded to include other parameters outside of our criteria. This review did not focus on the funding of CPTS in pharmacies; however, it is evident that cost is an important factor in considering such a service's feasibility, which could be a focus for future reviews.

Conclusion

Community pharmacists are seen as the most accessible health professionals [58] and are ideally placed to provide advice on both symptom presentations and OTC medication requests [61, 62]. Some have argued that their accessibility makes community pharmacy well suited to offer extended health services, providing convenient access points to those who are unable to use other services [58]. This review explored the potential for the future provision of more formally recognised triage services by evaluating the feasibility and the appropriateness of such services. From this review it is evident that the development and use of guidelines/protocols for the management of minor ailments within community pharmacies facilitates accurate assessment of a patient's condition with respect to whether a patient needs referral to another health care professional, and the urgency of this, or whether they can be safely treated in the pharmacy setting. Structured protocols along with adequate staff training would ensure the elicitation of a comprehensive and accurate patient history resulting in appropriate recommendations for the management of the condition. Such a service would be likely to reduce the burden on other health care providers. However, while we have highlighted the feasibility of such a service, we also acknowledge that a number of questions remain unanswered.

Abbreviations
CPTS: Community pharmacy triage services; ED: Emergency department; GP: General practitioner; IPA: International pharmaceutical abstracts; MAS: Minor ailments scheme

Acknowledgements
We would like to acknowledge the NZ Pharmacy Education and Research Foundation (NZPERF) and the Pharmacy Guild of NZ for the funding for two summer studentships that contributed to this work.

Funding
JM and RG received funding from the Pharmacy Guild of New Zealand and the New Zealand Pharmacy Education and Research Foundation for work on summer studentships which contributed to this paper. The views expressed in this paper do not necessarily reflect the views of these organisations, which had no involvement in the drafting of this paper.

Authors' contributions
LC: conception, extraction of data, analysis, interpretation, writing the review, revising and given final approval. JM: extraction of data, revising and given final approval. RG: extraction of data, revising and given final approval. TA: conception, revising and given final approval. MJ: conception, revising and given final approval. MM: conception, interpretation, revising and given final approval. JSha: conception, interpretation, drafting and revising and given final approval. JShe: conception, interpretation, drafting and revising and given final approval.

Competing interests
The authors declare that they have no competing interests.

References
1. Morris CJ, Cantrill JA, Weiss MC. GPs' attitudes to minor ailments. Fam Pract. 2001;18(6):581–5.
2. Bodenheimer T, Pham HH. Primary care: current problems and proposedsolutions. Health Aff. 2010;29(5):799–805.

3. Evans R et al. Apocalypse No : population aging and the future of health care systems. Social and Economic Dimensions of an Ageing Population, 2001. Research paper 59.

4. Anonymous. Public health and aging: trends in aging—United States and worldwide. JAMA. 2003;289(11):1371–3.

5. Cornwall J, JA. Davey. Impact of population ageing in New Zealand on the demand for health and disability support services and workforce implications New Zealand Institute for Research on Ageing (NZiRA) and the Health Services Research Centre (HSRC), Victoria University of Wellington. 2004. https://www.health.govt.nz/system/files/documents/publications/cornwallanddavey.pdf. Accessed 30 Sept 2016.

6. Baqir W, et al. Cost analysis of a community pharmacy 'minor ailment scheme' across three primary care trusts in the North East of England. J Public Health. 2011;33(4):551–5.

7. Bojke C, et al. Increasing patient choice in primary care: the management of minor ailments. Health Econ. 2004;13(1):73–86.

8. Merriam Webster dictionary. Full Definition of triage. Available from: http://www.merriam-webster.com/dictionary/triage. Accessed 30 Sept 2016.

9. Health, N.Z.M.o. Emergency department triage. 2011. Available from: http://www.health.govt.nz/our-work/hospitals-and-specialist-care/emergency-departments/emergency-department-triage. Accessed 30 Sept 2016.

10. Ministry of Health. Healthline. 2015. Available from: http://www.health.govt.nz/your-health/services-and-support/health-care-services/healthline. Accessed 30 Sept 2016.

11. Hassell K, et al. A pathway to the GP: the pharmaceutical 'consultation' as a first port of call in primary health care. Fam Pract. 1997;14(6):498–502.

12. Gauld NJ, et al. Widening consumer access to medicines through switching medicines to non-prescription: a six country comparison. PLoS One. 2014; 9(9):e107726.

13. Anonymous. Chloramphenicol eye drops approved as pharmacy medicine for treatment of bacterial conjunctivitis. Pharm J. 2005;274:697.

14. Gauld N. Improving access to urinary tract infection treatment: the reclassification of trimethoprim. SelfCare. 2012;3(6):115–20.

15. MINA study, Community Pharmacy Management of Minor Illness. Pharmacy Research UK, 2014.

16. ASMI Media Release. Available from: http://www.i2p.com.au/article/asmi-media-releases-september-2009. Accessed 30 Sept 2016.

17. Fielding S, et al. Estimating the burden of minor ailment consultations in general practices and emergency departments through retrospective review of routine data in North East Scotland. Fam Pract. 2015;32(2):165–72.

18. Proprietary Association of Great Britain. Making the case for the self care of minor ailments. 2009. Available from: http://www.selfcareforum.org/wp-content/uploads/2011/07/Minorailmentsresearch09.pdf. Accessed 30 Sept 2016.

19. Bednall R, et al. Identification of patients attending accident and emergency who may be suitable for treatment by a pharmacist. Fam Pract. 2003;20(1):54–7.

20. Welle-Nilsen LK, et al. Minor ailments in out-of-hours primary care: an observational study. Scand J Prim Health Care. 2011;29(1):39–44.

21. Bellingham C. How the minor ailments service works. Pharm J. 2004; 272(7284):115–6.

22. Mansell K, et al. Evaluating pharmacist prescribing for minor ailments. Int J Pharm Pract. 2015;23(2):95–101.

23. Chapman C, J Marriott, D. van den Bosch. The Nature, Extent and Impact of Triage Provided By Community Pharmacy in Victoria. Pharmacy Guild of Australia; 2010. http://guild.org.au/services-programs/research-and-development/archive—fourth-agreement/iig-008

24. Coelho RB, Costa FA. Impact of pharmaceutical counseling in minor health problems in rural Portugal. Pharm Pract. 2014;12(4):451.

25. Westerlund T, Andersson IL, Marklund B. The quality of self-care counselling by pharmacy practitioners, supported by IT-based clinical guidelines. Pharm World Sci. 2007;29(2):67–72.

26. Vella E, et al. Development of protocols for the provision of headache and back-pain treatments in Maltese community pharmacies. Int J Pharm Pract. 2009;17(5):269–74.

27. Philips Z, et al. The role of community pharmacists in prescribing medication for the treatment of head lice. J Public Health Med. 2001;23(2):114–20.

28. Martin Morales A, et al. Community pharmacy detection of erectile dysfunction in men with risk factors or who seek treatment or advice but lack a valid prescription. J Sex Med. 2013;10(9):2303–11.

29. Symonds T, et al. A feasibility study comparing pharmacist and physician recommendations for sildenafil treatment. J Sex Med. 2011;8(5):1463–71.

30. Mehuys E, et al. Self-medication of upper gastrointestinal symptoms: a community pharmacy study. Ann Pharmacother. 2009;43(5):890–8.

31. Westerlund T, et al. Evaluation of a model for counseling patients with dyspepsia in Swedish community pharmacies. Am J Health Syst Pharm. 2003;60(13):1336–41.

32. Marklund B, et al. Referrals of dyspeptic self-care patients from pharmacies to physicians, supported by clinical guidelines. Pharm World Sci. 2003;25(4):168–72.

33. Krishnan HS, Schaefer M. Evaluation of the impact of pharmacist's advice giving on the outcomes of self-medication in patients suffering from dyspepsia. Pharm World Sci. 2000;22(3):102–8.

34. Bilkhu P, et al. The management of ocular allergy in community pharmacies in the United Kingdom. Int J Clin Pharm. 2013;35(2):190–4.

35. Driesen A, Vandenplas Y. How do pharmacists manage acute diarrhoea in an 8-month-old baby? A simulated client study. Int J Pharm Pract. 2009; 17(4):215–20.

36. Rutter PM, Horsley E, Brown DT. Evaluation of community pharmacists' recommendations to standardized patient scenarios. Ann Pharmacother. 2004;38(6):1080–5.

37. Berger K, Eickhoff C, Schulz M. Counselling quality in community pharmacies: implementation of the pseudo customer methodology in Germany. J Clin Pharm Ther. 2005;30(1):45–57.

38. Schneider CR, et al. Provision of primary care to patients with chronic cough in the community pharmacy setting. Ann Pharmacother. 2011;45(3):402–8.

39. Kippist C, et al. How do pharmacists respond to complaints of acute insomnia? A simulated patient study. Int J Clin Pharm. 2011;33(2):237–45.

40. Watson MC, et al. Factors predicting the guideline compliant supply (or non-supply) of non-prescription medicines in the community pharmacy setting. Qual Saf Health Care. 2006;15(1):53–7.

41. Evans MJ, Gibbons AJ. Advice given in community pharmacies to patients with possible oral carcinoma. Br J Oral Maxillofac Surg. 2005;43(3):253–5.

42. Varela-Centelles P, et al. Oral cancer awareness at chemist's and herbalist's shops: new targets for educational interventions to prevent diagnostic delay. Oral Oncol. 2012;48(12):1272–5.

43. Scully C, Gill Y, Gill Z. How community pharmacy staff manage a patient with possible oral cancer. Br J Oral Maxillofac Surg. 1989;27(1):16–21.

44. Alkhatib L, et al. An evaluation of the reclassification of ophthalmic chloramphenicol for the management of acute bacterial conjunctivitis in community pharmacies in Western Australia. Int J Pharm Pract. 2015;23(2):111–20.

45. Hafejee A, Coulson IH. Community pharmacists' role in managing common skin problems. Br J Dermatol. 2006;155(6):1297.

46. Jiwa M, Spilsbury K, Duke J. Do pharmacists know which patients with bowel symptoms should seek further medical advice? A survey of pharmacists practicing in community pharmacy in Western Australia. Ann Pharmacother. 2010;44(5):910–7.

47. Ralph SG, Preston A, Clarke J. Over-the-counter advice for genital problems: the role of the community pharmacist. Int J STD AIDS. 2001;12(8):513–5.

48. Erni P, et al. netCare, a new collaborative primary health care service based in Swiss community pharmacies. Res Soc Adm Pharm. 2016;12(4):622–6.

49. Jiwa M, et al. Piloting and validating an innovation to triage patients presenting with cough to community pharmacies in Western Australia. Qual Prim Care. 2012;20(2):83–91.

50. Blenkinsopp A, Jepson M, Drury M. Using a notification card to improve communication between community pharmacists and general practitioners. Br J Gen Pract. 1991;41(344):116–8.

51. Hassell K, et al. Managing demand: transfer of management of self limiting conditions from general practice to community pharmacies. BMJ. 2001; 323(7305):146–7.

52. Parmentier H, et al. Community pharmacy treatment of minor ailments in refugees. J Clin Pharm Ther. 2004;29(5):465–9.

53. Chui WK, Li SC. Advice-giving on self-medication: perspectives of community pharmacists and consumers in Singapore. J Clin Pharm Ther. 2005;30(3):225–31.

54. Huibers L, et al. Safety of telephone triage in out-of-hours care: a systematic review. Scand J Prim Health Care. 2011;29(4):198–209.

55. Marklund B, et al. Computer-supported telephone nurse triage: an evaluation of medical quality and costs. J Nurs Manag. 2007;15(2):180–7.

56. Hanna LA, Hughes CM. 'First, do no harm': factors that influence pharmacists making decisions about over-the-counter medication: a qualitative study in Northern Ireland. Drug Saf. 2010;33(3):245–55.

57. Sheridan J, et al. Can I help you? A qualitative study of pharmacist and pharmacy assistant views on the role of pharmacy assistants in New Zealand. Int J Pharm Pract. 2011;19(4):228–35.

58. Gidman W, Cowley J. A qualitative exploration of opinions on the community pharmacists' role amongst the general public in Scotland. Int J Pharm Pract. 2013;21(5):288–96.

59. Testsafe. Care connect testsafe. 2011. Available from: http://www.testsafe.co.nz/Home.aspx. Accessed 30 Sept 2016.

60. Ministry of Health. Emergency department triage. Available from: http://www.health.govt.nz/our-work/hospitals-and-specialist-care/emergency-departments/emergency-department-triage. Accessed 30 Sept 2016.

61. Ngwerume K, et al. An evaluation of an intervention designed to improve the evidence-based supply of non-prescription medicines from community pharmacies. Int J Pharm Pract. 2015;23(2):102–10.

62. Simmons-Yon A, et al. Understanding pharmacists' experiences with advice-giving in the community pharmacy setting: a focus group study. Patient Educ Couns. 2012;89(3):476–83.

63. Maunder PE, Landes DP. An evaluation of the role played by community pharmacies in oral healthcare situated in a primary care trust in the north of England. Br Dent J. 2005;199(4):219–23. discussion 211.

64. Watson MC, et al. A cohort study of influences, health outcomes and costs of patients' health-seeking behaviour for minor ailments from primary and emergency care settings. BMJ Open. 2015;5(2):e006261.

8

Novel models to improve access to medicines for chronic diseases in South Africa: an analysis of stakeholder perspectives on community-based distribution models

Bvudzai Priscilla Magadzire[1][*] (iD), Bruno Marchal[1,2] and Kim Ward[3]

Abstract

Background: The rising demand for chronic disease treatment and the barriers to accessing these medicines have led to the development of novel models for distributing medicines in South Africa's public sector, including distribution away from health centres, known as community-based distribution (CBD). In this article, we provide a typology of CBD models and outline perceived facilitators and barriers to their implementation using an adapted health systems framework with a view to analysing how future policy decisions on CBD could impact existing models and the health system as a whole.

Methods: A qualitative exploratory study comprising in-depth interviews and non-participant observations was conducted between 2012 and 2014 in one province. Study participants consisted of frontline healthcare providers (HCPs) in the public sector and a few policy, supply chain and public health experts. Observations of processes occurred at two CBD sites. We conducted deductive analysis guided by the adapted framework.

Results: Models varied in typology ranging from formal (approved by the Department of Health) to informal (demand-driven) and with or without user-fees. Processes and structures also differed, as did HCPs' perceptions of what is appropriate. HCPs perceived that CBD models were largely *acceptable* to patients and *accommodating* of their needs. *Affordability* of services linked to charging of user-fees was a contested issue, requiring further exploration. CBD models operated in the absence of formal policy to guide implementation, and this, coupled with the involvement of non-health professionals, issues regarding medicines handling and storage; and limited patient counselling raised concerns about the quality of pharmaceutical services being delivered. Policy decisions on each of the health system elements will likely affect other elements and ultimately influence the structure and operational modalities of models. In anticipation of a future CBD policy, stakeholders cited the need for a *context specific* lens in order to harmonise with current implementation efforts.

Conclusion: A formal policy on CBD is required in an effort to standardise services for quality assurance purposes. Frontline HCPs should be involved in the development of such policy to ensure that existing arrangements already working well are not undermined. Further research will seek to contribute towards evidence-based development of policy and service delivery guidelines for CBD activities in South Africa.

Keywords: Community-based distribution, Access to medicines, Pharmaceutical policy, South Africa

* Correspondence: bmagadzire@gmail.com
[1]School of Public Health, University of the Western Cape, Private Bag X17, Bellville 7535, South Africa
Full list of author information is available at the end of the article

Background

South Africa shares with the rest of sub-Saharan Africa a high burden of chronic diseases, including HIV and non-communicable diseases [1]. This has led to an increasing demand for medicines for treatment of disease in a context of a weak health system [2]. The increased burden of disease has illuminated the need for the government to be more responsive to population needs and to ensure that people obtain health services (including accessing essential medicines) without suffering financial hardship. The latter are in line with principles of universal health coverage (UHC) [3].

The South African government released the National Health Insurance (NHI) White Paper in December 2015. This policy document discusses various health insurance modalities and reforms aimed at strengthening the country's health system. These include: expanding access to pharmaceutical products, a primary healthcare re-engineering strategy and establishment of an office of health standards compliance. Furthermore, it describes a vision of what is required for the successful implementation of NHI [4].

Against this background, we have witnessed a shift in the local access to medicines (ATM) domain, from a largely health facility-based approach to providing medicines for chronic diseases to novel community-based distribution (CBD) models, also referred to as alternative distribution or out-of-clinic models [5]. While the term "distribution" within the broader medicine supply chain context encompasses ordering, transportation and logistics management at various levels [6], its use in this article is confined to logistics activities to get patient-ready pre-packaged medicines to patients. This has been referred by some authors as the "last mile", where services are delivered to patients and often at the most vulnerable stage of distribution [7].

CBD models use community halls and similar gathering places as sites for medicine distribution, exploiting the proximity of these venues to patients' homes. Sometimes, they also include home deliveries. These models are geared towards addressing various supply- and demand-side barriers to accessing medicines [8]. Such barriers include: long waiting times, overburdened health centres which discourage patients from collecting medicines and reducing travel costs to distant health facilities. Furthermore, CBD models can allow for task-shifting to mid-level cadres or even to expert patients in order to address human resource shortages [9, 10]. The latter is facilitated by the choice of target beneficiaries, i.e. stable patients not requiring regular contact with a healthcare provider (HCP). Such patients can be sufficiently empowered to self-manage [11] and have six-monthly consultations. CBD is not only recognised in South Africa as an interesting solution to restricted access to medicines [12, 13], but in many other developing countries, [14–16] including Mozambique [5, 17–19], Zambia [20] and Kenya [21]. CBD models are driven by non-

governmental organisations (NGOs) in the majority of cases.

While CBD is gaining momentum in South Africa, the range of models and the pace of implementation are variable across provinces. This could be explained in part by the health system's governance structure, which allow provinces a fair degree of autonomy in the administration of health services [22]. The Western Cape is one province where CBD has been widely implemented. In this province, CBD falls under the umbrella of community-based services, an important component of the broader primary healthcare (PHC) platform that features in the provincial strategy for health, Healthcare 2030 [23]. CBD is facilitated by centralised dispensing of patient-ready medicine packages by a private distributor to health facilities [24–27]. These packages can easily be transported to CBD points.

This article draws on selected findings from a broad exploratory study commissioned by the Western Cape Department of Health (WCDoH) to improve access to medicines (ATM). The overall study sought to identify strategies to address the challenge of missed appointments among patients with chronic diseases in the metropolitan district of Cape Town [24]. We also sought to understand the structure of ATM strategies and the facilitators and barriers to effective implementation. We targeted frontline healthcare providers (HCPs), most of whom engage with patients on a regular basis. These stakeholders have a critical role in the attainment of policy outcomes yet their role is often overlooked [28, 29]. Our research showed that many HCPs identified CBD (among a few others) as an existing innovative strategy for ensuring that medicines reach patients. However, they also cited challenges, of which the most important was the lack of policy to govern CBD activities even though their implementation was actually underway. The implication was that certain issues related to CBD could be open to multiple interpretations. We discovered early on that governing CBD activities was far from being simple, given that these are "non-traditional" mechanisms for medicines distribution.

As the development of a CBD policy is a current priority in South Africa, in this article we seek to contribute to the policy-making process by exploring how CBD models currently operate in the Western Cape Province's local health system and identifying the perspectives of frontline HCPs regarding CBD models. In order to provide evidence that could inform policy design, we have adapted the health systems framework of van Olmen et al. (the framework) [30] as an analytical tool for the following reasons:

a) Its ability to assist us to identify and discuss the key elements of CBD models (e.g. medicines supply, human resources, infrastructure and population) and to draw the interconnections between the elements which will be of relevance to the design of CBD policy;

b) Its ability to frame CBD operations within the context of the broader health system;

c) The importance it attaches to values and principles in policy-making [22].

d) Its recognition of health systems as social systems which comprise people and organisations, and their interactions with others. As such, actors' values, interests, norms and relationships also influence the ultimate character of the system [31].

In this article we use the framework to provide a systematic description of CBD models and to illustrate how the configuration of the elements in each CBD model contributes to its effectiveness. Finally, we explore how our findings could inform the development of an impending CBD policy by drawing upon the perspectives of stakeholders.

Methods

Study design

This exploratory qualitative study was conducted between 2012 and 2014 in the metropolitan district of Cape Town, which has the greatest proportion of patients and the greatest pressure on health services in the Western Cape Province [24, 25].

Data collection

We used in-depth interviews, non-participant observations of two CBD sessions and document review as the data collection methods for this study.

Key informants

For this article, we drew from 45 in-depth interviews, which were conducted by the first author using a semi-structured interview guide. We purposively sampled informants who were most knowledgeable about the issues of interest from the following categories: (1) frontline HCPs, including doctors, nurses, pharmacists and pharmacist's assistants (PAs) from four PHC facilities, (2) policy makers, (3) sub-district and provincial managers from the WCDoH, (4) private sector pharmacists, (5) academics with expertise in pharmaceutical policy and public health and (6) NGO staff (Table 1). Interviews were conducted in English and each interview lasted about one hour. All the interviews were conducted at a place convenient for the respondents, i.e. their place of work. Where possible, interviews were recorded; alternatively, notes were taken. Three participants refused to be recorded as a matter of preference. Once no information was generated from the interviews and saturation was reached, no further interviews were conducted.

Table 1 Respondents' breakdown by professional category

Category	Number of respondents
National level policy maker in pharmaceutical regulation	1
Senior provincial directors and policy makers	5
Academic in public health	1
Provincial managers of the medicines supply chain	2
Mid-level managers (sub-structure pharmacists; primary healthcare managers)	4
Frontline health workers (clinicians, health promoters, NGO workers)	28
Private sector pharmacists	4
Total	45

Non-participant observations

The first author conducted observations on two occasions. The first session was for distribution of HIV treatment and another for distribution of medicines for non-communicable diseases (e.g. diabetes and hypertension). Both sessions took place in Khayelitsha, one of the largest townships in South Africa. During observations, the first author took note of patient-patient and patient-provider interactions and the process in general. Other items that were recorded included the queries that were posed by patients and any information related to patients' knowledge about their medication.

Document review

We reviewed guidelines and standard operating procedures for CBD in order to understand how the models are currently implemented [32, 33].

Data analysis

The recordings were transcribed verbatim and deductive analysis was applied. We sought for : (a) structure of CBD models, and used the main elements of the *analytical framework of van Olmen* et al. [30], (Fig. 1) which links the central elements required for models to function optimally i.e. *resources* (medicines, human resources, infrastructure, financing, monitoring and evaluation) to the performance of the service delivery platforms. All these elements require good *governance* (policies, regulatory frameworks) and *leadership*, taking into account the population's needs and demands [34] to attain ATM in terms of its different access dimensions or *outcomes*; i.e.: availability, affordability, accessibility, acceptability and quality) [35, 36] and ultimately improved health status and social and financial protection. Access outcomes can be broadly defined as follows:

- *acceptability*: fit between clients and providers' mutual expectations and appropriateness of care;

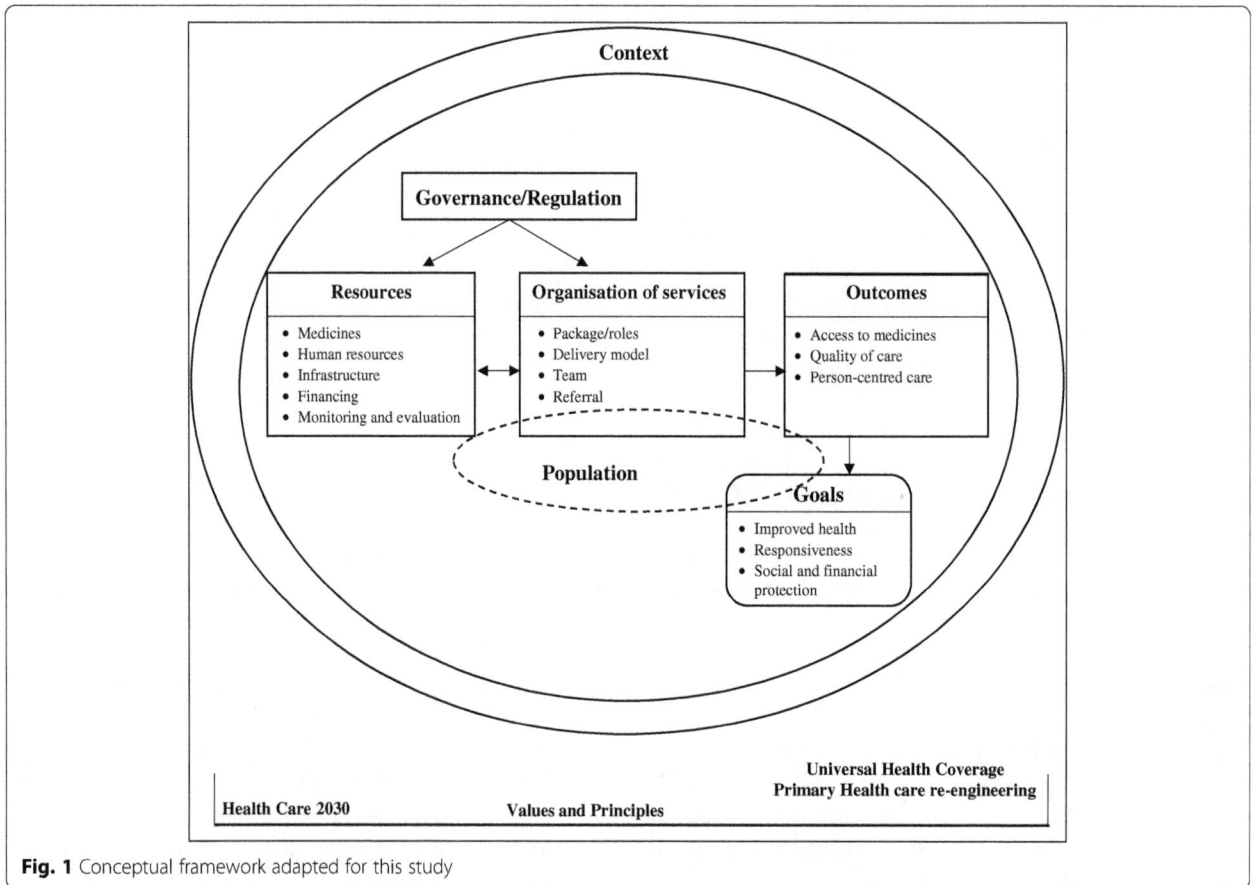

Fig. 1 Conceptual framework adapted for this study

- *accommodation*: fit between organisation of services and clients' practical circumstances;
- *availability*: fit between existing resources and clients' needs;
- *accessibility*: fit between physical location of healthcare and location of clients;
- *affordability:* fit between cost of care and ability to pay [35].

Outcomes are expressed both quantitatively and qualitatively by our adopted framework [30]. However, in the absence of objective outcome- and impact-level data for CBD models, we assessed selected outcomes only qualitatively, from the perspectives of informants. Accessibility is an inherent design feature of CBD models and as such this was not assessed. Using data from interviews and observations, we assessed how models were perceived by informants and patient engagement with CBD services. Our assumption was that if models increase ATM, this could be a proxy for utilisation. In addition, we considered *facilitators and barriers to effective implementation* and *context* factors because CBD models are embedded within a broader health system and these factors can influence outcomes and goals (Fig. 1). Quality was a cross-cutting issue

addressing the issues of scientifically and medically appropriate and good quality services. This is determined by aspects such as human resources and good quality medicines.

Data from document review and observations were used to triangulate key informant data.

The first author conducted the initial analysis (coding, retrieving of quotations representative of major themes and interpretation) using Atlas. TI version 7. Emerging themes were discussed with selected key informants through three feedback sessions (participant checking).

Results

This section starts by presenting an overview of how CBD services are organised (*Typology of CBD models*) then presents the remaining findings according to the elements of the framework (*human resources, medicines, infrastructure* and *population*). Finally, we present our findings related to *governance*, taking into account the implementation context.

Typology of CBD models

From the interviews with key informants, we found variation in focus and structure of CBD models implemented in the Western Cape Province. Regarding geographical spread, some areas had a single model while others had a combination of models. The mix of models available in an area was primarily dependant on the presence and mandate or interests of particular stakeholders whose activities tended to be geographically demarcated. However, they were all linked to nearby PHC facilities for medicines supply. In this article, we categorised them as formal and informal as explained below:

I. Formal: Models officially recognised and approved by the WCDoH. Services were provided free of charge to the patient. Formally recognised providers were expected to facilitate referrals and linkage to care for patients at risk who require consultation with the health provider. Some models were based on direct involvement of trained HCPs (i.e. nurses and/or post-basic pharmacists), while others were driven by community health workers (CHWs) with some basic health training, linked to NGOs.

II. Informal: Models driven by entrepreneurs with no basic training in health. They charged a service fee to the patient and were not officially recognised by the WCDoH. Informal providers could be described in two ways: either operating under the 'approval' of mid-level management or known anecdotally, but not easily identifiable. The latter operated on a small-scale and could not be easily distinguished from a relative or friend collecting medicines on behalf of the patient. At the time of research, service fees charged by the known informal providers ranged from ZAR10.00–20.00, which was equivalent to approximately US$1.00-2.00. It was unclear how informal providers market their services or initiate services in the absence of the approval of senior provincial leadership.

Patient enrolment in all the CBD models was facilitated by nurses and health promoters during club sessions (group-based education), and patients were asked to provide consent for their information to be supplied to the service provider of their choice. Table 2 shows the range of models that we identified at our study sites. We acknowledge that this list may not be exhaustive for the Cape Town metropolitan area.

Resources
Human resources
As illustrated in Table 2, task shifting from pharmacists to other HCPs and Non-Health Professionals (NHPs) is a common feature in CBD models. There was contention between participants about the involvement of NHPs and their permitted scope of practice.

Proponents for task-shifting in CBD models argued that this mechanism could address existing human resource shortages in the South African public sector by "de-medicalising" treatment to ensure sustainability of models. Informants cited a situation illustrating lack of sustainability of medicalised models: a clinical nurse practitioner was asked to urgently return to the health facility from a CBD site leaving patients unattended and necessitating their referral back to the health facility.

Another stakeholder (academic) argued that patient counselling by pharmacists, though desired, was in most cases impractical. The informant's own research showed that pharmacists in the Western Cape spend an average of only three minutes (range: 2–4 min) of face-to-face contact with a patient due to workload pressures. In light of these health workforce issues, stakeholders suggested the need for greater efforts towards empowering patients to manage their own therapy thereby reducing the need for regular contact with HCPs.

Those who opposed involvement of NHPs in CBD cited their lack of accountability to statutory bodies as a major concern in delivering pharmaceutical services. This is currently a grey area in the task-shifting discourse because

Table 2 Overview of models for community based distribution of medicines

Type of model	Classification	Human resources	Financing	Beneficiary population as per disease state
1. Distribution in community halls, churches, old-age homes or mobile clinics	Formal	Pharmacist's assistants, nurses	Health facility budget therefore government funding	HIV and/or NCDs
2. Distribution in small municipal clinics that do not offer NCD services	Formal	Pharmacist's assistants	Health facility budget therefore government funding	NCDs
3. Home delivery	Informal	Local social entrepreneurs	Out-of-pocket payments	NCDs
4. Home delivery or other community venues[a]	Formal	Community health workers[b]	A few organisations have international funding while the rest receive grants from the Department of Social Development (DSD) and other local businesses.	NCDs

[a]Places where the elderly meet for skills development and social activities, also termed Chronic Disease of Lifestyle clubs which the WCDoH identified through the DSD
[b]Attached to NGOs with service level agreements with the WCDoH

statutory bodies only regulate personnel who are registered with them.

Other concerns raised by participants related to the capacity of NHPs to: (i) conduct quality assurance (QA) processes (e.g. verifying medicines before handing them over to the patient), (ii) monitor therapeutic outcomes and (iii) link at-risk patients to appropriate care. These tasks are outside their scope of practice therefore, perhaps a more pertinent question is: which tasks should NHPs be expected to carry out? Many informants argued that QA processes should be ensured by the Chronic Dispensing Unit (CDU), a centralised dispensary responsible for dispensing and pre-packing of medicines in the public sector in this province. If performed optimally by ensuring minimal prescribing and dispensing errors, this would eliminate the need for checking parcels at the distribution point upon issue to patients. With QA processes out of the way, this would technically not be a full dispensing process, allowing NHPs to comfortably participate in the process.

It seemed even pharmacists who were responsible for checking the pre-packed medicine packages felt that the QA demands were time consuming and detracted from the intended benefits of both the CDU (which was established to reduce pharmacists' workload) and of CBD (which was established to take the pressure off health facilities and to improve access for patients).

While some informants mentioned that they would feel comfortable relying on CHWs to issue medicines that were already checked at the CDU, some clinicians were still reluctant. They suggested that CBD activities be placed under the responsibility of registered pharmacy mid-level workers known as pharmacist's assistants (PAs) as opposed to CHWs. A further suggestion was engagement of private-sector pharmacies to distribute public-sector medicines. In subsequent years, this model was proposed under the NHI scheme [37].

Medicines supply management

Our findings show that inefficiencies in procurement (a macro-level issue) affected medicines availability at the CDU where dispensing for CBD programmes takes place. As such, medicines omitted from parcels would require manual dispensing at health facilities, another reason why informants were sceptical about NHPs involvement as the final link to patients. As stated by a senior manager:

"I wouldn't like at this stage for community health workers to give medication, because, once in a while, something is missing, because of the out-of-stock situation. Now we got a serious situation as well...the Cape Medical Depot cannot always supply because of change of tender."

Another contentious issue raised was the handling and storage of "non-collected" medicines, i.e. parcels not collected by the patient on the appointment date. The handling of medicines by untrained personnel and their storage in transient unregistered sites casts doubt on the integrity of non-collected medicines and as such, these medicines are usually disposed of with resultant cost implications. Informants were of the opinion that some of these risks could be obviated if sites met minimum standards for medicine storage.

Infrastructure and logistics

Securing reliable venues for CBD activities emerged as another important aspect of CBD. During the time of our study, services were interrupted at one site because it was no longer available for CBD. The PA at the site expressed concern about the potential loss of confidence by patients experiencing service disruption. In addition to securing venues, opening times for the venues needed careful consideration. This often called for negotiation with the owners of the venue to ensure that times were suitable for the patients.

Reliable transportation for medicine delivery to CBD sites was also identified as a need. Government vehicles could be requested by PAs linked to formal CBD models, but this transportation mode was not accessible to CHWs who often walked to sites and carried the supplies. According to informants, the latter not only posed security risks and environmental risks for the medicines, but created inefficiencies for CHWs with home-based care duties who were often late for CBD activities. Informal providers used bicycles and this was also feared to potentially render medicines vulnerable to environmental risks.

Outcomes
Acceptability of CBD models and accommodation to clients' practical circumstances

We used our observation data related to patient-provider and patient-patient interactions during the CBD process to look into the *acceptability* of the models. Interactions between patients and providers and between patients were largely positive. Patients showed no restraint in engaging with the providers involved in CBD (both HPs and NHPs) even when they presented late for their appointments. In some cases, CHWs reported taking the initiative to deliver medicines to patients' homes when they failed to collect at community venues, a means of *accommodating* patients' practical circumstances. These deviations from formal processes were merely acts of goodwill facilitated by positive patient-provider relationships, but were noted to contribute to *acceptability*. Furthermore, CHWs reported using cost-effective social media methods such as the instant messaging application "WhatsApp" to remind patients of their appointments and to follow-up with those who missed appointments. In this regard, the close patient-provider interactions allowed for some degree of patient follow-up where there had been limited to no follow-up mechanisms in the health system. These experiences also reveal a form of grassroots innovation that could improve patient retention-in-care in the long-run.

Informants collectively felt that CBD models are suitable for patients who are empowered to take responsibility for the management of their illness. From observation during CBD operations, some patients were able to accurately identify their medicines, including identifying any missing medicines when there were medicines availability challenges.

Despite the positive aforementioned aspects, there were some concerns with stigma. At one site (a small municipal clinic which traditionally offered HIV services and was later also used as a distribution site for NCD medicines), patients on ART raised concerns about privacy because their appointments overlapped with patients enrolled in NCD programmes. With medicine collection points for ART being distinct, patients with HIV were easily identifiable and this was a huge concern for those who had not disclosed to family and friends. This raised questions about the appropriateness of integrating HIV and NCDs in the design of CBD models.

At a second site, providers also noticed similar reluctance from clients on ART. The pharmacist's assistant in charge of CBD at the site said:

"...we told them that it's only them who are going there; there are a lot of offices so no one will know why you are walking through that building, what you are going to do there..."

While in principle, patients should be offered the choice to collect medicines at CBD sites or at the health facility, in practice there seemed to be pressure to enrol all patients onto CBD models, because of the perceived benefits for both the health system and the patients. Asked if patients had a choice regarding their collection point, one PA stated *"...we don't prioritise that freedom".* In their view, once patients experienced the benefits of CBD, they appreciated the system and in most cases were no longer interested in the facility-based model.

Affordability to patients: to pay or not to pay for CBD services?

As stated earlier, the critical difference between the formal and informal CBD models was that the former provides services at no charge to the patient while the latter levies a user-fee. Many stakeholders grappled with the issue of paid services: some senior managers expressed disapproval of imposing out-of-pocket payments on the premise that medication was free and no direct charges should be introduced to the patients, while others feared that the absence of regulation on

levying fees could result in patient exploitation. Indeed, some patients had apparently mentioned to informants that the services were expensive for them but some HCPs still argued that paid services were demand-driven and that many patients were willing to pay for a service offering convenience. One nurse and PA were of the opinion that the elderly derived particular benefits since they often have impaired mobility, lack family and other support to collect medicine on their behalf and many stayed in areas that are not served by formal models. Also, the formal models had limited capacity to serve a large population. Some respondents felt that paid services offset the usual indirect costs for transport fees to the health facility and thus had no objection to charging fees for CBD services.

At the time of our study, one of the four study sites had no history of "fee-for" services, a second site still charged a fee and the remaining two sites had been mandated to cease services that attached a fee. Although some frontline HCPs approved of services levied for a fee at the second site, senior managers had strong reservations. However, HCPs reported that some patients still enquired about the service and attributed increased non-collection of medicines to the management's decision to stop these paid services. One pharmacist elaborated as follows:

"A few years ago, we had a courier service that was privately run and we had an objection from the government that it's unconstitutional to charge patients from a primary health care level. Then we stopped it. The patients benefited a lot from it and up to this day, patients are still asking "When is it coming back and why can't we have it back?", because they were prepared to pay. But the department said it is criminal for patients who can't afford the service. It didn't make sense to us but it came from the top level to be stopped basically, but it was working well and we were pushing almost 200 parcels a day from the facility." [Pharmacist]

In essence, views on paid services were quite divergent, with provincial managers expressing the need to safeguard patients against exploitation and with some frontline HCPs indicating that paid for services are demand-driven and should remain an option to patients.

Governance: Policy and regulatory issues

As stated earlier, for any service delivery model to function effectively, all health system elements require good governance in the form of policies and regulatory frameworks which consider the population's needs and demands.

At the time of this study, there was no policy to institute CBD models and guide the implementation efforts in the Western Cape. Stakeholders were not aware of policies in other parts of the world enabling the use of non-registered sites for distribution of medicines for chronic diseases and as an interim measure, they developed standard operating procedures (SOPs), based loosely on available pharmacy and health regulations. Stakeholder views on these SOPs varied. As one provincial manager explained:

> "... this (CBD) is new ... There was, like, really no definite law to guide the Pharmacy Council. So, whatever has happened has been an interpretation of the law by someone (provincial stakeholders) ..."

We were informed by a key actor during this study that some engagement between provincial and national stakeholders responsible for the policy making process had commenced by 2014. The South African Pharmacy Council (SAPC), which is the statutory professional body for pharmacy, together with the National Department of Health (NDoH) which has oversight of health activities and legislation, were cited as the two governance bodies responsible for drafting legislation. While recognising that CBD policy development is a national priority and that the process of policy-making can be slow, stakeholders insinuated that the process has not been altogether transparent. We found there was limited consultation of frontline HCPs on the issue and that no feedback on progress of the policy development process was given at this level. One senior manager had some information on the process and reported that a task team had been set-up and was steadily working on developing the policy.

Stakeholder perspectives on the future CBD policy

In general, informants envisaged that the policy will define organisation of CBD services to ensure the delivery of quality pharmaceutical services as defined by the Good Pharmacy Practice (GPP) standards [38]. There were some shared concerns that some aspects inherent to CBD models do not meet GPP standards, *inter alia*, medicines handling and storage and possible lack of patient counselling.

Some stakeholders justified the current structure of CBD services while others showed disfavour towards some aspects of CBD and offered suggestions for improved organisation and structure. Despite varying opinions on what the content of the CBD policy ought to be, a critical issue that was raised was the need for the policy to be *context specific and pragmatic*. There were concerns that existing CBD models could be jeopardised if the upcoming policy prescribed the use of qualified personnel (HCPs) and/or distribution from health sites only. It must be understood, however, that the call for flexibility is not akin to accepting sub-standard service. Rather, it is a call to be realistic regarding what is both *feasible and sustainable* in the local context. As one manager said:

> "...they (regulators) need to draft the legislation to reflect pharmaceutical services as they are delivered in 2015, and going forward not in 20 years ago and in 30 years ago. Medicines are not ordinary commodities. The integrity of the medicine has to be maintained... but our request collectively to council (SAPC) has been could one look at a framework where one could legally issue the medicines that are not on a health site... and have a set of norms and standards for the issuing of medicines ... as long as rules and standards are met and maintained and monitored."

Furthermore, the call for regulators' flexibility stemmed from the simple realisation that more diversification is required if the province (and indeed the country at large) is to truly expand ATM. A private-sector pharmacist elaborated on this aspect as follows:

> "I said to somebody from council (SAPC): we are trying to put down first world standards which is very noble, but we are a resource lacking third world, essentially, third world country. We have a component of first world, but ninety per cent is third world. We are a developing country. I hope it gets taken into consideration, because I think it's going to make implementation of a lot of what national health (insurance) wants to do almost impossible to start."

The quote above called into question the degree of alignment between the province's and country's goals of improving ATM and the focus by professional statutory bodies on what were sometimes perceived as rigid standards. There was also a prevailing view that perhaps professional bodies were minimally consulted in the development of CBD strategies and that subsequent disagreements are arising between policy stakeholders:

> "...how much dialogue is actually happening between national, what national (NDOH) is trying to bring through the National Health Insurance versus what Pharmacy Council (SAPC) is saying and the statutes to everybody in terms of best policy. I don't think they are on the same page as to what the best practice is. (private-sector pharmacist)

On a positive note, despite a lack of consensus among stakeholders on certain issues, there was notable commitment from the WCDoH leadership to engage with SAPC and eventually align with the future CBD policy. Stakeholders also anticipated that CBD implementation could eventually cost more than is currently envisaged if provinces have to invest in training personnel and adapting venues to meet requirements for medicine handling and storage for example.

Discussion

CBD models are regarded as a useful way to improve ATM in the Western Cape Province. In this article, we described a range of formal and informal CBD models present using the framework by van Olmen et al. [30]. The framework enabled us to illustrate how the configuration of the elements in each CBD model could contribute to its effectiveness and furthermore, to illustrate the interconnections between the CBD models and the wider health system elements, indicating how policy decisions on each of these elements will likely affect other elements. For example, the framework argues for the need to recognise patients' own contributions to their personal well-being [30]. Through our research, we noted demand-driven operations by informal providers in a context where senior managers were opposed to the idea. Some differences between formal and informal models were that the formal models are a health system response and therefore, at least in theory resourced and accountable to the system while informal models are grassroots driven, self-funded and with no accountability mechanisms to the health system. However, both have the same goal of improving ATM.

Another key lesson from the application of the framework is that it is the combination of different health system elements that makes a model work well. For example, a decision on the human resource cadre(s) could influence the structure and operational modalities of CBD models, particularly when task-shifting is

introduced and mechanisms for accountability and quality assurance become essential. Table 3 summarises what we identified to be facilitators and barriers associated with each CBD element in its current form, an approach we envisage will inform the policy debate.

Despite increased interest in CBD by stakeholders in the WC, medicines are governed by pharmaceutical policy, therefore, who handles them and how they are handled becomes a matter of regulatory interest. This dimension needs to be carefully navigated to ensure safety of the population. As there is currently no CBD policy, we explored how our findings could inform the development of a future policy, through knowledge of context needs and demands. Through this study, we have brought the voices of frontline HCPs to the policy discussion on ATM. As stated by Gilson & Raphaely, "*Policy actors are not just those officially tasked with policy development; they also include those with concern for particular policy issues or likely to be affected by policy developments...*" [39]. We identify HCPs as such because of their important role at the coal-face of the health services and as such as the actual implementers of policy.

We identified some lessons from this study which could inform the policy development process. First, reaching a consensus requires broad stakeholder consultation as part of the policy development process, which to our knowledge has not yet been conducted in this case. Despite some stakeholders being aware that the policy development process had commenced, we found that consultation

Table 3 Summary of how CBD elements facilitate or constrain CBD implementation

CBD element		Facilitators	Barriers
Medicines		o Centralised dispensing simplifies distribution process.	o Quality assurance processes must be fulfilled by HCPs prior to "last mile" distribution; o Stock-outs of medicines cripples CBD models; o Non-collected medicines cannot be re-dispensed.
Human resources	Community Health Workers	o Positive, close relationships with patients which can facilitate active follow-up when necessary.	o Not able to conduct quality assurance processes.
	HCPs	o Missing medicines from patient-ready parcels can be dispensed manually by the HCP at the CBD site.	o General shortage of HCPs undermine sustainability of deploying them to CBD sites.
	Informal providers	o Demand-driven therefore likely to suit beneficiary needs.	o No governmental oversight which could lead to financial exploitation of patients; o no accountability to professional statutory body which could compromise quality of pharmaceutical services.
Infrastructure and logistics		o Government vehicles available for transportation of medicines for some models.	o Poor transport systems for CHWs causing delays and posing security and environmental risks to medicines; o Availability of venues not always guaranteed.
Patient (population)'s engagement with CBD models		o Positive patient-patient; patient-provider relationships; o Some patients knowledgeable about their treatment regimen and proactive in addressing medicine-related concerns.	o Stigma associated with HIV still a reality.

and feedback on the progress of the process was not inclusive and that frontline HCPs who are responsible for implementing policies were not involved. Acknowledging that policy processes are in essence political, how much influence actors have might be contingent on their position in the political hierarchy, more than their knowledge and understanding of the issue [40]. Hence in this study, we have sought to elevate the voice of frontline HCPs, who possess knowledge and understanding of grassroots issues. This stakeholder group has been referred to as "street-level bureaucrats": they are tasked with policy implementation and often have to balance policy demands with the realities of their context [41]. Considering their perspectives during the policy development process could result in more responsive policies. As echoed by Morrow (2015), the process of formulating a pharmaceutical policy is as important as the policy document in ensuring collective ownership [42].

Second, the resistance by some stakeholders to aspects of CBD corroborates findings in other countries. Indeed, previous studies have shown that diversion from traditional ways of delivering pharmaceutical services and task shifting in the pharmaceutical sector in its different forms has in many instances met with resistance [43, 44]. Experiences of resistance to different CBD models were documented in Mozambique with the introduction of self-forming patient groups [19] and in Tanzania with the implementation of community retail drug shops, but this changed with time [45]. In Mozambique, as stakeholders gained knowledge and confidence in the model and the benefits became apparent, endorsement increased [19]. In Tanzania, retail drug shops which are a major source of medicines in rural and underserved areas also initially faced resistance, then catalysed development of policies. Of note, the Tanzania model illustrated that even informal providers can be assisted to comply with regulatory standards [45]. Whether or not this will become the experience of providers in our context, remains to be seen.

Implications for future research and the policy agenda
The current provincial [32, 33] and national [4] goals for UHC in South Africa include both CBD and a commitment to provision of quality services [46], presenting an opportunity to leverage the existing political window. However, while the need to develop a policy to govern CBD activities in South Africa is evident, it is uncertain what changes the anticipated policy will bring to existing models. As earlier indicated, many of our informants hoped that the introduction of policy will not pose a barrier to further implementation of current CBD models. This has been experienced in other contexts where innovation in community-based services began outside of public regulation [47]. We argue that despite the diverging stakeholder views, CBD must be assessed within

the lens of what it is endeavouring to achieve - sustainable ATM. The World Health Organisation (WHO) has recommended in other instances that implementing regulation targeted at innovative models should neither decelerate the speed at which action is already taking place nor usher in restrictions that may have a constraining effect on public health service delivery effort [48]. That said, there is need to conduct accurate assessments of the effectiveness of these models and to ensure that they are implemented in a way that ensures patient safety.

In addition, informal models present an additional set of challenges, i.e. the lack of accountability mechanisms and the potential financial burden on patients caused by paid services. While it is true that there are high poverty levels in this context, the paid option is voluntary. Perhaps the critical question is: "Why do patients choose to pay for medicines delivery when they can get a 'free' service?". Since we did not interview patients paying for this service as part of this study, we can only speculate that the parallel system tends to thrive because there is an opportunity cost related to the informal system, i.e. it offers benefits (e.g. the convenience of not having to take time off work, which could result in a cost of a different kind) that might not be present within the formal 'free' system. Future studies could assess whether this system imposes a financial or any other burden on patients. If it does, but has other benefits to patients, the next issue is whether the government can lend support to informal providers so that they operate at a lower or no cost to patients.

Finally, further research is required to identify how CBD models have been implemented in other settings and their cost to health systems. Therefore, as a follow-up study, we have designed a scoping review which aims to obtain systematic evidence about design and implementation of CBD models in low resource settings and hard to reach populations in high income countries. We intend to assess whether the issues raised in this article were identified and if so, how they were or could be managed or overcome.

Study limitations
A limitation of this study was the adoption of the analytical framework after data collection; therefore, not all components were addressed equally during interviews with stakeholders. This is particularly true for monitoring and evaluation of CBD models, an area that requires attention in future studies. Second, the lack of accurate data on outcomes imposed some limitation.

Conclusion
Improving medicines delivery is integral to attaining UHC and the introduction of CBD in South Africa is one mechanism to achieve this goal. To achieve the

intended benefits of CBD, frontline HCPs should be consulted in policy development and consideration should be given to similar models in other contexts. Further research will seek to contribute towards evidence-based development of policy and service delivery guidelines for CBD activities in South Africa within the frameworks of pharmaceutical policy and practice.

Abbreviations

ATM: Access to medicines; CHW: Community health worker; DSD: Department of Social Development; HCP: Healthcare provider; NGO: Non-governmental organisation; NHP: Non-health professional; PA: Pharmacists' assistant; PHC: Primary Healthcare; QA: Quality assurance; SOPs: Standard operating procedures; UHC: Universal Health Coverage; WHO: World Health Organisation

Acknowledgements

The authors wish to first thank the WCDoH for supporting the study through facilitating access to information. We would also like to acknowledge the input of our colleague during the early phases of manuscript development: Edwin Wouters. The content of the paper, however, remains the responsibility of the authors.

Funding

This research and involvement of co-authors was made possible by funding from the European Union Seventh Framework Programme Theme: Health-2009-4.3.2-2 (Grant no. 242262) under the title 'Accessing Medicines in Africa and South Asia [AMASA], which was concluded in 2013. Subsequent work was made possible by the first author's doctoral funding from the South African Research Chair Initiative (SARCHI) in Health Systems, Complexity and Social Change at the University of the Western Cape; African Doctoral Dissertation Fellowship (ADDRF); the SIPHI fellowship programme and the Third framework agreement programme, FA3-III (2014-2016).

Authors' contributions

BPM conceptualised the research, conducted the fieldwork and data analysis. All authors contributed to the conceptualisation of this manuscript. BPM drafted the first draft of this article. All authors contributed to the intellectual content of the article. BPM finalised the article. All authors read and approved the final manuscript.

Competing interests

The authors declare that they have no competing interests.

Author details

[1]School of Public Health, University of the Western Cape, Private Bag X17, Bellville 7535, South Africa. [2]Department of Public Health, Institute of Tropical Medicine, Antwerp, Belgium. [3]School of Pharmacy, University of the Western Cape, Bellville, South Africa.

References

1. Mayosi BM, Flisher AJ, Lalloo UG, Sitas F, Tollman SM, Bradshaw D. The burden of non-communicable diseases in South Africa. Lancet. 2009; 374(9693):934–47.
2. Schneider H, Blaauw D, Gilson L, Chabikuli N, Goudge J. Health systems and access to antiretroviral drugs for HIV in Southern Africa: service delivery and human resources challenges. Reprod Health Matters. 2006;14(27):12–23.
3. Bigdeli M, Peters D, Wagner A, editors. Medicines in Health Systems. Geneva: World Health Organisation; 2014.
4. National Department of Health. National Health Insurance for South Africa: Towards Universal Health Coverage. . Pretoria: NDoH; 2015.
5. Decroo T, Telfer B, Biot M, Maikere J, Dezembro S, Cumba LI, das Dores C, Chu K, Ford N. Distribution of antiretroviral treatment through self-forming groups of patients in Tete Province, Mozambique. J Acquir Immune Defic Syndr. 2011;56(2):e39–44.
6. Hayford K, Privor-Dumm L, Levine O. Improving Access to Essential Medicines Through Public-Private Partnerships. Baltimore: International Vaccine Access Center; 2011.
7. Ahmed S, Curry L, Linnander E. Project Last Mile: Applying Coca-Cola's Exper-se to Improve Delivery of Life-Saving Medicines.". New Haven: Yale Global Health Leadership Institute, Yale University, ; 2015.
8. Bigdeli M, Jacobs B, Tomson G, Laing R, Ghaffar A, Dujardin B, Van Damme W. Access to medicines from a health system perspective. Health Policy Plan. 2013;28(7):692–704.
9. Decroo T, Rasschaert F, Telfer B, Remartinez D, Laga M, Ford N. Community-based antiretroviral therapy programs can overcome barriers to retention of patients and decongest health services in sub-Saharan Africa: a systematic review. Int Health. 2013;5(3):169–79.
10. Decroo T, Van Damme W, Kegels G, Remartinez D, Rasschaert F. Are Expert Patients an Untapped Resource for ART Provision in Sub-Saharan Africa? AIDS Res Treat. 2012;2012:749718.
11. Van Olmen JK GM, Bermejo R, Kegels G, Hermann K, Van Damme W. The growing caseload of chronic life-long conditions calls for a move towards full selfmanagement in low-income countries. Glob Health. 2011;7:38.
12. Luque-Fernandez M, Van Cutsem G, Goemaere E, Hilderbrand K, Schomaker M, Mantangana N, Mathee S, Dubula V, Ford N, Herna MA, Boulle A. Effectiveness of Patient Adherence Groups as a Model of Care for Stable Patients on Antiretroviral Therapy in Khayelitsha, Cape Town, South Africa. PLoS One. 2013;8(2):e56088.
13. Wilkinson L. ART adherence clubs: a long-term retention strategy for clinically stable patients receiving antiretroviral therapy. S Afr J HIV Med. 2013;14(2):48–50.
14. Kredo T, Ford N, Adeniyi FB, Garner P. Decentralising HIV treatment in lower- and middle-income countries. Cochrane Database Syst Rev. 2013;(6): CD009987. doi10.1002/14651858.CD009987.pub2.
15. Mdege NC, Chindove S. Bringing antiretroviral therapy (ART) closer to the end-user through mobile clinics and home-based ART: systematic review shows more evidence on the effectiveness and cost effectiveness is needed. Int J Health Plann Mgmt. 2014;29:e31–47.
16. Wouters E, Van Damme W, van Rensburg D, Masquillier C, Meulemans H. Impact of community-based support services on antiretroviral treatment programme delivery and outcomes in resource-limited countries: a synthetic review. BMC Health Serv Res. 2012;12:194.
17. Rasschaert F, Decroo T, Remartinez D, Telfer B, Lessitala F, Biot M, Candrinho B, Damme W. Adapting a community-based ART delivery model to the patients' needs: a mixed methods research in Tete, Mozambique. BMC Public Health. 2014;14:364.
18. Rasschaert F, Barbara T, Faustino L, Tom D, Daniel R, Marc B, Baltazar C, Francisco M, Wim Van D. A Qualitative Assessment of a Community Antiretroviral Therapy Group Model in Tete, Mozambique. PLoS One. 2014;9:3.
19. Rasschaert R, Decroo T, Remartinez D, Telfer B, Lessitala F, Biot M, Candrinho B, Van Damme W. Sustainability of a community-based anti-retroviral care delivery model a qualitative research study in Tete, Mozambique. J Int AIDS Soc. 2014;17:18910.
20. Dube C, Nozaki I, Hayakawa T, Kakimoto K, Yamada N, Simpungwe JB. Expansion of antiretroviral treatment to rural health centre level by a mobile service in Mumbwa district, Zambia. Bull World Health Organ. 2010;88:788–91.
21. Khabala K, Edwards JK, Bienvenu B, Sirengo M, Musembi P, Kosgei RJ, et al. Medication Adherence Clubs: a potential solution to managing large numbers of stable patients with multiple chronic diseases in-informal settlements. Experience from Kibera, Nairobi Kenya. Trop Med Int Health. 2015;20:10. doi:10.1111/tmi.12539.
22. Schneider H, Schaay N, Dudley L, Goliath C, Qukula T. The challenges of reshaping disease specific and care oriented community based services towards comprehensive goals: a situation appraisal in the Western Cape Province, South Africa. BMC Health Serv Res. 2015;15:436.
23. Western Cape Government Health. Healthcare 2030: The Road to Wellness. Cape Town: WCGH; 2013.
24. Magadzire BP, Marchal B, Ward K. Improving access to medicines through

centralised dispensing in the public sector: A case study of the Chronic Dispensing Unit in the Western Cape Province, South Africa. BMC Health Serv Res. 2015;15:513.

25. Du Plessis J. The Chronic Dispensing Unit. S Afr Pharm J. 2008;75(9):46–7.

26. Du Toit J, Dames S, Boshoff R. Centralised Dispensing-An Affordable Solution. S Afr Pharm J. 2008;75(10):18–20.

27. Du Toit J. Improving accessibility to medicine: The "missing link". S Afr Pharm J. 2014;8(4):38–40.

28. Walt G. GL: Reforming the health sector in developing countries: the central role of policy analysis. Health Policy Plan. 1994;9(4):353–70.

29. Magadzire BP, Budden A, Ward K, Jeffery R, Sanders D. Frontline health workers as brokers: provider perceptions, experiences and mitigating strategies to improve access to essential medicines in South Africa. BMC Health Serv Res. 2014;14:520.

30. Van Olmen J, Criel B, van Damme W, Marchal B, van Belle S, van Dormael M, et al. Analysing Health System Dynamics. A Framework. Antwerp: ITG Press; 2012.

31. Sheikh K, George A, Gilson L. People-centred science: strengthening the practice of health policy and systems research. Health Res Policy Syst. 2014;12(1):19.

32. Western Cape Department of Health: Draft guidelines for Chronic ARV clubs. Undated.

33. Western Cape Government Health. Pharmacy Services Standard Operating Procedures: Down referral from CHC to NPO's. Cape Town: WCGH; 2012.

34. Rasschaert F, Pirard M, Philips MP, Atun R, Wouters E, Assefa Y, Criel B, Schouten EJ, Van Damme W. Positive spill-over effects of ART scale up on wider health systems development: evidence from Ethiopia and Malawi. J Int AIDS Soc. 2011;14 Suppl 1:S3.

35. Penchansky R, Thomas JW. The concept of access: definition and relationship to consumer satisfaction. Med Care. 1981;19(2):127–40.

36. The Right to Health Joint Fact Sheet [http://www.who.int/mediacentre/factsheets/fs323_en.pdf]. Accessed 25 May 2016.

37. National Department of Health. National Health Insurance for South Africa. Pretoria: Towards Universal Health Coverage; 2015.

38. South African Pharmacy Council: Good Pharmacy Practice in South Africa In. Edited by South African Pharmacy Council. Pretoria: South African Pharmacy Council; 2010.

39. Gilson L, Raphaely N. The terrain of health policy analysis in low and middle income countries: a review of published literature 1994–2007. Health Policy Plan. 2008;23(5):294–307.

40. Zulu JM, Kinsman J, Michelo C, Hurtig AK. Developing the national community health assistant strategy in Zambia: a policy analysis. Health Res Policy Syst. 2013;11(1):24.

41. Lipsky M. Street-Level Bureaucracy, 30th Ann. Ed.: Dilemmas of the Individual in Public Service. New York: Russell Sage; 2010.

42. Morrow N. Pharmaceutical policy Part 1 The challenge to pharmacists to engage in policy development. J Pharma Policy Pract. 2015;8:4.

43. Gray AG, T; Naidoo, Panjasaram.: Pharmacist's assistant: a case study of a mid-level worker option. SAHR.

44. Wiedenmayer KA KN, Charles J, Chilunda F, Mapunjo S. The reality of task shifting in medicines management- a case study from Tanzania. J Pharm Policy Pract. 2015;8:13.

45   Rutta E, Liana J, Embrey M, Johnson K, Kimatta S, Valimba R, Lieber R, Shekalaghe E, Sillo H. Accrediting retail drug shops to strengthen Tanzania's public health system: an ADDO case study. J Pharm Policy Pract. 2015;8(1):23.

46   Matsoso MF R. National Health Insurance: The first 18 months. SAHR. 2012.

47   Thoumi AU K, Drobnick E, Taylor A, McClellan M. Transformation Through Accountable Care Reforms Innovations In Diabetes Care Around the World: Case Studies Of Care Transformation Through Accountable Care Reforms. Health Aff. 2015;34(9):1489–97.

48   World Health Organisation. Task shifting. Global recommendations and guidelines. Geneva: WHO Document Production Services; 2008.

9

Engagement of the private pharmaceutical sector for TB control: rhetoric or reality?

Niranjan Konduri[*] [iD], Emily Delmotte and Edmund Rutta

Abstract

Background: Private-sector retail drug outlets are often the first point of contact for common health ailments, including tuberculosis (TB). Systematic reviews on public-private mix (PPM) interventions for TB did not perform in-depth reviews specifically on engaging retail drug outlets and related stakeholders in the pharmaceutical sector. Our objective was to better understand the extent to which the World Health Organization's (WHO) recommendation on engaging retail drug outlets has been translated into programmatic policy, strategy, and intervention in low- and middle-income countries.

Methods: The study included a content analysis of global-level documents from WHO and the Stop TB Partnership in five phases. A country-level content analysis from four data sources was performed. Global-level findings were tabulated based on key messages related to engaging retail drug outlets. Country-level findings were analyzed based on four factors and tabulated. National strategic plans for TB control from 14 countries with varying TB burdens and a strong private sector were reviewed.

Results: 33 global-level documents and 77 full-text articles and Union World Lung Health conference abstracts were included for review. Based on experience of engaging retail drug outlets that has emerged since the mid-2000s, in 2011 WHO and the International Pharmaceutical Federation released a joint statement on promoting the engagement of national pharmacy associations in partnership with national TB programs. Only two of 14 countries' national strategic plans had explicit statements on the need to engage their national pharmacy professional association. The success rate of referrals from retail drug outlets who visited an approved health facility for TB screening ranged from 48% in Vietnam to 86% in Myanmar. Coverage of retail drug outlets ranged from less than 5 to 9% of the universe of retail drug outlets.

Conclusions: For WHO's End TB Strategy to be successful, scaling up retail drug outlets to increase national coverage, at least in countries with a thriving private sector, will be instrumental in accelerating the early detection and referral of the 3 million missing TB cases. The proposed PPM pharmacy model is applicable not only for TB control but also to tackle the antimicrobial resistance crisis in these countries.

Keywords: Public-private mix, Tuberculosis, Pharmacists, Retail drug outlets, Private sector, Pharmacy associations

Background

There is no shortage of evidence that both regulated and unregulated private-sector retail drug outlets, also known as pharmacies, chemists, drug shops, drug sellers, drug vendors, or informal drug sellers, are often the preferred first point of contact for common health ailments due to their inexpensive services, ease of access, and lack of waiting times compared to public health facilities [1, 2],. There is substantial evidence regarding the health-seeking behavior of consumers, caregivers, and patients [3] related to childhood illnesses, malaria [4], sexually transmitted diseases [5], cough-like symptoms [6], prolonged cough [7], and tuberculosis (TB) [8, 9],. Systematic reviews on the role of private-sector retail drug outlets in the provision of health care [10] and their quality of services [11] and regulatory aspects [12] have examined this body of knowledge.

While 43 million lives were saved by TB treatment and care between 2000 and 2014, TB remains a scourge

* Correspondence: nkonduri@msh.org
Systems for Improved Access to Pharmaceuticals and Services (SIAPS) Program, Management Sciences for Health, 4301 N. Fairfax Dr. Suite 400, Arlington, VA 22203, USA

worldwide, and 9.6 million people contracted the disease in 2014 [13]. To end the TB epidemic by 2035, the World Health Organization's (WHO) End TB Strategy emphasizes tapping the full benefits of health policies and systems by engaging a much wider set of collaborators across government, communities, and the private sector. In 2013, WHO reported that 3 million people fail to get a quality-assured TB diagnosis each year and often seek care from multiple private-sector providers in their search for TB treatment. Private-sector retail drug outlets are a key ally in ensuring that patients are referred to appropriate and high-quality treatment providers in their neighborhood. WHO's first guideline on public-private mix (PPM) approaches for tuberculosis clearly spells out the range of interventions specifically needed for nonphysicians, such as private-sector retail drug outlets, pharmacists, and traditional healers [14]. However, the extent to which this specific recommendation has been translated into programmatic policy, strategy, and intervention in low- and middle-income countries is unclear.

A WHO review of PPM interventions found that TB detection increased between 10 and 36% with the successful treatment of 90% of new smear-positive pulmonary TB cases [15]. One systematic assessment examined the concept and practice of PPM and concluded that national TB programs (NTPs) need guidelines to make decisions on which type of provider to engage to meet the Stop TB Partnership's global objectives [16]. A recent systematic review evaluated the performance of PPM programs against six health system themes [17]. Given the broader PPM focus, these studies did not perform in-depth reviews specifically on engaging private-sector retail drug outlets in TB control. The latter represent a particular challenge for PPM interventions because they exist in large numbers and are often staffed by low-skilled employees whose clients are looking for a quick remedy. Meanwhile, the PPM schemes ask the retail drug outlets to focus on referrals that bring no inherent benefit to the drug seller and sometimes resistance from the client.

To better understand the evolution of the recommendations concerning the engagement of private-sector retail drug outlets in TB control, we performed a content analysis of documentation from global agencies. We also reviewed and examined whether retail drug outlet engagement in TB control is merely rhetoric reflected in global guidelines and practiced in a handful of settings or reality reflected in country policy and practice. We examined whether NTPs, at least in countries with a large private sector, have embraced retail drug outlets and implemented interventions to engage them as part of their PPM strategy.

Methods
Global-level content analysis
We conducted the search in five phases. First, we reviewed all resources, tools, and publications available on WHO's PPM web page. We also reviewed relevant documents from WHO's Global TB program and Stop TB Partnership web pages. We performed a content analysis of all relevant documents for recommendations and manually scanned all documents to verify statements related to the purpose of this review. Second, we reviewed the publicly available WHO and Stop TB Partnership PPM subgroup meeting notes, or the agendas in the absence of meeting notes, from 2002 to 2015. We applied the search terms "pharmacy" and "pharmacist." Third, we reviewed WHO's annual global TB reports from 2000 to 2015 for the search terms "PPM", "public-private partnerships", "pharmacy", "pharmacist", "chemist", and "private sector." Fourth, we reviewed annual reports, strategic plans, and key Stop TB Partnership documents sourced from WHO's website from 2003 to 2015. Fifth, we reviewed 15 meeting reports and recommendations from WHO's Strategic and Technical Advisory Group for Tuberculosis from 2001 to 2015. In all instances, we hand searched additional documents mentioned or described in these documents and added them for review as appropriate.

Country-level content analysis
We searched PubMed and Google Scholar using free words at the time of this review (see Additional file 1 for search terms). For PubMed, an advanced search was used to find additional articles with the terms included in the title or abstract. We hand searched the bibliographies of relevant articles and contacted study authors for additional clarification. All articles were screened by one reviewer (ED) and verified by another (NK). Article inclusion criteria were those articles related to retail drug outlets and could be a commentary, an assessment of the situation, or an intervention. All other articles that had other PPM components or described such things as health-seeking behavior or diagnostic delays were excluded. Because we anticipated that there would be very few studies or articles that focused on retail drug outlets and TB control or included them as part of a broader PPM intervention, we expanded our search through three sources. First, we searched the abstract books of the Union World Conference on Lung Health published by the *International Journal of Tuberculosis and Lung Disease* from 2004 to 2014. We searched abstracts for the following terms: "pharmacy", "pharmacist", "chemist", "shops", and "seller". Second, we collected available national TB strategic plans or action plans specifically from countries with high TB burden and focused on 14 such countries where the private expenditure for health

was at least 45% or more of the total health expenditure and assessed country policy on PPM in relation to private pharmacy engagement [18]. Third, we retrieved the estimated number of licensed and unlicensed retail drug outlets relative to the country population against the TB burden for 13 of 14 countries (excluding India) to permit comparisons. The latter analysis was performed to assess public health implications of the relative level of scaling up PPM interventions involving retail drug outlets.

In this review, we consistently use the term "retail drug outlets" to reflect the various terms used in the literature, including drug seller, drug shop, medicine store, private pharmacy, chemist, informal drug seller, patent drug vendor, patent medicine vendor, and accredited drug dispensing outlet. However, during the multistage search process, we used these varying terms to identify relevant documents. From a regulatory standpoint, in the majority of the countries, outlets are generally classified into two categories. Category I includes those outlets that are legally allowed to sell only non-prescription medicine, also known as over-the-counter drugs, while Category II includes those outlets that are legally allowed to sell prescription medicines. In practice, there may often be no distinction in terms of what is being sold, but many other legal requirements are maintained.

Results
Global documentation: WHO and the Stop TB Partnership
A total of 33 global-level documents were reviewed. The content analysis of 16 key documents from the WHO and Stop TB Partnership websites is presented in Table 1. Pharmacists were first included as part of the formal definition of private providers in WHO's 2001 emerging policy framework to involve private practitioners [19]. A summary of the notes and presentations from eight Stop TB Partnership PPM meetings is shown in Table 2. Aspects of private pharmacy engagement were addressed in 2002, 2006, and from 2010 to 2014 in 11 Stop TB PPM subgroup meetings. The PPM subgroup dedicated significant time during the 2011 subgroup meeting to discussing and sharing experiences on anti-TB drugs and the private sector and engaging pharmacists. This meeting resulted in a concrete recommendation to the Directly Observed Treatment Short Course (DOTS) Expansion Working Group and the Stop TB Coordinating Board to disseminate widely the WHO/International Pharmaceutical Federation (FIP) joint statement on promoting the engagement of pharmacy associations and drug regulatory bodies in national partnerships to stop TB.

A summary of related information from WHO's nine annual Global TB reports is shown in Table 3. The momentum on overall PPM approaches gained traction

between 2005 and 2010, and emerging results were shown in the 2011 and 2012 reports. No annual reports from the Stop TB Partnership, including those from TB REACH grants, had any information or statements that were significantly related to the purpose of this review.

Country-level findings
PubMed identified 32 unique articles for the search terms that were used, and seven articles that had a retail drug outlet component were included for review. The Google Scholar search identified 62 unique articles related to TB in the private sector, and five relevant articles were included for review. Among the Union World Conference on Lung Health abstracts between 2004 and 2014, we found 65 relevant abstracts for review. Including the 12 full-text articles sourced from PubMed and Google Scholar and 65 Union abstracts, a total of 77 relevant articles and abstracts representing 18 countries were analyzed based on four factors and tabulated (Additional file 2). Of the 18 represented countries, 11 were in Asia, five in Africa, and two in Latin America. India (17) had the most articles and abstracts included in this review, followed by Cambodia (9). Among the 77 articles and abstracts, 52 were interventions involving retail drug outlets, and 24 were assessments concerning any aspect of retail drug outlets, such as sales of anti-TB drugs and knowledge of providers. Only one abstract described a regulatory component concerning the restriction of anti-TB drugs involving key stakeholders, including the national medicines regulatory authority.

Only 15 of the 52 intervention-related articles and abstracts reviewed explicitly documented the specific number or percentage of referrals of presumptive TB cases from retail drug outlets or resulting smear-positive TB cases (Table 4). All other articles and abstracts had grouped numbers or percentages of referrals among all private providers in their overarching PPM interventions, making it difficult to obtain data on the contribution of referrals specifically among retail drug outlets. Between 2003 and 2014, there was no substantial progression or variation in the number of referrals regardless of the country setting. The success rate of referred patients who visited an approved health facility for TB screening varied from 48% in Vietnam in 2003 to 86% in Myanmar in 2014.

Of the 14 selected high-burden TB countries where the private expenditure for health was at least 45% of the total health expenditure, the most recent versions of national strategic plans for TB control were available for all but two. Of the 14 countries reviewed, the national strategic plans of 12 formally included retail drug outlet engagement primarily for referral of persons suspected of having TB (Table 5). Only Bangladesh and Indonesia had explicit statements on the need to engage their local

Table 1 Key Documents from the WHO and Stop TB Partnership Websites

Key documents	Key messages related to engaging private-sector retail drug outlets	Gaps
TB patients and private providers in India (1997) [44]	Exclude anti-TB drugs from private channels. Prescriber-oriented education in private drug-distribution channels. Delegation of TB control responsibilities to non-governmental organizations. Public-private collaboration for the delivery of documented TB cures.	No recommendation of engaging "drug retailers" despite documenting evidence of their TB drug dispensing practices.
Global Plan to Stop TB (2001–2005) [45]	DOTS strategy implementation specified for private practitioners, non-governmental organizations, hospitals, clinics, prisons, industry, and military.	No explicit mention of engaging private pharmacies.
Legislation and Regulation for TB Control (2001) [46]	Create an effective partnership with private-sector physicians to implement national guidelines on TB control. Envisage the regulation of a drug supply for TB exclusively through the public health system.	No mention of engaging private pharmacies.
Emerging policy framework for involving private practitioners (2001) [19]	First WHO document to include "private pharmacists" as part of the formal definition of private providers to be engaged in TB control. Global assessment in 23 countries focused on private physicians. Captured evidence on patient health-seeking behavior in pharmacies and unrestricted availability of anti-TB drugs.	Options for engagement prioritized only for physicians. Restriction on TB drug availability in the private sector specified without engagement of wholesalers and private pharmacies.
Improving TB Drug Management. Accelerating DOTS Expansion (2002) [47]	In the context of analyzing TB drug management practices and to inform decision-making, recommendations were made to monitor private pharmacies or private clinics if they are an important source of anti-TB drugs.	None
Expanded DOTS Framework (2002) [48]	Involve private-sector health providers for case detection and DOTS implementation.	No specification of private pharmacies as part of the private sector.
Expanding DOTS in a changing health system (2003) [49]	Considerations on how best to ensure standardized, high-quality, affordable drugs through all providers, including private pharmacies, will be necessary.	Engaging private pharmacies to ensure an uninterrupted supply of high-quality drugs was briefly considered in the context of the role of private providers. There was no mention of engaging private pharmacies from the perspective of patient case detection and referral.
PPM DOTS Practical Tool (2003) [50]	"Pharmacists" was mentioned several times throughout the document, including considerations on how to engage them. A sample referral form for non-physicians was included to encourage adaptation and use depending on the local context.	None
PPM Guidelines (2006) [51]	The guideline clearly lists the importance of engaging pharmacists, drug shops and non-physicians so that the poor and vulnerable can receive appropriate care and referrals. Interventions include identifying persons suspected of having TB, collecting sputum samples, making referrals, notifying/recording cases, and supervising treatment. Pharmacy associations were listed among various PPM stakeholders for engagement at the national level.	None

Table 1 Key Documents from the WHO and Stop TB Partnership Websites *(Continued)*

DOTS Expansion Working Group Strategic Plan (2006) [52]	The term "PPM DOTS" has evolved to represent a comprehensive approach to involve all relevant health care providers in DOTS. PPM-DOTS targets a wide range of audiences as well as private health care providers not yet sufficiently linked to NTPs. Private pharmacies were included among a variety of private providers.	None
Second Global Plan to Stop TB (2006) [53]	Promotes the wider and more strategic use of existing strategies for TB control with an explicit mention of engaging "private pharmacies" and the "informal health sector" for introducing or scaling up PPM-DOTS.	None
9th WHO STAG-TB Meeting (2009) [54]	Special session on policy change for improved quality and rational use of anti-TB drugs. Recommended to schedule anti-TB drugs as restricted with special reporting requirements for pharmacies and prescribers. WHO must develop approaches to engage pharmaceutical companies, professional associations, and pharmacies to curb unethical practices and promote rational use of anti-TB drugs.	None
PPM Scale up (2010) [55]	Non-physicians and private pharmacies were included as part of a PPM task-mix strategy. Pharmacists may be able to identify persons with TB-like symptoms, collect sputum samples, refer suspects, notify or record cases, and supervise treatment.	None
Third Global Plan to Stop TB (2011) [56]	There is good evidence that PPM approaches can increase the percentage of people who are diagnosed and receive high-quality treatment by between one-quarter and one-third, with health care providers, such as pharmacists, traditional healers, and private practitioners, often serving as the first point of contact for people with TB symptoms.	None
Role of pharmacists in TB care and control (2011) [57]	The WHO/FIP joint statement recommended engaging pharmacists and national pharmacy associations in TB control.	None
Engaging all providers for drug-resistant TB (DR-TB) (2015) [58]	Non-physicians, such as private pharmacists, are currently engaging in PPM for TB care and control. They can be similarly engaged in patient-centered care for DR-TB, such as by providing DOTS and identifying and reporting side-effects of second-line drugs. Pharmacists can also provide education to family members on infection control and strategies to prevent and manage stigma.	None

pharmacy professional association. This review found that, over the last two decades, the role of retail drug outlets has evolved from pilot projects and guidance in global documents to formal incorporation into country plans.

None of the 14 countries' national strategic plans explicitly establish targets for engaging private-sector retail drug outlets or necessarily prioritize urban or rural outlets. The public health contribution of retail drug outlets to TB case finding depends on the number of retail drug outlets in the country, the population, the relative TB burden, the percentage of engaged pharmacists who refer patients, and the percentage of clients with symptoms who are successfully counseled for

Table 2 Stop TB PPM Subgroup Meetings

Year	Aspects related to private-sector retail drug outlets
2002	Involvement of pharmacies was listed as an innovative approach. Incentives for pharmacy involvement in referrals and treatment.
2006	Pilot experience on engaging private pharmacies in Cambodia and drug vendors in Vietnam was mentioned.
2008	WHO Activities in the Americas Region: The experience of NTPs in engaging private pharmacies and traditional medicine is scarce. Mexico has an agreement with the national pharmacy association. Constraints in the Americas include limited knowledge of the role and coverage of the private sector, including private pharmacies. Donor perspective: USAID supported the following activities Cambodia: pharmacy staff and traditional healer training and referral systems. Ethiopia: training and referral systems for private pharmacies.
2010	Cambodia reported progress on engaging private doctors and pharmacists: 12,577 suspects were referred, 6,403 were evaluated, and 1,418 TB cases were identified (2005–2008). An analysis of patient health-seeking behavior helped to design the intervention. Ghana reported progress on working with regulatory authorities to restrict access to anti-TB drugs and to require private pharmacies to refer all persons suspected of having TB to the NTP.
2011	The terms "pharmacy" and "pharmacist" were mentioned 19 times in the meeting report and discussed frequently, as reflected in numerous presentations. The PPM secretariat was recommended to support the documentation and dissemination of innovative approaches, such as engaging pharmacists in TB care and control. NTPs and Ministries of Health were recommended to work with national pharmacy associations to tap the role of pharmacists in early case detection and improving TB treatment and care.
2012	One of the expected outcomes of the subgroup meeting was to produce practical tools on social franchising for and engaging pharmacies in TB care.
2013	Reported progress made on designing guidance and tools to engage private pharmacies.
2014	The meeting provided recommendations to address the knowledge gap on income sources and amounts for chemists to inform the types of incentives that might work. PPM programs must enforce regulation for the rational use of anti-TB drugs and accreditation systems for collaborating providers.

Table 3 WHO Annual Global TB Reports

Year	Private-sector pharmacy aspects
2005	Cambodia: Based on the findings of a 2002 study on the prevalence of health care-seeking behavior in the private-sector, Cambodia launched a pilot project to engage private practitioners and pharmacies. Kenya: Diagnostic and treatment services projects to engage all providers, including pharmacies, are ongoing.
2007	Cambodia: Planned activities include mapping the locations of private pharmacies and recording the training of non-NTP staff. The Philippines: Achievements include initiating operational research projects in PPM, including collaboration with pharmacies. South Africa: Achievements include engaging pharmacists, private-sector general medical practitioners, traditional health practitioners, community care givers, and community-based organizations in the referral and support of TB patients.
2008	Afghanistan: Achievements include conducting a study on the role of private pharmacies in the treatment of TB in the central region of Afghanistan. Planned activities include developing training modules for private practitioners and private pharmacies to engage all care providers. Kenya: Achievements include sensitizing pharmacists and additional private practitioners on TB to encourage the referral of TB suspects for diagnosis.
2010	Countries have prioritized different types of care providers, including pharmacies in Cambodia, private hospitals in Nigeria, public hospitals in China and Indonesia, social security organizations in Mexico, and prison services in Kazakhstan.
2011	In 20 countries for which data were available, PPM contributed approximately 20 to 40% of all notifications in 2010 in the geographical areas in which PPM was implemented (no specific data for pharmacies). The role of pharmacists in TB care and control was discussed, including a box summary outlining the WHO/FIP joint statement.
2012	Intensified efforts by NTPs to engage the full range of care providers using PPM initiatives are also important; in most of the 21 countries that provided data, 10 to 40% of national notifications were from non-NTP care providers (no specific data for pharmacies).
2013	No specific information pertaining to private-sector pharmacy engagement.
2014	No specific information pertaining to private-sector pharmacy engagement.
2015	In India, patients receive e-vouchers for standardized medications to be redeemed at no charge from private chemists.

referral by the pharmacist. Figure 1 compares 13 of 14 countries of comparable size (excluding India) for the first three of these factors (see Additional file 3 for data sources). This figure highlights different situations within countries. Cambodia, for example has a relatively low incidence of TB cases compared to other countries but very high per capita TB burden, with one retail drug outlet serving an average of 2,225 people. Consequently, based on the 77 articles and abstracts reviewed (Additional file 2), the coverage of retail drug outlets ranged from less than 5 to 9% of the universe of retail drug outlets in a given country.

Discussion

The findings from this review demonstrate one aspect of the evolution of PPM in TB diagnosis, care, and treatment over time. Despite the inclusion of private

pharmacists in the 2001 WHO document, "Involving private practitioners in tuberculosis control: Issues, interventions and emerging policy framework," evidence of the engagement of this cadre of private-sector health providers appeared slowly over the following decade. For example, in 2004, the Union World Conference on Lung Health contained no abstracts that met the inclusion criteria for this review; however, by 2014, there were 14 qualifying abstracts. A similar trend was observed in global guidance documents. The term "private sector" was mentioned in the first WHO annual TB report in 2000; however, it wasn't until 2003 that the terms "public-private mix" and "public-private partnership" first appeared in WHO's annual TB report. Notably, 2003 was also the first year that the annual report included the term

Table 4 Number of Referrals or Smear-positive Cases from Retail Drug Outlets over Time

Country	Year	Number of retail drug outlets	Number of referrals	% screened among referrals	Smear-positive cases
Vietnam	2003	150	310	48% (149)	10
Bolivia	2005	70	41	27% (11)	3
Philippines	2005	no data	2,334	no data	no data
Philippines	2005	no data	1,550	37% (575)	83
Cambodia	2008	683	4,230	79% (3,356)	1,769
India (Tamil Nadu)	2010	402	101	no data	no data
Philippines	2011	119	942	11% (99)	14
India (2 cities)	2012	80	23	No data	8
Burkina Faso	2013	131	821	44% (361)	17
India (Andhra Pradesh)	2013	60	117	89% (104)	6
Myanmar	2013	99	224	65% (145)	18
India (Tamil Nadu)	2014	550	382	66% (252)	130
India (Andhra Pradesh)	2014	177	871	91% (792)	90
Myanmar	2014	212	no data	no data	53
Myanmar	2014	263	2,335	86% (2,013)	395

"pharmacies." The PPM subgroup meetings of the Stop TB Partnership showed a similar trend. While the first subgroup meeting took place in 2002, it was not until 2006 that "pharmacies/pharmacists," "chemists," and "seller" were included. Since that first inclusion, at least one of these terms has been in every meeting report or related document.

Need for tailored strategies to increase national coverage
The findings of this review have several implications for the potential role of retail drug outlets in TB diagnosis, care, and treatment. The primary finding is that a variety

of articles and abstracts in varying geographic locations have demonstrated that retail drug outlets are willing and able to contribute to TB control efforts, as shown by the number of referrals (Table 4). However, given the diversity of the private sector in high-TB-burden countries and the reality that NTP budgets are stretched across competing priorities, a number of considerations are warranted as countries decide whether to scale up the engagement of retail drug outlets nationwide. None of the 77 reviewed articles and abstracts mentioned or described attempts to scale up retail drug outlet

Table 5 NTP Strategy or Action Plans

	% of private expenditure on health[a]	National strategic plan version	Private retail drug outlet engagement in strategy	Professional pharmacy association engagement in strategy[b]
Cambodia	79.5	2014–2020	X	
Afghanistan	78.8	2013–2017	X	
Nigeria	76.1	2015–2020	X	
Myanmar	72.8	2016–2020	X	
Philippines	68.4	2013–2016	X	
India	67.8	2012–2017	X	
Bangladesh	64.7	2015–2020	X	X
United Republic of Tanzania	63.7	2010–2015	X	
Pakistan	63.2	2015-2020	X	
Indonesia	61.0	2015–2019	X	X
Kenya	58.3	2015–2018	X	
Vietnam	58.1	2011–2015	X	
Uganda	55.6	2015–2020		
Democratic Republic of the Congo	46.9	2014–2017		

[a]Private expenditure on health as a percentage of total expenditure on health. WHO (2013) [18]
[b]Only if 'pharmacy association' was explicitly mentioned in the strategy instead of the generic term 'professional association'

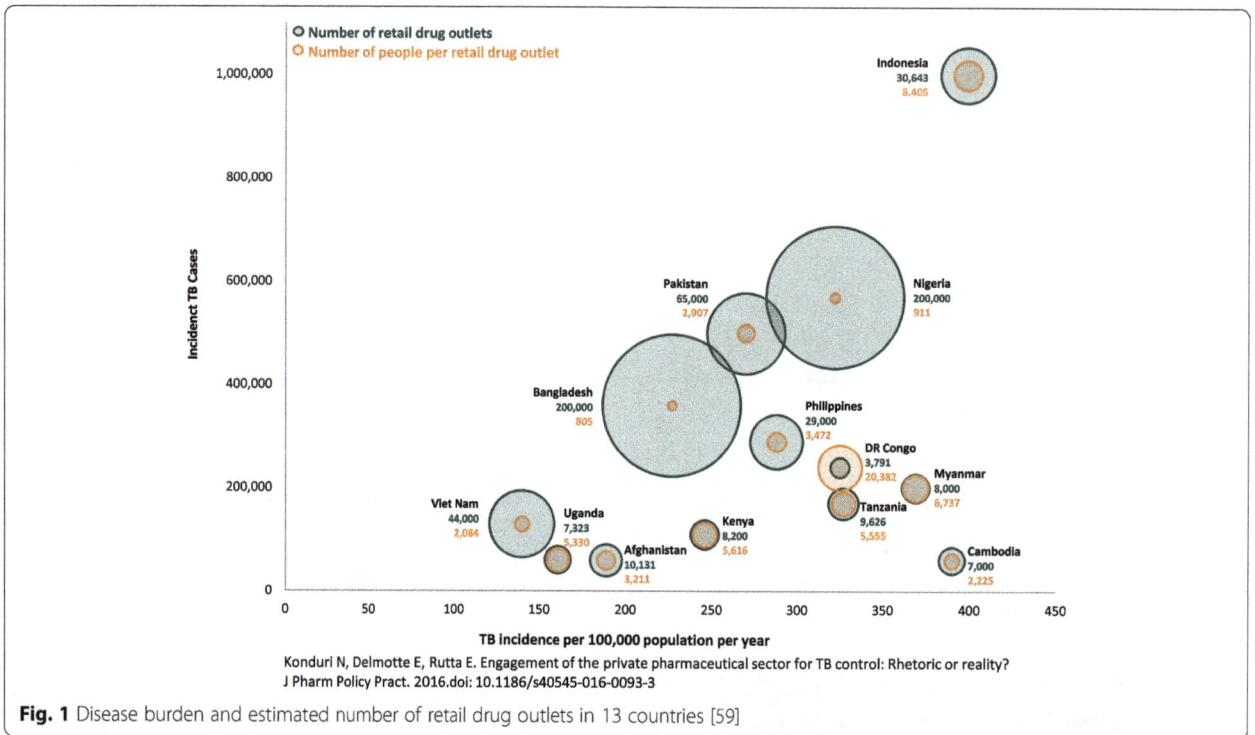

Fig. 1 Disease burden and estimated number of retail drug outlets in 13 countries [59]

engagement to increase national coverage. Pakistan had established progressive annual targets not only for engaging retail drug outlets but also for referrals and smear-positive TB cases to be detected [20].

For example, even if staff at between 10,000 and 20,000 of the drug outlets in Bangladesh or Nigeria are trained in rational antimicrobial dispensing and the referral of persons suspected of having TB, it is unlikely to have the desired public health effect, given that this comprises only 5 to 10% of the total universe of outlets. However, in most of the countries reviewed (appendix 2), the number of retail drug outlets engaged tend to be several hundred or over a thousand, which is a more manageable number to engage for quality improvement and regulatory efforts. Therefore, in Fig. 1, a large green circle (large number of outlets) means the retail drug outlet intervention is somewhat daunting and may need to rely on changing structures and incentives rather than on individual engagement, while a large brown circle (large number of clients per outlet) means that there are some useful economies of scale in engaging individual outlets. Figure 1 illustrates the reality not only for TB but also for the public health implications of irrational dispensing of antibiotics and the threat of antimicrobial resistance. Indonesia, which has a very high relative TB burden compared to Bangladesh, Nigeria, and Pakistan, has comparatively fewer retail drug outlets (30,643) that serve an average of 8,405 people per outlet, illustrating a different scenario that requires tailored strategies for maximum impact. India has an estimated 850,000 retail drug outlets.

Through a public-private partnership with various entities, approximately 9% of the outlets (*n* = 75,000) in 12 selected districts across four states of India were engaged over a four-year period and accounted for nearly one-third of India's 1.2 billion people and one-third of its smear-positive TB cases [21, 22],. This partnership reported that approximately 10 to 15% of suspected cases referred by 7,000 pharmacists over two years were found to be positive and placed on treatment. Clearly, this example illustrates not only the success of engaging retail drug outlets but also the need for steady scale up to increase national coverage. Figure 1 highlights the numbers problem that is common for PPM interventions in general but most acute for retail drug outlet interventions [23].

Need for data on costs and number of unique referrals
This review also highlighted current gaps among the 77 articles and abstracts reviewed. For example, while many of the articles and abstracts described the potential returns of engaging retail drug outlets, none of the 12 full-text articles described the necessary inputs in terms of cost. TB programs that may need to prioritize among various PPM interventions must have an understanding of the estimated costs and cost effectiveness of each intervention [24, 25],. Such estimates, if modeled from pilot or small-scale initiatives, would allow TB programs to use a set amount of funding to determine which intervention would return the greatest output in terms of presumptive TB cases referred and

ultimately confirmed. For example, one program estimated an implementation cost of $176,635 related to engaging retail drug outlets in two regions of Tanzania to inform the NTP on a scale up strategy [26]. Another factor that may impact the cost effectiveness of such an engagement is the extent to which retail drug outlets serve as the first point of care for individuals with TB-like symptoms in a given country [27, 28],. While in some countries these providers are a first point of contact for communities, in others, different points of private care may be more common, such as private clinics or hospitals. For NTPs to better prioritize interventions, an estimate of the expected cost and return is needed. At a minimum, data on the costs to engage the retail drug outlet and the resulting additional yield in new cases are needed.

As shown in Table 4, there is a great need for data on the number of unique referrals (i.e., persons suspected of having TB or TB-like symptoms) provided by retail drug outlets as opposed to an aggregate number of referrals provided by all PPM providers. Such data would allow countries to compare the relative potential and benefit of engaging various actors within the realm of PPM. Data on periods of longer than two years on the number of referred persons who eventually visited an approved diagnostic clinic and were confirmed as smear-positive TB are also needed. Further studies are needed to examine the affordability and sustainability of incentive mechanisms, such as phone credit, compared to moral persuasion [29, 30].

Role of national pharmaceutical associations

Retail drug outlets do not operate in isolation and have linkages with wholesalers, distributors, and retail associations. While the majority of the 52 reviewed interventions primarily trained retail drug outlets to provide referrals, there are opportunities to engage other stakeholders as part of a multi-pronged intervention. A country's national pharmaceutical association must be engaged to tap into its network of pharmacy professionals and provide policy guidance to identify educational, managerial, and regulatory approaches to engage retail drug outlets. Cambodia, India, and the Philippines, for example, have involved their local pharmacy associations significantly in advocacy and mobilization among their member networks of retail drug outlets [21, 31, 32]. In our review of the national strategic plans of selected countries, only Bangladesh and Indonesia explicitly made statements of intent to engage professional pharmacy associations. While Cambodia, India, and the Philippines have engaged professional pharmacy and retail drug outlet associations, an explicit statement was not found in any of their updated 2015–2020 national strategic plans. It cannot be assumed that the engagement of professional associations is automatic because changes in program leadership and/or fluctuations in funding levels can influence priorities. Major knowledge gaps often found among retail drug outlets, such as the etiology of the disease, awareness of public-sector programs, and referrals to accredited private clinics, can be addressed by leveraging partnerships with the national pharmacy association.

For PPM interventions involving retail drug outlets, the intervention design needs to consider the different players and their roles and align incentives for each stakeholder (Fig. 2). In the short term, the focus may be to train staff at retail drug outlets to identify common presenting signs and symptoms of TB and refer patients to facilities where they can be properly diagnosed and managed. However, in the long term, more stakeholders need to be sensitized to exert their role. A country's national pharmaceutical association can work with pharmacy schools to revise their curricula to ensure that pharmacy assistants and pharmacists have the requisite knowledge on TB and the rational use of antimicrobials. Pharmacy schools are a major resource not only for any baseline assessments and evaluation activities but also for engaging pharmacy students to collect data, monitor retail drug outlet performance, recognize real-world challenges and stimulate thinking on options for policy and practice [33]. None of the 77 articles and abstracts reviewed explicitly mentioned engagement with pharmacy schools. Although there is paucity of such documented experiences, the Philippines Pharmacy Association produced an instructors' manual for revising pharmacy school curricula to incorporate content on TB control and the role of pharmacy professionals and retail drug outlets [34]. In addition, the Indian Pharmaceutical Association involved pharmacy students to act as TB community educators [35].

Role of national medicines regulatory authority

Among the 77 articles and abstracts reviewed, only one from Ghana documented a restriction on sales of anti-TB drugs without a formal legal ban. In countries with a large presence of local anti-TB drug manufacturers and where sales of anti-TB drugs are not legally prohibited, reaching and engaging these manufacturers and their wholesalers and distributors is a key to success. In collaboration with the national medicines regulatory authority, the NTP can work with local TB drug manufacturers to engage their sales representatives to promote the recommended WHO first-line medicines instead of loose, single TB tablets, to encourage dispensers to screen and refer those patients who present with persistent cough, and to not sell antimicrobials or anti-TB drugs until a proper diagnosis is made. Given the influence that wholesalers and distributors have on the retail sector, these actions could have a tremendous effect, particularly in countries with a large private-sector market [36]. For example, in Mumbai, India, certain retail drug outlets were

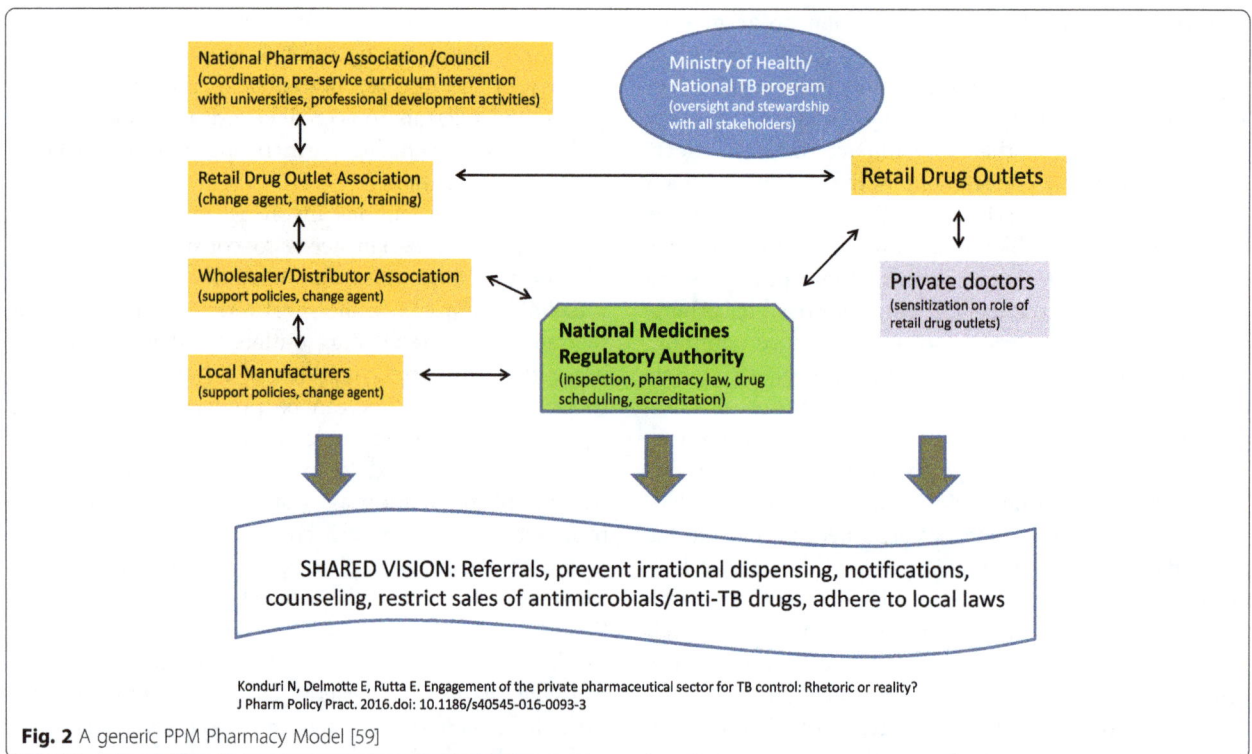

Konduri N, Delmotte E, Rutta E. Engagement of the private pharmaceutical sector for TB control: Rhetoric or reality? J Pharm Policy Pract. 2016.doi: 10.1186/s40545-016-0093-3

Fig. 2 A generic PPM Pharmacy Model [59]

accredited and recognized to serve as DOTS providers rather than perceiving this engagement as a loss of business.

The national medicines regulatory authority must be involved in relevant stakeholders meetings and training sessions involving retail drug outlets and related professional associations. Presenting a unified approach will ensure that all key stakeholders share a vision of improved early case identification and referral, reduced inappropriate antimicrobial and TB medicine sales, better contributions to overall TB notifications, and adherence to regulations and laws. In countries where an outright regulatory ban on the import and sale of anti-TB drugs is possible, consistent enforcement is key to preventing a recurrence because of the availability of anti-TB drugs in retail drug outlets [37]. In other settings, such as India, which issued a regulation in 2014 to limit over-the-counter sales of not only anti-TB drugs but also specific antimicrobials, enforcement is not sufficient, and incentives among all stakeholders must be aligned [38]. Recent systematic reviews of retail drug outlets and of the quality of pharmacy services in Asia found limited evidence of interventions related to regulatory enforcement and profit motives among private retail drug outlets [39, 40],. Therefore, it is important to place the PPM pharmacy model intervention within the larger PPM intervention package, particularly in countries with a high to moderate TB burden and a large proportion of the population receiving private-sector care [41]. It may be appropriate for referrals to be organized within private-sector providers, such as doctors, general practitioners, chest physicians, specialists,

or clinics/hospitals, which may be where patients prefer to seek treatment. In most cases, the NTP may already be working with private-sector providers, such as general practitioners and hospitals.

Given the limited resources and competing priorities within the NTP, a long-term strategy could be for the Ministry of Health, particularly in countries with a large private sector to address other disease programs and invest in the PPM pharmacy model with links to the primary care system. Interventions that are comprehensive, such as Tanzania's accredited drug dispensing outlet model, could be a good investment in the long run for TB and other diseases, such as diarrhea and malaria, and for family planning services [42].

Limitations of this review

This review primarily focused on the role of private-sector retail drug outlets in TB control. It is possible that we may have missed some papers that did not use the terms in our search methodology. For example, community pharmacies in Bangladesh are called "village doctors" and are sensitized to refer patients suspected of having TB [43]. Because we excluded studies that were primarily focused on health-seeking behaviors of patients, we may have missed content related to the situation assessment of retail drug outlets and possible information on referrals. In addition, the relative scarcity of full-text articles on this topic compared to conference abstracts may have induced bias in the interpretation of past work involving retail drug outlets and the referral of persons suspected of having TB. The content of the abstracts varied widely in the extent of information available, and we did not have access to posters or presentations that may contain some detail on the content. The primary authors attempted to contact at least 20 selected authors of the 65 reviewed abstracts for further clarification and to seek posters or presentation files but heard back only from 6 authors. We did not perform any formative review of other Union regional conference materials or of grey literature from international development partners working with NTPs. We may have also missed presentations made at other conferences related to private-sector health care. Finally, we excluded other studies that may have documented experiences of retail drug outlets for other health conditions, such as malaria, family planning and reproductive health, and HIV. Despite these limitations, our paper has value in blending information from global and country documentation related to the objectives of this review.

Conclusion

For the End TB Strategy to be successful, prioritizing and harnessing the power of private-sector retail drug outlets will be instrumental in accelerating the early detection and referral of the 3 million missing cases. The proposed PPM pharmacy model could become a scalable reality and make a significant contribution by harnessing both short-term solutions such as systematically engaging retail drug outlet dispensers and long-term solutions like partnerships with pharmacy schools and pharmacy associations that is long overdue in many countries. For decades, we have known about the potential of retail drug outlets but their level of engagement has not been commensurate with the TB burden and rapid growth of the private health sector. To successfully scale up PPM pharmacy models and reach ambitious targets, the international TB community must tailor interventions to the size and reach of each country's retail drug outlet network, particularly in settings with a thriving private sector.

In addition, from a public health and pharmaceutical policy perspective, the crisis of antimicrobial resistance is unlikely to be adequately addressed through a disease-specific framework. Country authorities must recognize the community's well-documented preference for seeking services from retail drug outlets and make a concerted effort to increase coverage of retail drug outlet engagement across the health system.

Abbreviations

DOTS: Directly observed treatment short course; FIP: International Pharmaceutical Federation; NTP: National TB programs; PPM: Public-private mix; TB: Tuberculosis; USAID: United States Agency for International Development; WHO: World Health Organization

Acknowledgements

The authors are grateful to Dr. William Wells of USAID and Dr. Mukund Uplekar of the World Health Organization, Global TB Program, for their review of this manuscript. They provided thoughtful comments and advice to greatly strengthen the previous version of the manuscript. Dr. Sameh Saleeb of the USAID SIAPS Program, Management Sciences for Health, is appreciated for providing management support to ensure final production of this manuscript. We thank Dr. Kanjinga Kakanda of Management Sciences for Health for helping to source estimates of private-sector retail drug outlets from specific countries. Susan Gillespie of Management Sciences for Health is thanked for providing professional editorial support.

Funding

This work was made possible by the generous support of the American people through the US Agency for International Development (USAID, Washington DC, USA) Cooperative Agreement Number AID-OAA-A-11-00021. No funding bodies had any role in the study design, data collection, analysis, or decision to publish. The findings and conclusions in this article are those of the authors and do not necessarily represent the views of Management Sciences for Health, the Systems for Improved Access to Pharmaceutical and Services Program, USAID, or the US Government.

Authors' contributions

NK conceived of, designed, and led the review. NK and ED contributed substantially to the development and implementation of study methods, literature review and content analysis. NK and ED jointly prepared the first draft of the manuscript. ER contributed to analysis and interpretation of study findings, writing of the manuscript and synthesizing key messages. All authors read and approved the final version.

Authors' information

Emily Delmotte and Edmund Rutta were employed with Management Sciences for Health at the time of manuscript development.

Competing interests

The authors declare that they have no competing interests.

References

1. Khan MM, Grübner O, Krämer A. Frequently used healthcare services in urban slums of Dhaka and adjacent rural areas and their determinants. J Public Health. 2012;34(2):261–71.
2. Sudhinaraset M, Ingram M, Lofthouse HK, Montagu D. What is the role of informal healthcare providers in developing countries? a systematic review. PLoS One. 2013;8(2):e54978.
3. Kiwuwa MS, Charles K, Harriet MK. Patient and health service delay in pulmonary tuberculosis patients attending a referral hospital: a cross-sectional study. BMC Public Health. 2005;5:122.
4. Lalchhuanawma R, Murhekar MV. Health-seeking behaviour for febrile illness in malaria-endemic Kolasib district, Mizoram, India. Int Health. 2012;4(4):314–9.
5. Chalker J, Chuc NT, Falkenberg T, Do NT, Tomson G. STD management by private pharmacies in Hanoi: practice and knowledge of drug sellers. Sex Transm Infect. 2000;76(4):299–302.
6. Tumwikirize WA, Ekwaru PJ, Mohammed K, Ogwal-Okeng JW, Aupont O. Management of acute respiratory infections in drug shops and private pharmacies in Uganda: a study of counter attendants' knowledge and reported behaviour. East Afr Med J. 2004;Suppl:S33–40. PMID:15125114.
7. Ukwaja KN, Alobu I, Nweke CO, Onyenwe EC. Healthcare-seeking behavior,

treatment delays and its determinants among pulmonary tuberculosis patients in rural Nigeria: a cross-sectional study. BMC Health Serv Res. 2013;17:13–25.

8. Mesfin MM, Newell JN, Walley JD, Gessessew A, Madeley RJ. Delayed consultation among pulmonary tuberculosis patients: a cross sectional study of 10 DOTS districts of Ethiopia. BMC Public Health. 2009;9:9–53.

9. Hoa NB, Tiemersma EW, Sy DN, Nhung NV, Vree M, Borgdorff MW, Cobelens FG. Health-seeking behavior among adults with prolonged cough in Vietnam. Trop Med Int Health. 2011;16(10):1260–7.

10. Smith F. Private local pharmacies in low- and middle-income countries: a review of interventions to enhance their role in public health. Trop Med Int Health. 2009;14(3):362–72.

11. Smith F. The quality of private pharmacy services in low and middle-income countries: a systematic review. Pharm World Sci. 2009;31(3):351–61.

12. Wafula FN, Miriti EM, Goodman CA. Examining characteristics, knowledge and regulatory practices of specialized drug shops in Sub-Saharan Africa: a systematic review of the literature. BMC Health Serv Res. 2012;27:12–223.

13. World Health Organization. Tuberculosis Fact Sheet No. 104. Geneva: World Health Organization; 2015.

14. WHO. Engaging all health care providers in TB control. Guidance on implementing public-private mix approaches. Geneva: World Health Organization; 2006.

15. Lönnroth K, Uplekar M, Blanc L. Hard gains through soft contracts: productive engagement of private providers in tuberculosis control. Bull World Health Organ. 2006;84(11):876–83.

16. Malmborg R, Mann G, Squire SB. A systematic assessment of the concept and practice of public-private mix for tuberculosis care and control. Int J Equity Health. 2011;10(1):49.

17. Lei X, Liu Q, Escobar E, Philogene J, Zhu H, Wang Y, Tang S. Public-private mix for tuberculosis care and control: a systematic review. Int J Infect Dis. 2015;34:20–32.

18. WHO. Global Health Observatory data repository. 2014. http://apps.who.int/gho/data/node.main. Accessed 14 Dec 2016.

19. WHO. Involving Private Practitioners in Tuberculosis Control: Issues, Interventions, and Emerging Policy Framework. Geneva: World Health Organization; 2001.

20. Qadeer, E. and Rutta, E. Setting Targets for Private Retail Pharmacies Engagement in TB in Pakistan. May 2014. Presented at Public Private Mix (PPM) Models for the Sustainability of Successful TB Control Initiatives. Washington: USAID and World Bank.

21. Lilly MDR-TB Partnership. Creating champions of change. Enrolling community pharmacists in a national tuberculosis control initiative. The Lilly MDR-TB Partnership; 2014. https://lillypad.lilly.com/WP/wp-content/uploads/Creating-Champions-of-Change.pdf. Accessed 14 Dec 2016.

22. Revised National TB Control Programme Annual Status Report. TB India 2015. Central TB Division. Ministry of Health and Family Welfare.

23. Wells WA, Uplekar M, Pai M. Achieving systemic and scalable private sector engagement in tuberculosis care and prevention in Asia. PLoS Med. 2015; 12(6):e1001842.

24. Mahendradhata Y, Probandari A, Ahmad RA, Utarini A, Trisnantoro L, Lindholm L, van der Werf MJ, Kimerling M, Boelaert M, Johns B, Van der Stuyft P. The incremental cost-effectiveness of engaging private practitioners to refer tuberculosis suspects to DOTS services in Jogjakarta, Indonesia. Am J Trop Med Hyg. 2010;82(6):1131–9.

25. Ramaiah AA, Gawde NC. Economic evaluation of a public–private Mix TB project in Tamil Nadu, India. J Health Manag. 2015;17(3):370–80.

26. Kakanda K, Delmotte E, Rutta E, Mwatawala S, Valimba R. Engaging private retail drug outlets in early tuberculosis case finding in Tanzania: final report. Submitted to the US Agency for international development by the systems for improved access to pharmaceuticals and services (SIAPS) program. Arlington: Management Sciences for Health; 2014.

27. Grover M, Bhagat N, Sharma N, Dhuria M. Treatment pathways of extrapulmonary patients diagnosed at a tertiary care hospital in Delhi, India. Lung India. 2014;31(1):16–22.

28. Ukwaja KN, Alobu I, Nweke CO, Onyenwe EC. Healthcare-seeking behavior, treatment delays and its determinants among pulmonary tuberculosis patients in rural Nigeria: a cross-sectional study. BMC Health Serv Res. 2013;13:25.

29. Glish L, Sinhradsvong L, Phanalasy S, Chanthalangsy P, Stankard P, Gray R. Tuberculosis case detection via private pharmacies in Lao PDR. In Abstract Book: 44th World Conference on Lung Health of the International Union Against Tuberculosis and Lung Disease. Paris: Int J Tuberc Lung Dis. 2013;p. S339.

30. USAID. Public Private Mix (PPM) Models for the Sustainability of Successful TB Control Initiatives. May 2014. Washington, DC.

31. PATH. Public-private mix. Involving pharmacies and other providers in TB control – a Cambodia case study. 2011. https://www.path.org/publications/files/CP_cambodia_ppm_tb_cs.pdf. Accessed 14 Dec 2016.

32. Philippine Tuberculosis Initiatives for the Private Sector Final Report. Chemonics International. 2006. USAID Contract No. 492-C-00-02-00031

33. SIAPS. Baseline study of private drug shops in Bangladesh: findings and recommendations. Submitted to the US Agency for international development by the systems for improved access to pharmaceuticals and services (SIAPS) program. Arlington: Management Sciences for Health; 2015.

34. Mortera L, Vianzon R. Private-public partnerships towards achieving TB control in the Philippines, Presentation made at 1st Forum of National Partnerships to Stop TB in the WHO Western Pacific and South-East Asia Regions, Seoul, Republic of Korea. 2012.

35. Gharat M. Tuberculosis awareness campaign on 24th March by Indian Pharmaceutical Association's Students' Forum. 2012. http://www.fip.org/www/index.php?page=news_publications&news=newsitem&newsitem=44. Accessed 14 Dec 2016.

36. Wells WA, Ge CF, Patel N, Oh T, Gardiner E, Kimerling ME. Size and usage patterns of private TB drug markets in the high burden countries. PloS ONE. 2011;6:e18964.

37. WHO. Joint program review of Cambodia's National Tuberculosis Program. 2012.

38. Gazette of India. Schedule H1. Ministry of Health and Family Welfare. http://www.cdsco.nic.in/writereaddata/588E30thAug2013.pdf. Accessed 14 Dec 2016.

39. Miller R, Goodman C. Performance of retail pharmacies in low- and middle-income Asian settings: a systematic review. Health Policy Plan. 2016. doi: 10.1093/heapol/czw007

40. Hermansyah A, Sainsbury E, Krass I.Community pharmacy and emerging public health initiatives in developing Southeast Asian countries: a systematic review. Health Soc Care Community. 2015. doi: 10.1111/hsc.12289

41. Stop TB Partnership. The paradigm shift 2016–2020, Global plan to END TB. 2016.

42. Rutta E, Liana J, Embrey M, Johnson K, Kimatta S, Valimba R, Lieber R, Shekalaghe E, Sillo H. Accrediting retail drug shops to strengthen Tanzania's public health system: an ADDO case study. J Pharm Policy Pract. 2015;25:8–23.

43. Hamid Salim MA, Uplekar M, Daru P, Aung M, Declercq E, Lönnroth K. Turning liabilities into resources: informal village doctors and tuberculosis control in Bangladesh. Bull World Health Organ. 2006;84(6):479–84.

44. WHO. TB Patients and Private For-Profit Health Care Providers in India. Geneva: World Health Organization; 1997.

45. Stop TB Partnership. Global Plan to Stop TB. Phase 1: 2001 to 2005. Geneva, Switzerland.

46. WHO. Good Practice in Legislation and Regulations for TB Control: An Indicator of Political Will. 2001. Geneva, Switzerland

47. Management Sciences for Health, WHO and Stop TB Partnership. Improving TB Drug Management: Accelerating DOTS Expansion. 2002. Geneva, Switzerland.

48. WHO. An Expanded DOTS Framework for Effective Tuberculosis Control. 2002. Geneva, Switzerland.

49. WHO. Expanding DOTS in the Context of a Changing Health System. 2003. Geneva, Switzerland.

50. WHO. Public-Private Mix for DOTS Practical tools to help implementation. 2003. Geneva, Switzerland.

51. WHO. Engaging all health care providers in TB control: Guidance on Implementing Public-Private Mix Approaches. 2006. Geneva, Switzerland.

52. WHO and Stop TB Partnership. DOTS Expansion Working Group Strategic Plan 2006–2015. Geneva, Switzerland.

53. Stop TB Partnership and WHO. The Global Plan to Stop TB, 2006–2015. Geneva, Switzerland.

54. WHO. Strategic and Technical Advisory Group for Tuberculosis (STAG-TB). Report of the ninth meeting. 9–11 November 2009. Geneva, Switzerland.

55. WHO. Public-Private Mix for TB Care and Control: A Toolkit. 2010. Geneva, Switzerland.

56. Stop TB Partnership and WHO. The Global Plan to Stop TB, 2011–2015. Geneva, Switzerland.

57. WHO and International Pharmaceutical Federation. Joint Statement: The Role of Pharmacists in Tuberculosis Care and Control. 2011. Hyderabad, India.

58. WHO. Framework for the engagement of all health care providers in the management of drug resistant tuberculosis. The END TB Strategy. 2015. Geneva, Switzerland.

59. Konduri N, Delmotte E, Rutta E. Engagement of the private pharmaceutical sector for TB control: Rhetoric or reality? J Pharm Policy Pract. 2016. doi: 10.1186/s40545-016-0093-3

Civil society engagement in multi-stakeholder dialogue: a qualitative study exploring the opinions and perceptions of MeTA members

Gemma L. Buckland-Merrett[*], Catherine Kilkenny and Tim Reed

Abstract

Background: The Medicines Transparency Alliance (MeTA) is an initiative that brings together all stakeholders in the medicines market to create a multi-stakeholder dialogue and improve access, availability and affordability of medicines. Key to this multi-stakeholder dialogue is the participation of Civil Society Organisations. A recent MeTA annual review, identified uneven engagement of civil society organisations in the multi-stakeholder process. This study was designed to explore the engagement of Civil Society Organisations in the MeTA multi-stakeholder process and the factors influencing their participation.

Methods: Participants were drawn from a convenience sample of key MeTA informants attending a MeTA global meeting in Geneva in 2014. Study participants consisted of members of MeTA, which included representatives from government, the private sector and civil society. In-depth semi-structured face-to-face interviews were conducted to identify perceptions around the barriers to civil society engagement in the multi-stakeholder process. Interviews were guided by a conceptual framework exploring the three main themes of the political environment, relative stakeholder strength and agenda setting/gatekeepers. Interviews were structured to enable additional themes to emerge and be explored. Fifteen interviews were conducted. The interviews were audio recorded, transcribed verbatim and analysed using a general inductive approach. All interviewees provided written informed consent.

Results: Findings were captured within three main overarching themes: the political environment, relative stakeholder strength and agenda setting/gatekeepers, with the opportunity for additional themes to emerge in the interviewing process. The study conformed these three themes were important in the engagement process. Participants reported that civil society engagement is particularly limited by those who set the agenda. It was largely seen that the political environment was the significant factor that enabled or disabled all others. The findings counter the argument that CSO barriers to engagement are predominantly due to capacity issues.

Conclusions: This study enriches previous findings by providing insights into civil society participation in multi-stakeholder dialogue, specifically the MeTA initiative. The development of more rigorous and systematic accountability mechanisms in order to maintain the legitimacy of decision-making processes and establish more equal power relations would significantly benefit the engagement of civil society organisations. The results inform practical recommendations for MeTA and future multi-stakeholder programmes tasked with improving policy on the access, availability and affordability of medicines.

Keywords: Multi-stakeholder dialogue, Partnerships, MeTA, Civil society engagement

* Correspondence: Gemma@haiweb.org
Health Action International, Overtoom 60 (2), 1054 HK Amsterdam, The Netherlands

Background

Globally, one in three people lacks access to essential medicines [1]. Moreover, when access does exist, medicines can be too expensive, counterfeit or sub-standard, wrongly prescribed or out of stock in the nearest health centre. The pharmaceutical market and medicine supply chains are at the root of these problems; poor information on price and quality, promotion of medicines, distorted competition, corrupt practices and irrational use of medicines [2]. Understanding information about the medical supply chain within health systems is essential to identify how problems should be tackled and by whom. The Medicines Transparency Alliance (MeTA) was established in 2008 as a response to this. MeTA is premised on the idea that making information about medicine supply chains available for analysis by major stakeholder groups will lead to an improved understanding of the problems. This in turn will foster a greater incentive to pioneer change, greater responsibility and accountability upon those needed to instigate change and will lead to increased access to medicines for the most vulnerable sectors of society. In order to achieve its overall goal, MeTA pursued three key objectives; to better inform pharmaceutical policies, to improve practice and to enable multi-stakeholder participation [3]. MeTA sought to improve the access, availability and affordability of medicines for seven countries where access is currently limited (Ghana, Jordan, Kyrgyzstan, Peru, the Philippines, Uganda and Zambia).

At the country level MeTA was developed in response to respective political and social contexts. Whilst being a global alliance, countries were encouraged to shape their structures, priorities and work programmes within existing frameworks to ensure the project would be country led and as sustainable as possible. Each of the pilot countries has organised a Multi-stakeholder Forum, a Council and a Secretariat. One of the most fundamental elements of MeTA in each pilot country was the creation of the national MeTA Councils as multi-stakeholder groups. It was vital that governments, the private sector and civil society organisations (CSOs) were actively engaged as stakeholders in each MeTA council. This created an 'issue network'; *"a relatively open network of antagonistic actors"*, with a mutual aim, who have expert knowledge and build relationships through information exchange but may subsequently have very different policy ideals [4–8].

The combination of transparency and multi-stakeholder groups may have been used before [9], but applying this model to the area of medicines and health policy was a unique strategy. Indeed, transparency around medicines policy is not a new concept, MeTA's aim was to creating a multi stakeholder alliance, to generate evidence and translate evidence into policy and practice [10]. Crucially, for CSOs participating in MeTA they were being invited to engage in an area where they

had previously found themselves on the margins. Indeed, the involvement of CSOs in policy decision making in general is often limited [10]. The CSOs participating in MeTA consist of community, patient, health, consumer, good governance and transparency groups, media, and faith-based organisations - a network of stakeholders acting in the space between individuals, the state and the private sector. It is, generally accepted that an engaged civil society is central to true democratic legitimacy and promoting accountability [11–14]. Civil Society Organisations (CSOs) have a long history of involvement on health and access to essential medicines, consumer protection and promotion of transparency, including many national as well as international groups. In-country CSOs are focused on health in different ways – as service providers, advocates for rights, or providers of care and support for people with specific health problems. The inclusion of CSOs as one of the three stakeholder groupings in the MeTA pilot was therefore entirely appropriate. However, in a recent MeTA annual report, despite highlighting the considerable advances MeTA has made since the initial pilot phase, reports of obstacles preventing full engagement between CSOs and other stakeholders, were described [15].

To date, little research has been done to explore the full range of factors that cause variation in the ability of CSOs to engage meaningfully in policy development or multi-stakeholder platforms. In the literature, causes of the unequal engagement of civil society are positioned as largely stemming from within civil society as opposed to external factors. Indeed, the most cited factor in determining civil society engagement is the availability of technical capacity [16, 17]. However, for MeTA the barriers to CSO engagement were not perceived as issues arising primarily from poor technical capacity. The issues appeared to be more driven by the domestic, social and political context. Few scholars have tackled the question of what accounts for the variation in civil society engagement beyond capacity issues. Explanations are likely to be insufficient if they do not engage with the reality of the multi-stakeholder process and the dynamics which push and pull decisions and issues both inside and outside of CSOs in different directions. This 'push and pull' can be conceptualised as issue emergence and the twin steps of the construction and acceptance of problems as issues. The construction of issues, which consists of definition and framing of a problem, is a key part of issue networks and are logically prior to decisions on issues and solutions championed by networks. This process demonstrates that a stakeholder is responsible for a particular issue and issue acceptance occurs when the issue is championed by at least one major player in the wider network [18, 19]. However, where some actors have more power over decision-making than others, it is likely that CSO perspectives fade into the background if they contradict the policy plans of these gatekeepers. Equally, where the political environment does not welcome the inclusion of civil society opinions (e.g. where engagement is sporadic or where government officials have their own agendas) the likelihood of issue acceptance is threatened. In the case of MeTA, issue acceptance occurs at the internal level of MeTA and at the level of MeTA-government relations.

Despite the limited literature, a number of questions are raised which recognise the influence of factors external to CSOs, such as a highly political policy environment, fear of political opposition and government suspicion [20–22]. Indeed, this resonates with views from a recent CSO meeting, where, *"relative stakeholder strength, local cultural issues* (e.g. *history of democratic process) and agenda setting/threats"* were seen as the key barriers to CSO engagement [15]. In order to explore this issue in more depth this study interviewed MeTA members about their knowledge and experiences of engaging in policy development and multi-stakeholder platforms. Exploring the barriers to CSO participation in MeTA will not only aid in understanding how the policy dialogue can be improved around medicines policy but it will also contribute to the wider discourse on the role of CSOs in multi-stakeholder engagement [20].

Methods
Key informants
This study adopted a qualitative approach and was undertaken at the MeTA Global Meeting in November 2014 in Geneva, Switzerland. A list of attendees at the MeTA Global Meeting was obtained prior to the meeting. Participants for the study were sampled purposively based on the following criteria: interviewees must be part of the MeTA alliance (representatives of one of the three stakeholder groups from the participating countries of the alliance), must regularly attend meetings and must speak English or have a translator available. Based on this selection criterion, fifteen participants were recruited for the study and were sent information regarding the study. This included a participant information sheet, which provided an overview of the research study and processes and a research consent form that participants could complete to indicate their interest in participating. This information was also passed on by the researcher conducting the interviews directly prior to the interview itself. Participants were advised that they could withdraw from the study at any time.

Interviews
A series of face-to-face, semi-structured interviews was undertaken. To ensure consistency, interviews were conducted by the same interviewer. Questions were developed following a review of the relevant literature [1–19] and by identifying suggested key barriers to civil society

engagement in the 2014 MeTA annual review. These questions informed a conceptual framework developed to ascertain what actors perceived as barriers to civil society engagement. The conceptual framework focused questions on three main themes: (1) local political environment (2) power imbalances and (3) agenda setting/gatekeepers. Additional questions were used to obtain information about civil society representative's experiences of multi-stakeholder engagement and their perception of the ways in which they were encouraged or discouraged to voice their opinions. In all interviews, questions were asked about the power relationships between stakeholders within and outside of MeTA and factors which facilitated or inhibited civil society influence on policy change. Questions were asked in English (using a translator where necessary) and were open-ended in order to allow discussions to be led by interviewees as opposed to the interviewer. Demographic information, including sector and country of employment were recorded at the time of the interview. Interviews took place at a quiet location close by to the Global Meeting. Fifteen interviews were conducted, at which stage data saturation was reached. Most interviews were around 50 min in duration (range: 20–50 min). Face to face semi-structured interviews were chosen over qualitative methods due the opportunity to take advantage of social ques and allow for additional themes to emerge. Synchronous communication also gives the advantage of spontaneous answers and direct reaction on answers. All participants were interviewed in the same location to provide a private space for people to partake honestly to enhance the validity of the study.

Data analysis
After each interview, the interviewer made field notes and this information was used to describe how each interview was conducted and to note issues or comments not sufficiently captured by audio recordings. This information aided interpretation of data. All interviews were audiotaped with the consent of participants. Interviews were transcribed verbatim and the transcripts were checked against the audio recordings. The full transcripts used in the subsequent analysis process. To ensure anonymity, names, place of work, or any other identifying information was removed, and a unique code number was assigned to each transcript. Analysis of data was undertaken by the research team via a staged process to ensure reliability. In the first instance, transcripts were read after each interview to inform further interview questions in order to enable continuous comparison of new and previous interview content. The data were analysed using the general inductive approach (GIA) [21] using the thematic framework as a guide. GIA is a thematic analysis approach with both deductive and inductive features. In GIA, while the

general (or overarching) themes are derived from the research objectives (deductive feature), more specific categories/themes arise from the data (inductive feature) [21]. NVivo 10 software (QSR International) was used to support the analysis process. Identification and interpretation of quotes was carried out by two separate members of the research team.

Results

Of the 15 individuals who participated, four were MeTA country co-ordinators (with civil society backgrounds), two were representatives of the private sector and the remaining nine MeTA members were representatives from civil society. Participants selected represented the following countries; Jordan, Peru, Kyrgyzstan, Zambia, Uganda, Philippines, Ghana. Key findings from the research are presented below.

The political environment as a barrier to CSO engagement

Despite advances in political freedoms, some MeTA groups operate in political contexts which constrain civil society work and engagement in policy processes. The majority of respondents spoke of the importance of the wider political context to civil society's ease or difficulty engaging policy. A history of civil society engagement with government in a democratic setting was seen as a clear advantage by all respondents, whereas a lack of this was thought to correspond with difficulties in civil society participation:

The lack or presence of political will has the power to disable or enable our [civil society's] ability to act and political will has been seriously lacking in Peru...there is no real history of dialogue between our government and civil society and the government do not want to listen to different perspectives. [P3]

Regular consultations between civil society and the state were seen as a significant advantage to engagement to civil society representatives in all countries. However, in some countries, consultations with the ministry of health were reported to largely take the form of the provision of evidence for policy change as opposed to providing insight on policy issues. Some actors expressed doubts as to what meaningful action could arise from these consultations. Similarly, the 'good will' demonstrated by allowing civil society to participate in consultative stages of the policy process was reported to not translate into further policy action, leaving civil society representatives feeling marginalized:

Sometimes, it feels like our participation inside and outside of MeTA is just tokenism...we talk and talk

and talk but whether anything materializes...well, let's see. [P2]

A civil society representative from Peru explained that, while it was originally intended for civil society to provide the government with opinions and recommendations, civil society consultations have been blocked by ministers:

"...so in the access to essential medicines programme called Farmacise, *civil society are supposed to provide the government with opinions...recommendations. But the government has blocked that. They don't want to listen to them specifically in that area. It has been closed for civil society participation so far. That is the big concern in Peru right now."* [P1]

Unpredictable government engagement with MeTA was also highlighted as a barrier to civil society engagement, as securing government representatives' presence and input was seen as integral to getting MeTA perspectives represented in policy:

In Ghana, we had a challenge with the secretariat. That's finished now. There was a secretariat that was not performing. There today, not there tomorrow. The new one is better, he gives time. [P9]

In some cases, government officials perceived the presence or voices of CSOs as diminishing or undermining the authority of the state. Perceived former civil society 'interference' in policy was also seen as a source of tension by a civil society representative from Ghana, who believed that this had led to government officials being less receptive to civil society opinions. In Kyrgyzstan, civil society has an excellent relationship with the ministry of health but there are tensions between civil society and the Department on Drug Provision and Medical Equipment in the Kyrgyz Republic (DRA). DRA officials were described as a strong barrier to civil society's ability to influence policy, insofar as it was suggested that they had resorted to defamation of MeTA online. It was suggested that previous civil society recommendations to the ministry of health may be behind this. Tensions with the ministry of health were highlighted in Jordan, where civil society representatives described facing strong pushback and exclusion, most recently concerning negotiations to drive down the price of a Multiple Sclerosis treatment by 50%. According to one civil society representative, sometimes giving civil society a hearing in consultations was used as a way to silence them and prevent civil society action:

The fight is mainly with the Ministry of Health. The ministry make many promises of policy and price

*changes to CSOs... some believe that the minister of
health is stalling and creating delays, cancelling
meetings last minute and making promises which are
not delivered...they don't just say no as if they did we
could bypass them and go directly to the royal court.*
[P2]

Power imbalances

Power imbalances outside of MeTA were described as
greatly influencing which actors had a say in policy
decisions by the majority of respondents. Government
officials were reported to have the strongest voice in
Uganda. In Ghana, the government were reported to
have the most power inside of MeTA, with this
imbalance exacerbated by something of a representa-
tional monopoly within MeTA. Until recently, there
was only one civil society representative inside MeTA,
remedied only after a visit from international
members:

*Thankfully, during a visit from international members
from the WHO and HAI it was agreed that one person
was not sufficient to represent all of the civil society
members of MeTA...that proposal sparked resistance
from the leadership but the number of representatives
was increased to two.* [P5]

In Kyrgyzstan the main perceived barrier to civil society engagement was the DRA's unchecked power; generally, the DRA was thought to have more influence than
the ministry of health on policy and were reported to
marginalise the private sector:

*[T]hey [the DRA] can do whatever they want and no
one can stop them; if they hate a group or business
they can put a lot of pressure on them... They cannot
talk about this openly or they will be punished: they
just try to use civil society because the regulatory
agency have such huge power and can put huge
pressure on them.* [P13]

Conversely, in Peru, Zambia, Ghana and Jordan,
respondents voiced the opinion that the private sector
not only had a stronger voice than civil society outside
of MeTA but was also more powerful than governments. This manifested in a number of ways, for
example by having the power to appoint or remove
government officials or influence policy by leveraging
their profits and influence: One respondent also
highlighted the unchecked power of procurement
officers, who had the power to procure certain medicines and supplies, influencing buying patterns of
medicines procurement for their own profit.

Gatekeepers and agenda setting

Where civil society positions did not correlate with the
government's own agenda, ministers' own policy agendas
were often identified as a strong factor in inhibiting or
enabling civil society participation outside of MeTA. In
most countries, the strength of government depended
on the relative importance of certain issues to ministers.

The active involvement of government officials inside
the MeTA process was widely seen as greatly beneficial
to raise the profile of issues with governments. However,
although having members of government in powerful
positions within MeTA was reported to increase engagement, many respondents expressed ambivalence. Where
government engagement within MeTA was necessary to
influence policy, sporadic engagement from government
officials represented a hurdle to civil society engagement,
as in Ghana and Uganda:

*The strength of the ministry of health in Uganda
barrier to things getting done because if they are not at
the table you have to find a way of getting them to the
table; if they are not in meetings...for example, this
meeting, we feel that it makes our jobs harder.* [P11]

Concerns about having government representatives in
powerful positions within MeTA were raised by a participant, who emphasised possible conflicts of interest
and difficulties in ensuring that some stakeholders do
not have unchecked power:

*For example, there might be changes in policy that
work towards the interests of the government or the
private sector. If the government is the leading member
of the MeTA council, how can this be balanced? Who
will balance it? How can you be critical if you need
them to sign off on every policy change? So I think that
would be a difficult position. Where will people go if
they have problems with the government? I don't know
what the dynamics would be like [sic] there, if that
would be the system.* [P2]

In some cases the disproportionate influence of government officials outside of MeTA was reported as influencing which conversations were conducted within
MeTA. Some respondents referred to powerful individuals within MeTA having their own policy agendas and
using their position to influence which positions MeTA
could take.

*It makes a difference in what we can say...because
they are the ones who are listened to, they are the ones
who are consulted by government....If there are
agitations of any kind the president of the Ghana
association is the last person who needs to be*

consulted. So he keeps quiet, you bring the draft to him...he has the final decision...if he does not like a point he just sends it back. [P5]

Some interviewees emphasised being non-confrontational and avoiding making demands in order to be heard. Where power imbalances were reported to be minimal, this simply took the form of all stakeholders "agreeing to disagree" [P2]. In Kyrgyzstan it was noted that, due to tensions with the DRA, civil society members are careful to mediate their interactions with the DRA. Conversely, respondents in countries where engagement was low reported taking care when approaching government officials, as they were thought to have a large amount of power in the policy process within and outside of MeTA. Their presence not only influenced the agenda but also how debates were conducted. For example, in Zambia gaps in services can be highlighted by civil society, but not expressed as being the result of government shortcomings:

Our approach is not confrontational. When we speak with government...if all we do is point fingers and accuse them of things, nothing happens. We have to engage in more...civil ways. [P8]

Capacity

Interview responses revealed key variations and similarities in the factors viewed as facilitating and inhibiting civil society participation. Contrary to the existing literature, capacity was not seen as a barrier to engagement, it was however frequently referenced and therefore an overview of respondents' views of capacity is also presented.

While room for further civil skills strengthening with regards to policy was recognised every interviewee stated that technical capacity to engage in the area of medicines policy as part of MeTA was strong: In all countries, capacity was thought to be strengthened through the inclusion of members with previous technical or policy experience due to the skills and recognition they brought to MeTA:

We have the capacity. We have members who are trained in health and have had advocacy training, Master's degrees, we have retired medical and pharmaceutical officers. All of these things help us to be taken seriously. [P5]

Representatives from all countries noted that civil society engagement had been strengthened through capacity-building activities run by MeTA. A civil society respondent from Uganda stated that whereas previously the Ugandan government had accused civil society of *"just being noisy"*, now the government is aware that civil society within

MeTA *"use evidence to get the change that we want"*. A similar view was expressed by a civil society representative from Jordan, where civil society did not previously possess the technical skills for evidence-based advocacy. Outside of MeTA, views of civil society capacity were not always positive. For example, a respondent from Zambia expressed a belief that members of professional associations did not necessarily believe that civil society had the capacity to engage in policy. A civil society respondent reported that heads of hospitals also had doubts about civil society capacity and perceived civil society as interfering with their day to day functioning:

Heads of hospitals, they get a certain level of responsibility and autonomy with their budgets...they have a lot of freedom in how they spend it. They don't want anyone messing up their good life, so they say, "Who are these people? What do they know about medicines"? [P10]

A number of respondents expressed the opinion that, while capacity is an important factor in engaging with policy, it was not the strongest predictor of civil society success in the multi-stakeholder process; barriers were most often perceived in getting powerful stakeholders to engage once a certain level of capacity had been achieved:

It doesn't matter how high our capacity is. At the end of the day, if we cannot engage with government in a way they appreciate it just doesn't work. [P15]

Discussion

This research explored the opinions and perceptions of civil society organisations in the MeTA multi-stockholder dialogue process. Furthermore, the study used MeTA as a case study to confirm the factors which limit civil society engagement in multi-stakeholder dialogue. These findings advance our understanding of multi-stakeholder dialogue within the medicines policy arena and provide further insights into how we can effectively foster transparent and open information sharing to create improved policy surrounding access to medicines. The study used in-depth interviews to explore three key themes relevant to the variations seen in CSO engagement within MeTA; (1) local political environment (2) power imbalances and (3) agenda setting/gatekeepers. The study also allowed for the emergence of new themes in order to gain a deeper understanding and identify where improvements might be made.

Prior research has shown that a lack of civil society capacity can seriously impact civil society's ability to engage with policy [16]. However, capacity-building strengthening activities carried out by MeTA did not have any effect on engagement [15]. Despite stating that they had good technical capacity, many civil society representatives did not perceive themselves as well-positioned to influence policy. Capacity was not identified as a current barrier to civil society engagement by any respondent in this study. This was the case not only in countries where civil society engagement is strong, but also in those countries where engagement was reported to be comparatively weak in a recent MeTA annual review [15].

Of the three main themes explored, political environment was deemed especially important, and the ultimate deciding factor for effective collaboration. In countries where government's commitment to policy change in the area of access to medicines is strong, civil society find dialogue and collaboration more consistent and productive than CSOs do in those countries where commitment and multi-stakeholder engagement is weak. In addition, where governments offer an open consultation process to civil society, engagement is higher than in political systems in which governments regularly block policy consultations or changes proposed by civil society.

Unequal power dynamics and relative stakeholder strength outside of MeTA were seen to hamper civil society engagement on a number of levels. Firstly, where the private sector has more influence than civil society due to a higher degree of political currency in consultations or the ability to leverage monetary resources, civil society are disadvantaged. The powerful position of other stakeholders such as procurement officers, hospital heads and government officials were also cited as an issue. Ultimately, wherever political will was lacking or the private sector had a disproportionate influence on the direction of policy, civil society are disadvantaged. Power imbalances strongly influence the extent of ownership felt by actors over issues or solutions which emerge within MeTA. Actors have varying levels of power within MeTA and power imbalances were evident, particularly where civil society were underrepresented or only involved in consultative processes. Issue networks themselves do not have policy goals; these arise from actors within the network and some actors have more power than others in the issue formation process. Furthermore, if issue definition involves demonstrating that a party is responsible for a certain situation and proposing credible solutions, a culture of having to be careful in 'blaming' government officials for previous mistakes may stand in the way of truly participatory engagement for civil society [18].

The issue of gatekeepers and agenda setting as a barrier to policy engagement was most commonly raised regarding government officials and the position they hold within MeTA. Indeed, it is suggested that in countries with a less hospitable political environment to civil society, issue adoption often occurs when the issue is championed by one major player in the broader network [17]. Gatekeepers are seated in powerful positions within MeTA due to their power to lend credibility, sources or pathways to a raised 'issue'. These benefits were widely discussed and seen as integral to MeTA's policy influencing activities. However, gatekeepers can also block the entry of policy issues into the policy process; gatekeepers have *"powerful demonstration effects, signalling that certain causes are important"* [19]. If gatekeepers disagree with civil society positions, this represents a significant disadvantage for civil society, insofar as their views may be silenced [23]. Here, it is likely that the policy suggestions most likely to reach policy makers are those most well-aligned to the positions already held by the policy maker or the wider government department. Conversely, the position of civil society is at its strongest within MeTA when the process of issue formation was closest to the principle of collaborative governance [24, 25]. That is, where stakeholders representing different interests make policy decisions or recommendations to a final decision-maker who does not substantially change consensus recommendations.

There is a sophisticated academic debate on the 'democratic deficit' in global policy-making and the approaches necessary to make public policy-making more accountable [26]. Despite this, issues of accountability were rarely, if ever, explicitly discussed during the interviews. It is argued that multi-sectoral networks should be embedded in a pluralistic system of accountability, making use of a combination of accountability, as outlined by Benner and colleagues [27]. For example, they may employ measures of "internal accountability" (oversight committees) or "reputational accountability" (naming and shaming) [27]. It is likely that more rigorous and systematic accountability mechanisms are needed within MeTA in order to maintain the legitimacy of decision-making processes. Overall, further research into the power structure of local MeTA councils and meetings would be useful in order to identify the conditions under which stakeholders act collaboratively. This study suggests that, particularly where government officials are serving as chairs, clear guidelines to government engagement within MeTA should be formulated in order to ensure that proper checks and balances are put in place. This would represent a step towards ensuring that no one actor has the power to sign off on policy changes within MeTA. It is unclear whether any government officials involved with MeTA have been systematically trained in civil society relations but, although actors would still be confined by the overarching political environment, such training may prove useful in ensuring that there is enough space for diversity of opinion and debate both within and outside of MeTA. Furthermore, clearly defined goals and specific expected outputs should be designed by each MeTA country group in order to focus and motivate MeTA members and ensure accountability. In this way, actors may be more open to the strategies of other sectors if these strategies appear useful for achieving agreed upon goals. It may be useful to complement this with some frank discussion about perceptions of power relations within and outside of MeTA, the various sources of influence around the table and the strategies needed to address any problematic power differentials. This may involve the use of professional facilitation or introduction of specific measures to *"level the playing field"* through, for example, formalised power-sharing rules, or increased representation of "weaker" stakeholder groups.

The qualitative nature of the study means that this research draws heavily on the personal experiences of civil society members. While this is an advantage insofar as we have gained an in-depth understanding of their perceptions of the multi-stakeholder process, a reliance on personal reflections limits this paper's reach to some extent by relying on respondents' ability to recall events or actions. The possibility of participants wanting to shine a favourable light on the work of their own organisations should also be considered, as should wishes not to offend country governments by portraying them as unresponsive. Furthermore, the use of convenience sampling in selection of study participants may lead to bias due to the fact any civil society members attending the conference in Geneva may possibly be more engaged in the policy process than other civil society counterparts.

In reality, actors in a network may come together because of disagreements over the presence of a solution to certain issues. The practice of collaboration has long demonstrated that multi-stakeholder partnerships and relationships are often fraught, with many facing significant setbacks in delivering the resources or outcomes originally stated. Even where preliminary milestones have been achieved, multi-stakeholder groups often still experience collaborative inertia which can have significant effects on outputs [27]. In light of these challenges, MeTA serves as an interesting case study to explore how civil society are encouraged or prevented from voicing opinions and influencing policy in a meaningful way without assuming shared agendas.

Conclusion

This study enriches the current understanding of civil society engagement in multi-stakeholder dialogue, by providing ginsights into the opinions and perceptions of CSO's participating in a multi-stakeholder alliance, MeTA, aimed at improving access to medicines policy. The studies confirms that the political environment, relative stakeholder strength and gatekeepers have a significant role in CSO engagement within the MeTA issue network. However, it was largely seen that the political environment was the one factor that enabled or disabled all others. In this case, the findings counter the argument that CSO barriers to engagement are predominantly due to capacity issues. It is evident that there is no one-size-fits-all template for civil

society engagement: any interventions in these relationships must be tailored to their specific contexts and goals. However, for MeTA it is likely that the use of more rigorous and systematic accountability mechanisms in order to maintain the legitimacy of decision-making processes and establish more equal power relations would significantly benefit the engagement of CSOs. This study provides a significant starting point for a discussion about potential barriers and solutions for improving transparency, accountability and evidenced-based policy making in improving access to medicines through multi-stakeholder dialogue.

Abbreviations
CSO: Civil Society Organisation; DRA: Drug Regulatory Authority; MeTA: Medicines Transparency Alliance; NGO: Non-governmental organisation; WHO: World Health Organization

Acknowledgements
Not applicable.

Funding
No external funding has been received for this study.

Authors' contributions
GBM analysed and interpreted the final data and was the primary contributor in writing the manuscript. CK carried out the interviews and contributed to the writing of the manuscript. GBM, CK and TR all contributed to the intellectual content of the manuscript. All authors read and approved the final manuscript.

Competing interests
The authors declare that they have no competing interests.

References
1. Ahmadiani S, Nikfar S. Challenges of access to medicine and the responsibility of pharmaceutical companies: a legal perspective. Daru. 2016;24:13.
2. Leisinger KM, Garabedian LF, Wagner AK. Improving access to medicines in Low and middle income countries: corporate responsibilities in context. South Med Rev. 2012;5(2):3–8.
3. The Medicines Transparency Alliance. http://www.medicinestransparency.org. Accessed 10 Apr 2016.
4. Rosenblum NL, Lesch CHT. In: Michael E, editor. Civil society and government. London: Oxford University Press; 2011. p. 8.
5. Huxham C, Vangen S. Realizing the advantage or succumbing to inertia? Organ Dyn. 2004;33:190–201.
6. Peels R, Develtere P. Civil society involvement in international development cooperation: in search for data. Soc Indic Res. 2009;93:331–49.
7. Keast R, Mandell M. Network theory in the public sector: building new theoretical frameworks. New York: Routledge; 2013.
8. Heclo H. Issue networks and the executive establishment: government growth in an age of improvement. In: King A, editor. The new American political system. Washington: American Enterprise Institute; 1978. p. 104.
9. Bäckstrand K. Multi-stakeholder partnerships for sustainable development: rethinking legitimacy, accountability and effectiveness. Eur Environ. 2006;16:290–306.

10. Allard G, Martinez CA. The influence of government policy and NGOs on capturing private investment. 2008. http://www.oecd.org/investment/globalforum/40400836.pdf Accessed 15 Jan 2015.

11. Putnam R. Making democracy work. Princeton: Princeton University Press; 1993.

12. Putnam R. Bowling alone: the collapse and revival of American community. New York: Simon & Schuster; 2000.

13. Fox J. Civil society and political accountability: propositions for discussion. 2000. http://kellogg.nd.edu/faculty/research/pdfs/Fox.pdf. Accessed 29 January 2015.

14. Armstrong K. Inclusive governance? Civil society and the open method of co-ordination. In: Smismans S, editor. Civil society and legitimate European governance. Cheltenham: Elgar, Edward Publishing, Inc; 2006. p. 42–67.

15. MeTA. MeTA annual review 2014. 2014. http://www.medicinestransparency.org/fileadmin/uploads/MeTA_Annual_Review_2014_APPROVED.pdf. Accessed 29 Jan 2015.

16. Court J, Mendizabel E, Osborne D, Young J. How civil society can be more effective. 2006. http://www.odi.org/sites/odi.org.uk/files/odi-assets/publications-opinion-files/200.pdf. Accessed 15 January 2015.

17. Curren Z. Civil society participation in the PRSP: the role of evidence and the impact on policy choices. 2005. http://www.odi.org/sites/odi.org.uk/files/odi-assets/publications-opinion-files/8271.pdf. Accessed 29 January 2015.

18. Keck M, Sikkink K. Activists beyond borders. Cornell: Cornell University Press; 1998.

19. Bob C. The marketing of rebellion. Cambridge: Cambridge University Press; 2005.

20. Fowler A. NGOs as agents of democratization: an African perspective. J Int Dev. 1993;5:325–39.

21. Thomas DR. A general inductive approach for analyzing qualitative evaluation data. Am J Eval. 2006;27(2):237–46.

22. Brown L. Organizational barriers to NGO strategic action. Lok Niti. 1988;5:1–11.

23. Hanlon J. New missionaries in Mozambique. London: Mimeo; 1990.

24. Marres N. Net-Work Is Format Work: Issue Networks and the Sites of Civil Society Politics. In Dean J, Asherson J, Lovink G, editors. Reformatting Politics: Networked Communications and Global Civil Society. Routledge, London; 2006. p. 3–19. 4

25. Vangen S, Huxham C. Introducing the theory of collaborative advantage. In: Osborne S, editor. The New public governance? Emerging perspectives on the theory and practice of public governance. London: Routledge; 2010. p. 163–4.

26. Smith M. The global diffusion of public policy: power structures and democratic accountability. Territory Politics Governance. 2013;2:118–31.

27. Benner T, Reinicke T, Witte W. Multisectoral networks in global governance: towards a pluralistic system of accountability. Gov Oppos. 2004;39:191–210.

11

Antibiotic knowledge, attitudes and behaviours of Albanian health care professionals and patients

Susanne Kaae[1*], Admir Malaj[2] and Iris Hoxha[2]

Abstract

Background: The inappropriate use of antimicrobials is a problem worldwide. To target future interventions, a thorough understanding of the reasons behind this current behaviour is needed. Within the EU, the culture of antimicrobial use has been intensely studied, but this is not the case in non-EU southeastern European countries, despite the frequent use of (broad-spectrum) antibiotics (ABs) in this region. The aim of this study was to explore AB knowledge, attitudes and behaviours of health care professionals (HCPs) and patients in one southeastern European country, Albania.

Methods: In total, 16 semi-structured interviews were carried out with four groups of interviewees: physicians, community pharmacists, and patients with and without AB prescriptions. Interviews were used to investigate participants' recent practices with four specific antibiotics for upper respiratory tract infections, along with their typical behaviours, knowledge and attitudes towards the use of antimicrobials. A directed content analysis was applied.

Results: The patients showed little awareness of the differences between viruses and bacteria; however, they often self-diagnosed, which led them to request ABs from pharmacies without a prescription. Pharmacists felt pressured to give in to patients' demands. All of the participants (including HCP) showed suboptimal beliefs about illness severity as they all believed that 'flu complications', i.e. flu/cold symptoms that persisted after 2–3 days, should be treated with ABs. Physicians usually had no rapid tests to guide them in their practice; however, they were not concerned about this fact. HCPs acknowledged AMR, but only a few of them seemed to consider its risk in their daily practice.

Conclusions: Patients had high levels of trust in and desire for ABs, and HCPs did not often negotiate with patients' demands. Suggested initiatives to improve the prudent use of ABs in Albania include higher reimbursement for prescribed antibiotics (to reduce illegal sales), academic detailing as well as implementing public awareness campaigns.

Keywords: Antibiotics, Albania, Interviews, Antibiotic knowledge, Attitudes, Practices, Patients, Pharmacists, Physicians

Background

Antimicrobial agents, such as antibiotics (ABs), have dramatically reduced the number of deaths from infectious diseases during the 70 years since their introduction. However, due to the inappropriate use of this type of medicine, many micro-organisms have become resistant to antibiotics [1]. This problem is estimated to cause 25,000 deaths annually in the EU. The costs incurred by drug-resistant infections amount to an estimated €1.5 billion annually due to increases in healthcare expenditures and productivity losses [1].

To combat antimicrobial resistance (AMR), the WHO Regional Office for Europe has initiated several programmes for both EU and non-EU member states. One programme engages in surveillance of drug consumption in the non-EU countries of southeastern Europe. The published results from 13 countries in this geographical

---

* Correspondence: susanne.kaae@sund.ku.dk

[1]Department of Pharmacy, Section for Social and Clinical Pharmacy, Faculty of Health and Medical Sciences, University of Copenhagen, Universitetsparken 2, 2100 København Ø, Denmark

Full list of author information is available at the end of the article

area show some indication of inappropriate AB use. Specifically, the findings suggest little consumption of narrow-spectrum penicillin and high consumption of ABs, such as penicillin combinations, third-generation cephalosporins and long-acting macrolides, causing an increased risk of AMR [2].

To support interventions that decrease inappropriate AB consumption, a qualitative multi-country study was collaboratively launched in 2014 by non-EU countries in southeastern Europe, the Health Technology and Pharmaceuticals group of the WHO, the Regional Office for Europe and qualitative researchers from the Section of Social and the Clinical Pharmacy, University of Copenhagen (SSC) [3]. The aim of the qualitative AMR study was to explore AB knowledge, attitudes and behaviours of health care professionals (HCPs – i.e., both physicians and community pharmacists) and patients in each country as a means to target more effective future interventions in the area.

To date, AB knowledge, attitudes and behaviours are factors that have been demonstrated to influence the use of ABs, particularly in western societies. For example, it has been shown that inappropriate prescribing is driven by physicians' perceptions that patients expect AB prescriptions, fear of disease progression and fear of losing patients to competitors [4–8]. Most HCPs recognize the risk of AMR; however, they are significantly more likely to perceive AMR as a national problem rather than one being affected by their own practice [8, 9]. Contradictory attitudes towards AB prescribing have also been identified among non-western physicians [8]. Furthermore, lack of awareness of appropriate AB use is widespread among patients. One survey found that on average only 48% of EU residents could correctly state that ABs are ineffective against the cold and flu, and participants with low levels of education were more likely to have misconceptions about ABs [10].

In contrast to most western European countries, many eastern European countries are prone to the often illegal sale of over-the-counter (OTC) ABs in community pharmacies; however, some uncertainty exists about the actual extent of the problem. A systematic review published in 2011 found that northeastern European countries, such as Lithuania, Poland and Romania, have a high frequency of OTC sales of ABs (approximately 30%), whereas others have suggested that only approximately 8% of the ABs used in this region are obtained without a prescription [11]. Furthermore, there are indications that OTC sales of ABs have in fact decreased in countries such as Lithuania due to legislation in this area [12]. The review from 2011 also reported that approximately 6% of ABs are sold OTC in some countries in southeastern Europe, i.e., Croatia, Slovenia and Slovakia [13], while other studies have suggested that

approximately 50% of ABs are sold OTC in this region [2]. This estimate was supported by a study carried out in Bosnia–Herzegovina in 2010, where 58% of the visited pharmacies illegally sold ABs without a prescription [14].

One southeastern European country that is a part of the qualitative WHO AMR research project is Albania. Albania gained independence in 1912 and is a former communist country with a distinct culture. Albania has a GNP of €10.0 billion (2014), which has constrained the basic education of the public [15], and one-third of its population (2.8 million inhabitants in total) are not covered by a public health insurance policy [16]. Only physicians have the right to prescribe medication and AB should according to law be obtained by prescription only. In recent years, Albania has experienced a rapid increase in the number of community pharmacies, which has challenged the implementation of inspections [17]. The country does not produce or import penicillin V; additionally, specific guidelines for the use of ABs do not exist.

Several of these factors are assumed to contribute to high and inappropriate AB consumption in Albania. This assumption has partly been demonstrated by studies showing that illegal OTC sales of ABs occur in 80% of Albanian pharmacies and that the use of broad-spectrum and penicillin combinations is common practice [18, 19].

It has been argued that interventions addressing physicians' prescribing practices related to ABs must encompass context-specific actions [20]. Thus, to inform policymakers and other stakeholders of the specific reasons behind the current use of ABs in Albania, the aim of this study was to investigate the AB knowledge, attitudes and behaviours of patients and HCPs in the country.

Methods

Qualitative semi-structured interviews were selected as the most adequate method to investigate AB knowledge, attitudes and behaviours of patients and HCPs in order to collect detailed accounts of participants' individual experiences and perceptions regarding AB use in order to understand the culture around this phenomenon in-depth [21].

Four types of interviewees were included, as they were all believed to provide valuable insight into the existing culture of AB use: patients/adults who had used ABs with a prescription, patients/adults who had used/purchased ABs illegally without a prescription, community pharmacists (both admitting to legal and non-legal sales of ABs) and physicians working in the primary care system. Despite the fact that physicians and community pharmacists are the legal and professional gatekeepers to patients' access to ABs, the influence of patients on for example physicians' AB prescribing practices has been demonstrated in previous studies [7, 22]. Therefore, it was considered important to incorporate these groups in this study.

The study was restricted to investigate AB use for upper respiratory tract infections (URTIs) for several reasons. First, the majority of ABs prescribed in ambulatory care are used to treat respiratory tract infections, and viruses can cause up to 80% of all URTIs [23, 24], making it an accessible and relevant case for studying inappropriate as well as common uses of ABs. Second, restricting the area of research would allow for more homogenous data, thereby increasing the possibility of identifying stronger patterns. Further, four specific ABs were followed: amoxicillin-clavulanic acid, azithromycin, ciprofloxacin and ceftriaxone. This decision was made to ensure the comparability of the data and also because these specific ABs had been shown to be used inappropriately in the region of southeastern Europe, posing a particular public health risk, as most were broad-spectrum ABs [2].

Seven general research questions were established in relation to investigating and addressing AB knowledge, attitudes and behaviours: the process of diagnosis, how and why a specific AB was selected, where and how ABs were purchased, the patients' use of ABs, satisfaction with the AB process along with AB knowledge and AB attitudes. The questions were operationalized as open questions in interview guides with some variation between the four groups of interviewees [3]. Hence, pharmacists for example were only interviewed about experiences pertaining to his/her pharmacy practice along with his/her knowledge and attitudes and thus not interviewed about how diagnosis is carried out by physicians or how patients used the purchased AB (please see Additional file 1).

In terms of interview technique, to allow for as detailed accounts as possible, patients were asked to answer the different questions specifically in relation to the most recent occurrence within the last 3 months (to reduce memory bias) in which they had one of the four specific ABs prescribed to them or sold to them at the pharmacy counter for a URTI. Likewise, HCPs were asked to describe two or three consultations during the last week in which they had prescribed or sold a specific AB for a URTI. Hence, this technique of referring to recent specific incidents was applied to generate coherent and detailed narratives of interviewees' experiences with ABs [25]. For example, a full description of how patients purchased an AB in a pharmacy without a prescription would inevitably also contain aspects of the patients' knowledge and attitudes towards ABs. Additionally, the narrative would likely include both their and the pharmacists' behaviour and social interactions [3]. The

narratives of the different groups of interviewees could further be compared and used to supplement each other to achieve a more complete picture of how ABs were used in daily life. All of the groups were additionally asked if they had other previous experiences with AB use, and if so, they were asked whether those instances were similar to the specific recent account they had just provided.

The semi-structure of the interviews was thus defined by a pre-developed interview guide with open questions to generate narratives and probing during the interviews according to the achieved answers.

Two interviewers from Albania completed a two-day training course led by two researchers from an established Social Pharmacy research group from the University of Copenhagen. Both of these researchers had substantial experience with conducting semi-structured interviews [26]. The training of the Albanian data collectors included how to conduct the semi-structured interviews in compliance with the specific requirements of the qualitative AMR project.

Since the study was considered exploratory, being the first of its kind in Albania, a convenience yet purposive sampling strategy was used [27]. Specifically, the snowball sampling technique was used in which the Albanian researchers asked people in both their professional and private networks if they knew of patients and HCPs who fit the inclusion criteria. To reduce selection bias, the researchers attempted to ensure heterogeneity with respect to age, gender and education.

The participants were verbally informed about the aim of the project, and all participants provided verbal consent to proceed. The appointments were agreed upon in advance for two reasons: to ethically allow participants to withdraw and to ensure that enrolled patients had begun their AB treatment before being interviewed about their medicine use. The interviews were not recorded due to the culture in Albania in which many people do not feel confident when recorded. Instead, extensive hand-written notes were taken. Most of the interviews were thus conducted by both interviewers, allowing one interviewer to concentrate on taking notes. Two patient interviews revealed that the recent use of ABs was for a URTI affecting the child of the interviewee and not themselves; these interviews were still included, as they were considered to be useful for addressing the study's research questions.

To ensure feasibility as well as research quality, 16 semi-structured interviews in total were conducted and included in the analysis (four within each interviewee group). Kvale recommends 15 interviews plus/minus 10 interviews when conducting semi-structured interviews in to order to produce validated results [21].

Analysis

The first step of the analysis involved directed content analyses [28], in which answers from each of the transcripts/notes pertaining to the general research questions were extracted, i.e., relevant answers were deductively identified. In the second step, one participant's answers were compared with those from other participants within the same group to derive a general understanding of how that group used or thought about ABs. In the third step, the understanding of each interviewee group was compared with the other groups both with regard to knowledge, attitudes and behaviour. Hence, to arrive at a more complete picture of typical AB behaviour, attitudes and knowledge, the developed understanding of each group of interviewees was compared and contrasted with other groups. The identified patterns were then (re-)organized into the initial categories of knowledge, attitudes and behaviour.

Researchers from Albania and a researcher (first author) from the SSC carried out the first step separately, compared their results in a consensus meeting, and then finalized the last steps of the analysis together. This procedure was considered to be optimal for ensuring high validity since the Albanian researchers could identify certain cultural aspects of AB use, whereas the SSC researchers coming from other cultures could identify other aspects.

Results

The 16 interviews were conducted between the winter of 2014 and the spring of 2015. The overall demographics of the participants are shown in Table 1. Of the 16 participants, 12 were females with patients aged 30 to 59 years (including two mothers of three children between 2 and 6 years of age). The HCPs ranged in age from 27 to 45 years.

Knowledge

The patients expressed their belief that ABs fight infection, yet most were unsure exactly how they do so. Only a few patients distinguished between bacterial and viral infections.

The pharmacists stated that ABs should not be used when OTC medicines such as paracetamol and syrups were sufficient. Otherwise, with the exception of one pharmacist who said that ABs should not be used for viral symptoms, the pharmacists provided no clear responses regarding AB recommendations. With regard to the physicians, the majority described how ABs should be used to treat complicated bacterial or viral infections.

Most of the HCPs acknowledged that AB resistance exists, and several had observed some situations where patients returned due to a lack of AB efficiency. However, at the same time, some HCPs appeared to question the seriousness of AB resistance. With the exception of

Table 1 Participant demographics

Patients with prescription		
Age	Gender	Education/work
30	Male	Secondary education
Mother of boy of 6 years of age	Female	Higher education
Mother of children of 2 and 4 years of age	Female	Higher education
41	Female	Secondary education

Patients without prescription		
Age	Gender	Education/work
36	Female	Higher education
28	Female	Post graduate education
47	Female	Higher education
59	Male	Secondary education

Community pharmacists			
Age/experience	Gender	Location of practice	Size of practice
30–7 years of experience	Female	Urban area	70–100 customers per day
27–4 years of experience	Female	Urban area	100–150 customers per day
29–6 years of experience	Male	Urban area	40–60 customers per day
31–8 years of experience	Female	Urban area	50 customers per day

Physicians			
Age/experience	Gender	Location of practice	Number of consultations
36–9 years of experience	Female	Urban area	10–20 patients per day
45–20 years of experience	Male	Urban area	15–30 patients per day
28–4 years of experience	Female	Rural area	10 patients per day
42–15 years of experience	Female	Urban area	20–25 patients per day

one HCP, the HCPs did not specify any actions in their daily professional practice in which they took this knowledge into consideration.

As no national clinical guidelines on ABs exist in Albania, the HCPs stated that their basis for AB knowledge and AB-related practices came from continuing educational activities, such as materials on the internet, visits from pharmaceutical company representatives, discussions with colleagues, and their formal education.

Attitudes

A common understanding between all interviewee groups existed that if a patient suffered from flu/cold symptoms for 2–3 days and OTC medicines had not cured the symptoms within this period, then patients needed stronger medication to recover, i.e., ABs. Most of the interviewees described a condition that they referred to as 'flu complications'.

The patients and HCPs both seemed to have a high level of trust in ABs, particularly amoxicillin-clavulanic acid and azithromycin. The patients appeared to believe that their symptoms could always be cured. In addition, the physicians and pharmacists described the need to give guarantees to patients that the medicines would work and the blame patients placed on HCPs if their conditions were not cured.

A pressure to satisfy patients was thus felt by both physicians and pharmacists. If patients were not satisfied, then they threatened to choose another pharmacy or physician whom they believed could better help them. Both groups of HCPs admitted that this could lead to professional practices that were not always optimal. The pharmacists especially expressed feeling pressured by patients to sell ABs OTC as if they refused patient would then turn to another pharmacy. Hence, situations in which patients requested specific ABs without prescriptions were common. However, the physicians did not express receiving pressure to prescribe ABs in this way because if patients truly wanted ABs, then they would obtain them directly from the pharmacy.

Behaviour

In addition to the concept of treating 'flu complications' with ABs, both the patients and HCPs also described several situations in which ABs were prescribed or sold to prevent further worsening of flu or cold symptoms, e.g., patients who were busy at work.

As described, many patients turned directly to pharmacies to obtain ABs without a prescription. For most interviewees, including physicians, this type of practice seemed to be an accepted behaviour. The patients turned directly to pharmacies for multiple reasons; for example, their symptoms were perceived to be manageable. In these situations, some patients would request a specific AB with which they had previous positive experiences, or they would request a general AB. A pattern of self-diagnosis was thus identified. Patients mainly sought physicians when they had severe symptoms, symptoms that they had not previously experienced or if the situation concerned their children.

In situations where patients requested a general AB, the pharmacists would inquire about the patients' former experiences with ABs when deciding what action to take. To ensure the effectiveness of the AB, several pharmacists often selected broad-spectrum ABs.

Regarding physician practices, it was observed that diagnostic tests were usually not available at public clinics. The physicians also described that the test results often took several days to receive. Therefore, physicians instead relied on their clinical observations, which they believed to be sufficient in most cases, to make a proper diagnosis. Several physicians, however, expressed that they would like to use rapid tests.

It also seemed to be common practice for physicians to ask patients if they could afford to pay beyond the public reimbursement scheme, which would allow physicians to prescribe a wider range of ABs – including some injectable broad-spectrum ABs.

Discussion

Several factors were identified that arguably could lead to an increased risk of AMR. The patients showed little awareness of the differences between viruses and bacteria; however, they often self-diagnosed, which led them to request ABs from pharmacies without a prescription. Especially community pharmacists felt pressured to give in to patients' demands. Pharmacists often chose broad-spectrum ABs to ensure the treatment's effectiveness. All of the participants (including HCP) showed incorrect beliefs about illness severity as they all appeared to believe that 'flu complications', i.e. flu/cold symptoms that persisted after 2–3 days, should be treated with ABs even preventatively. Physicians' attitudes and practices were also found problematic. Hence, physicians usually had no rapid tests to guide them in their practice; however, they were not concerned about this fact. Further, HCPs acknowledged AMR, but only a few of them seemed to consider its risk in their daily practice.

Limitations

A relatively small number of people were interviewed within each interviewee group with regard to the typical AB culture thereby challenging the validity of the results. However, due to the specific design of the study, comparisons between the four groups' were applied. These comparisons allowed researchers to identify relatively consistent patterns across the groups, and hence only consistent patterns are reported in this paper.

As qualitative research in general, this study points to issues of relevance to the investigated topic and we can therefore not draw conclusions as to whether the results are transferable to all patients and HCPs in the country including the frequency and extent of the observed tendencies. Several of our results have been confirmed by quantitative studies in the country, including the results related to the common practice of selling ABs without a prescription in community pharmacies in Albania and the practice of buying ABs outside the national reimbursement scheme, which underlines the argument that relevant aspects to AB use culture have been identified in this study [18, 19].

The results might be biased as most interviews were conducted in cities, and rural AB practices might differ from these patterns. Additionally, as the participants were recruited through snowballing sampling; some participants were remotely acquainted with the researchers, why they may have exhibited more rational AB behaviour or having higher knowledge about ABs than the general population of patients and HCPs. However, all of the interviewed pharmacists admitted to illegally selling ABs (perhaps due to not recording the interviews), which showed that this type of behaviour was also captured in the sample. The snowball sampling strategy further proved suboptimal since it led to the recruitment of a few patients who did not fit all of the initial inclusion criteria. The challenges of not recording the interviews were the loss of details and a generally higher risk of misinterpreted results due to only having (selective) notes.

Despite these limits, the specific aim of using qualitative methods to explore AB knowledge attitudes and behaviours appears to have been achieved, as several patterns potentially leading to irrational use of AB were identified.

Reasons behind inappropriate behaviour

The patients often self-diagnosed, and thus the practice of purchasing ABs without a prescription was common. Physicians and especially pharmacists gave in to patient demands despite not always being comfortable doing so. This was a very unfortunate finding since HCPs are the final gatekeepers to the prudent use of ABs.

According to recent literature, pharmacists sell AB illegally OTC (although recognising that this is against the standards set by regulatory authorities) for three overall reasons: commercial interests, feeling pity for/ wanting to help the patient or finding it counterproductive to resist patient demand for AB as they could easily then obtain the AB in another pharmacy [29–31]. Pharmacists in Albania seem in particular influenced by the latter i.e. to think that refusing patient to have AB OTC will have no effect why they eventually gave in and sold ABs.

In this study, one of the reasons for patients' strong desire for ABs (and therefore pressure on pharmacists to dispense) was the belief that ABs could relieve them of bothersome symptoms. This high level of patient trust in ABs has likewise been reported in other countries, and a study conducted in Russia and Lithuania found that prescribing ABs for URTI has become an integral and even common practice for these types of infections [6].

Another strong 'belief precursor' found in this study for high AB consumption in Albania was the widely recognized however overestimated condition of 'flu complications' in terms of severity and need of AB treatment.

Although western physicians also justify prescribing ABs according to symptom severity and duration, ABs were prescribed for 'flu complications' of shorter durations and for less serious symptoms than, for example, conditions called 'toxic' by British physicians [32]. Patients in western countries have likewise been demonstrated to endure symptoms of RTI for more than 2–3 days before seeking the help of a health care professional [33].

Prescribing ABs as a preventive measure was also observed in this study. This practice has also been reported in the West but likely to a lesser degree and mostly in specific situations. For example, a German study showed a 23% increase in the prescription of ABs on Fridays [34]. This finding was confirmed by a Norwegian study in which physicians tended to prescribe more ABs right before the weekend to help their patients avoid queues at emergency departments over the weekend [35].

The specific Albanian case

The differences in Albanian HCPs' quick decisions to prescribe and sell broad-spectrum ABs might be explained by this study's findings showing that HCPs shared patients' high level of trust particularly in broad-spectrum ABs and the common idea of 'flu complications'. This was supported by the results, which showed that some of the HCPs lacked pharmacological knowledge about ABs. Hence, physicians in other countries appear to disagree more often with their patients when prescribing ABs, and they then try to negotiate with patients to find a solution, than what was observed in this study [22].

Another reason for irrational prescribing or dispensing of broad-spectrum AB might pertain to diagnostic uncertainty, which was reported by Albanian pharmacists and likewise reported by physicians in western countries [4]. Whereas many physicians in western countries report relying on delayed prescribing, adhering to guidelines or use a variety of clinical tests as a way to reduce uncertainty [8, 35–37], Albanian pharmacists often choose broad-spectrum ABs as a strategy to reduce uncertainty, i.e., playing it safe. In contrast, Albanian physicians expressed very little diagnostic uncertainty despite the lack of rapid tests, which is an attitude that has also been shown among physicians from other non-western countries [8].

In Sweden it was found that physicians, who used less structured approaches to diagnose the cause of sore throat, were more concerned about differential diagnoses to and complications of the observed condition compared for example to physicians strictly adhering to guidelines or using clinical tests in a structure manner [36, 37]. If this understanding is general and also pertains to Albanian physicians using unstructured diagnostic approaches, it could explain why Albanian physicians find it necessary often to prescribe AB in these situations which then leads to irrational prescribing.

To target AB behaviours linked to insufficient knowledge and inappropriate attitudes, the underlying culture and social infrastructure have to be taken into account. In Albania, this could include paying attention to the current lack of access to primary care services, as 1/3 of the Albanian population are not entitled to free medical consultations. Reimbursing all or most of the price of regular AB prescriptions could be considered, because at the current time, reimbursements for ABs with a prescription reduce the total price only by approximately 12%, giving patients little financial incentive to seek a prescription from a physician. However, physicians in Lithuania have now suggested the opposite i.e. no reimbursement for ABs at all, as they believe reimbursement leads to higher consumption [12]. Hence, using reimbursement as a regulatory mean to control use of ABs can be challenging.

Other initiatives might include launching public campaigns to raise the public's awareness about taking ABs in 'special' cases, as this has proven successful in other countries [8]. A restructuring of the microbial test system could also be introduced to provide results to physicians earlier [7, 38], although not all of the physicians in this study seemed to believe that rapid tests were necessary. Academic detailing helping physicians to reflect on their own practices could promote an adjustment to this attitude [7, 8], especially as continuing medical education activities are lacking. Currently in Albania, while a continuing education (CE) system for physicians, dentists and pharmacists exists, it is not well structured, and the responsibility falls on the HCP to seek annual credits on CE activities and select the type and field of CE activity in which to participate. Hence, the CE system in Albania is not prioritizing what are the professional needs that HPs have to fulfil. Finally, it is essential that laws regarding the prescribing and dispensing of ABs, are enforced.

Conclusions

A multitude of reasons for the inappropriate use of antibiotics in Albania was identified. Patients' exhibited high level of trust in ABs and subsequently requested AB prescriptions or illegally purchasing them over-the-counter, even for flu-like symptoms lasting for 2–3 days. Health care professionals did not appear to negotiate with patients' demands; pharmacists preferred to play it safe using broad-spectrum antibiotics, and physicians were overly confident in their ability to diagnose infections without rapid tests. Especially pharmacists were found to give in to selling antibiotics because they did not believe that they could change the current system.

Suggested initiatives in the future include introducing higher reimbursement for prescribed antibiotics, academic detailing to avoid misunderstanding of proper antibiotic use and public awareness campaigns.

Abbreviations
ABs: Antibiotics; AMR: Antimicrobial resistance; HCP (including physicians and community pharmacists): Health care professional; OTC: Over-the-counter; SSC: Section of Social and Clinical Pharmacy, University of Copenhagen; URTI: Upper respiratory tract infection

Funding
The Health Technology and Pharmaceuticals group of the WHO, Regional Office for Europe covered different expenses in relation to the study (for example, travel costs of the different researchers) including fees for some specific tasks that were conducted by researchers from the Section for Social and Clinical Pharmacy, University of Copenhagen. The WHO group provided input on the design of the study but did not take part in the data collection, the data analysis/interpretation or in writing the manuscript.

Authors' contribution
SK developed the idea, design and data collection instruments of the project; AM and IH revised the developed materials, AM and IH translated the materials into Albanian and collected the data; AM and IH translated the transcript-notes into English; SK, AM and IH carried out the analysis together; SK wrote the draft for the manuscript; AM and IH revised the manuscript; SK, AM and IH have all read and approved of the final manuscript.

Competing interests
The authors declare that they have no competing interests.

Author details
[1]Department of Pharmacy, Section for Social and Clinical Pharmacy, Faculty of Health and Medical Sciences, University of Copenhagen, Universitetsparken 2, 2100 København Ø, Denmark. [2]Faculty of Pharmacy, University of Medicine Tirana, Albania, Fakulteti Farmacise, Rr. Dibres 371, 1000 Tirana, Albania.

References
1. EuropeanCommission. Antimicrobial resistance. Health and Food Safety; 2015. http://ec.europa.eu/dgs/health_food-safety/amr/index_en.htm. Accessed 31 Aug 2015.
2. Versporten A, Bolokhovets G, Ghazaryan L, et al. Antibiotic use in eastern Europe: a cross-national database study in coordination with the WHO Regional Office for Europe. Lancet Infect Dis. 2014;14:381–7.
3. Kaae S, Sporrong SK, Traulsen JM, et al. Experiences from a pilot study on how to conduct a qualitative multi-country research project regarding use of antibiotics in Southeast Europe. J Pharm Policy Pract. 2016;9(20). doi:10.1186/s40545-016-0069-3.
4. Rodrigues A, Roque F, Falcao A, et al. Understanding physician antibiotic prescribing behaviour: a systematic review of qualitative studies. Int J Antimicrob Agents. 2013;41:203–12.
5. Lopez-Vazquez P, Varquez-Lago J, Figueiras A. Misprescription of antibiotics in primary care: a critical systematic review of its determinants. J Eval Clin Pract. 2012;18:473–84.
6. Jaruseviciene L, Radzeviciene-Jurgute R, Lazarus JV, et al. A study of antibiotic prescribing: the experience of Lithuanian and Russian GPs. CEJ Med. 2012;7(6):790–9.
7. Tonkin-Crine S, Yardley L, Little P. Antibiotic prescribing for acute respiratory

tract infections in primary care: a systematic review and meta-ethnography. J Antimicrob Chemother. 2011;66:2215–23.

8. Rezal RS, Hassali MA, Alrasheedy AA, et al. Physicians' knowledge, perception and behaviour towards antibiotic prescribing: a systematic review of the literature. Expert Rev Anti Infect Ther. 2015;13(5):665–80.

9. Giblin T, Sinkowitz-Cochran R, Harris P, et al. Clinicans' perceptions of the problem of antimicrobial resistance in health care facilities. Arch Intern Med. 2004;164:1662–8.

10. EuropeanCommission. Antimicrobial resistance. Special Eurobarometer 407. 2013. http://ec.europa.eu/health/sites/health/files/antimicrobial_resistance/docs/ebs_407_en.pdf. Accessed 30 Aug 2015.

11. Safrany N, Monnet DL. Antibiotics obtained without prescription in Europe. Lancet Infect Dis. 2012;12:182–3.

12. Jaruseviciene L, Jurgute RR, Bjerrum L, et al. Enabling factors for antibiotic prescribing for upper respiratory tract infections: Perspectives of Lithuanian and Russian general practitioners. Ups J Med Sci. 2013;118:98–104.

13. Morgan D, Okeke I, Laxminarayan R, et al. Non-prescription antimicrobial use worldwide: a systematic review. Lancet Infect Dis. 2011;11:692–701.

14. Markovic-Pekovic V, Grubisa N. Self-medication with antibiotics in the Republic of Srpska community pharmacies: pharmacy staff behavior. Pharmacoepidemiol Drug Saf. 2012;21:1130–3.

15. Decision of Council of Minister.No.695. Për miratimin e kuadrit makroekonimik e fiskal të rishikuar për periudhën 2016 – 2018 [Approval of the macroeconomic and fiscal framework for the period 2016 - 2018, revised]. 2015.

16. Law no. 10383. Për sigurimin e detyrueshëm të kujdesit shëndetësor në Republikën e Shqipërisë", i ndryshuar [Compulsory health care in the Republic of Albania, revised] 2011.

17. Decision of Council of Minister.No. 24. Për miratimin e structures dhe mënyrës së funkdionimit e organizimit të Agjencisë Kombëtare të Barnave dhe Pajisjeve Mjekësore [Approval of the structure of functioning and organizing of the National Agency for Medicines and Medical Devices] 2015.

18. Hoxha I, Malaj A, Malaj L. Antibiotic use in Albania between 2011 and 2012. J Infect Dev Ctries. 2015;9(1):94–8.

19. Hoxha I, Malaj A, Tako R, et al. Survey on how antibiotics are dispensed in community pharmacies in Albania. Int J Pharm Pharm Sci. 2015;7(7):449–50.

20. Currea GC, Siersma VD, Lopez-Valcarcel BG, et al. Prescribing style and variation in antibiotic prescriptions for sore throat: cross-scetional study across six countries. BMC Fam Pract. 2015;16(7):1–8.

21. Kvale S. Interviews: an introduction to qualitative research interviewing. 1st ed. London: Sage Publications; 1996.

22. Strandberg EL, Brorsson A, Hagstam C, et al. I'm Dr Jekyll and Mr Hyde: Are GPs' antibiotic prescribing patterns contextually dependent? A qualitative focus group study. Scand J Prim Health Care. 2013;31:158–65.

23. Heikkinen T, Järvinen A. The common cold. Lancet. 2003;361:51–9.

24. Barton E, Spencer R. URTIs: recommended diagnosis and treatment in general practice. Prescriber. 2011;22(8):23–36.

25. Groleau D, Young A, Kirmayer L. The McGill Illness Narrative Interview (MINI): An interview schedule to elicit meanings and modes of reasoning related to illness experience. Transcul Psychiatry. 2006;43(4):671–91.

26. Kaae S, Traulsen J. Qualitative methods in pharmacy practice research. In: Pharmacy Practice Research Methods (ed Z-U-D Babar). Springer: Heidelberg; 2015. p. 49–68.

27. Bowling A. Research methods in health - investigating health and health services. 2nd ed. Berkshire: Open University Press; 2002.

28. Hsieh H, Shannon S. Three approaches to qualitative content analysis. Qual Health Res. 2005;15(9):1277–88.

29. Gebretekle GB, Serbessa M. Exploration of over the counter sales of antibiotics in community pharmacies of Addis Ababa, Ethiopia: pharmacy professionals perspective. Antimicrob Resist Infect Control. 2016; 5(2). doi:10.1186/s13756-016-0101-z.

30. Ghiga I, Lundborg C. 'Struggling to be a defender of health' - a qualitative study on the pharmacists' perceptions of their role in antibiotic consumption and antibiotic resistance in Romania. J Pharm Policy Pract. 2016;9(10). doi:10.1186/s40545-016-0061-y.

31. Salim AM, Elgizoli B. Exploring the reasons why pharmacists dispense antibiotics without prescription in Khartoum state, Sudan. Int J Pharm Pract. 2017;25:59–65.

32. Kumar S, Little P, Britten N. Why do general practitioners prescribe

antibiotics for sore thorat? Grounded theory interview study. Br Med J. 2003; 326(138):1–6.

33. Dekker A, Verheij TJ. Velden AWvd. Inappropriate antibiotic prescription for respiratory tract indications: most prominent in adult patients. Fam Pract. 2015;32(4):401–7.

34. Kuehlein T, Szecsenyi J, Gutscher A, et al. Antibiotic prescribing in general practice–the rhythm of the week: a cross-sectional study. J Antimicrob Chemother. 2010;65:2666–8.

35. Høye S, Frich JC, Lindbæk M. Delayed prescribing for upper respiratory infections: a qualitative study of GPs' views and experiences. Br J Gen Pract. 2010;60:907–12.

36. André M, Gröndal H, Strandberg E, et al. Uncertainty in clinical practice - an interview study with Swedish GPs on patients with sore throat. BMC Fam Pract. 2016;17(56). doi:10.1186/s17875-016-0452-9.

37. Hedin K, Strandberg E, Gröndal H, et al. Management of patients with sore throats in relation to guidelines: An interview study in Sweden. Scand J Prim Health Care. 2017;1502–7724 (Online). doi:10.3109/02813432.2014.972046.

38. Rezal RS, Hassali MA, Alrasheedy AA, et al. Prescribing patterns for upper respiratory tract infections: a prescription-review of primary care practice in Kedah, Malaysia and the implications. Expert Rev Anti Infect Ther. 2015; 13(12):1547–56.

12

Comparison of medicines management strategies in insurance schemes in middle-income countries

Warren A. Kaplan[1], Paul G. Ashigbie[1], Mohamad I. Brooks[1,2] and Veronika J. Wirtz[1*]

Abstract

Background: Many middle-income countries are scaling up health insurance schemes to provide financial protection and access to affordable medicines to poor and uninsured populations. Although there is a wealth of evidence on how high income countries with mature insurance schemes manage cost-effective use of medicines, there is limited evidence on the strategies used in middle-income countries. This paper compares the medicines management strategies that four insurance schemes in middle-income countries use to improve access and cost-effective use of medicines among beneficiaries.

Methods: We compare key strategies promoting cost-effective medicines use in the New Rural Cooperative Medical Scheme (NCMS) in China, National Health Insurance Scheme in Ghana, Jamkesmas in Indonesia and Seguro Popular in Mexico. Through the peer-reviewed and grey literature as of late 2013, we identified strategies that met our inclusion criteria as well as any evidence showing if, and/or how, these strategies affected medicines management. Stakeholders involved and affected by medicines coverage policies in these insurance schemes were asked to provide relevant documents describing the medicines related aspects of these insurance programs. We also asked them specifically to identify publications discussing the unintended consequences of the strategies implemented.

Results: Use of formularies, bulk procurement, standard treatment guidelines and separation of prescribing and dispensing were present in all four schemes. Also, increased transparency through publication of tender agreements and procurement prices was introduced in all four. Common strategies shared by three out of four schemes were medicine price negotiation or rebates, generic reference pricing, fixed salaries for prescribers, accredited preferred provider network, disease management programs, and monitoring of medicines purchases. Cost-sharing and payment for performance was rarely used. There was a lack of performance monitoring strategies in all schemes.

Conclusions: Most of the strategies used in the insurance schemes focus on containing expenditure growth, including budget caps on pharmaceutical expenditures (Mexico) and ceiling prices on medicines (all four countries). There were few strategies targeting quality improvement as healthcare providers are mostly paid through fixed salaries, irrespective of the quality of their prescribing or the health outcomes actually achieved. Monitoring healthcare system performance has received little attention.

Keywords: Health insurance, Drugs, Middle-income countries, China, Indonesia, Ghana, Mexico, Universal health coverage

* Correspondence: vwirtz@bu.edu
[1]Department of Global Health, Boston University School of Public Health, Crosstown Center, Room CT-363, 801 Massachusetts Avenue, Boston, Massachusetts 02118, USA
Full list of author information is available at the end of the article

Background

Over the last decade international agencies and individual countries have shown commitment to promote universal health coverage (UHC), defined as: "[...] ensuring that all people have access to needed promotive, preventive, curative and rehabilitative health services, of sufficient quality to be effective, while also ensuring that people do not suffer financial hardship when paying for these services" [1].

The World Health Organization (WHO) defines a series of necessary conditions to achieve UHC, one of which relates to medicines - "Access to essential medicines and technologies to diagnose and treat medical problems." Various authors have described in more detail how to define access and how to measure it [2, 3]. Nonetheless, how to balance medicines access, affordability, quality and sustainability of supply, has played a relatively minor role in discussions regarding UHC and the necessary conditions needed to achieve it [4]. Medicines management is critical to successful implementation of UHC but, until recently, few studies exist guiding policy development and implementation in low and middle-income countries.

Accordingly, we employ a case-based approach to study what strategies payers use to promote cost-effective use of medicines. We have chosen four insurance schemes in Mexico, China, Ghana and Indonesia, which provide coverage for poor and/or underserved populations. We compare the medicines management strategies to promote cost-effective use of medicines in these insurance schemes and discuss challenges in their implementation.

Methods

Selection of the countries

We chose four countries (China, Indonesia, Ghana and Mexico) which (1) are at different stages of development with regard to UHC of their population; (2) have different funding arrangements (e.g. social health insurance (SHI) or tax-based systems), and (3) are from different geographical regions. In addition, we also considered country income level and whether the health service providers are public or private.

Literature review and stakeholder interviews

We carried out a desk review of relevant peer-reviewed and grey literature related to UHC and medicines published between 2000 and 2013 for each of the four countries. To complement our review we conducted interviews with stakeholders (3 in China; 4 in Ghana, 1 each in Indonesia and Mexico) involved in developing medicines coverage policies or affected by these policies. We sought the perception of these stakeholders regarding relevant publications as well as administrative documents describing the medicines- related aspects of the health benefit or insurance programs. We also asked them specifically to identify publications discussing the unintended consequences of medicines coverage and pharmaceutical management policies in place.

Conceptual framework for analysis

Analytically, the medicines and finance policies used to balance access, affordability, quality and sustainability were divided into the following five broad categories [5]: (1) selection, (2) procurement, (3) contracting, (4) utilization management, and (5) monitoring member satisfaction, and purchasing and prescribing patterns.

For each of these broad categories, the public and private sectors have often-times competing interests with regard to UHC [4]. These interests are: (1) keeping costs affordable, (2) ensuring availability of quality generic and innovator products, (3) improving equitable access, and (4) ensuring appropriate use.

Results

Brief summary of scaling up health insurance coverage in each country studied

Table 1 describes the countries included and their respective characteristics as of 2014. They represent a range of insurance coverage from 39% in Ghana to approximately 100% for Mexico and China. Two countries have UHC with only government revenue funding (Indonesia, Mexico), two a mix of government revenues and beneficiary contribution (Ghana, China). Each country is from a different WHO Region. Two countries are lower-middle (Indonesia, Ghana) and two are upper-middle income countries (Mexico, China). An overview of the demographic, health and health care related indicators of the four countries chosen can be found in Appendix.

China

In China, three major health insurance programs cover specific groups: rural residents under the New Rural Cooperative Medical Scheme (NCMS), urban employees under the Urban Employees Basic Medical Insurance (UE-BMI), and unemployed urban residents under the Urban Residents Basic Medical Insurance (UR-BMI). We note that in early 2016, China announced the decision to merge the UR-BMI and NCMS schemes [6]. There will be unified coverage, a fund pooling mechanism, a benefits package and reimbursement rates, a basic medical insurance drug list, unified selection of health providers, and fund management. For the purpose of this retrospective study, only the NCMS will be analyzed as no evaluation has been made of the combined UR-BMI and NCMS schemes. Various experiments are also taking place at lower levels, giving the entire Chinese insurance system a very dynamic nature. The NCMS incorporates voluntary enrollment and coverage of catastrophic illnesses. Apart from these two requirements, the design and implementation of the program is

Table 1 Countries selected as case studies and the characteristics as of 2014

Country	Development stage of UHC[a] % population covered in the entire country[a]	Funding arrangement (year of inception)[b]	Geographical region (WHO region)	Country income level	Provider mix[b]
China	90%	NRCMS (2003): Premiums and federal and local government subsidies URBMI (2007): Premiums and government subsidies	WPR	UMIC	NRCMS: Largely private contractors URBMI: Largely public
Indonesia	40–63%	JAMKESMAS (2004): Government revenues	SEAR	LMIC	Jamkesmas: Nearly exclusively public
Ghana	39%	NHIS (2004): Social Health Insurance	AFR	LMIC	NHIS: Mixed public/private providers
Mexico	80–100%	SP (2003): Premiums and taxes	AMR	UMIC	SP: Nearly exclusively public

[a]The percentage of the population covered varies by data source and method of estimating coverage; hence, we report for some countries a range. Percentage coverage is based on most recent reporting or 2014, whichever is later

[b]This information refers to the reform program that specifically targets the poor population: NRCMS New Rural Coorperative Medical Scheme, URBMI Urban Residence Basic Medical Insurance, MoHME Ministry of Health and Medical Education, NHIS National Health Insurance Scheme, RHI Rural Health Insurance, SP Seguro Popular

Region: WPR Western Pacific Region, SEAR South-east Asian Region, AFR African Region, AMR Region of the Americas, EMR Eastern Mediterranean Region

left to local governments. An extensive survey in Western and Central China found the most common model of NCMS combines a medical savings account (MSA) and high-deductible catastrophic insurance for inpatient services. Eighty percent of the 10 RMB premium (about 1.5 USD as of this writing), is put into an MSA to pay for outpatient visits and can be shared among household members. The government's 20 RMB subsidy plus the remaining 2 RMB premium are pooled to cover inpatient hospital expenses above a certain deductible. The amount of the deductible varies by locale, with the majority of them above 400 RMB. Besides the deductible, patients still have to pay 40–60% of covered inpatient expenses. The benefit package also caps the benefit payment at 10,000–20,000 RMB. NCMS risk-pooling is at the county level, not the village level.

Indonesia

In 2005, the Askeskin program provided basic health coverage and medicines to the poor. This health insurance program was later expanded to include the near-poor in 2007 and renamed as Jamkesmas. The Jamkesmas program in 2012 had over 76 million beneficiaries – a third of the national population – and was the largest health insurance scheme in Indonesia [7]. Two other social health insurance schemes also existed in Indonesia: Askes was targeted to civil servants and had 17 million beneficiaries while Jamsostek enrolled 5 million employees in the private sector [7]. Combined, the three social health insurance programs covered 40% of the Indonesian population in 2012. However, the analysis in this study only looked at the Jamkesmas program from 2012–2013 and its medicines related benefits. We note that the Indonesian government enacted the Badan Penylenggara Jaminan Sosial (BPJS) law (Law No. 24/2011) in 2011 which was intended to unify all social health insurance programs under one

not-for-profit administrator in 2014. The Indonesian government rolled out the Jaminan Kesehatan National (JKN) program on January 1, 2014, with the ambition to achieve national UHC by January 2019 [8].

Ghana

In 2003, the National Health Insurance Authority (NHIA) was established as the regulator and the implementer of all health insurance schemes in the country (National Health Insurance Scheme (NHIS)). The NHIS is primarily financed by a 2.5 percentage top up of the Value Added Tax (National Health Insurance Levy) and a 2.5% levy of social security contributions made by formal sector employees (involuntary payroll deductions), and premiums paid by informal sector workers [9]. Both public and private health facilities are accredited to provide services under coverage by the NHIS. More than 50% of all patients, whether using the NHIS or not, seek care from the private sector [10]. These private institutions include for-profit standalone pharmacies and licensed chemical sellers, for profit hospitals and clinics and not-for-profit health providers (mission hospitals). Mission health facilities which account for a substantial proportion of district hospitals in the country are usually described as private not for profit but their health workers are on government employee payroll and they also benefit from government programs meant for the public sector. In total, government support to overall expenditure of mission health facilities budget is 34–35%; the remaining is internally generated. In terms of service delivery mission institutions provide 30% of inpatient care and 20% of outpatient care (personal communication from key informant). Apart from the NHIS there are a small number of private insurers which also offer insurance packages with medicines benefits to well-to-do clients and are outside the scope of this study which will focus on NHIS.

Mexico

In 2000 around 50% of the population did not have health insurance, mostly those working in the informal sector or the self-employed [11]. In the past, the entitlement of health insurance had been defined by employment status with those in formal employment and their dependents covered by social security [12]. With the creation of the national health insurance program called *Seguro Popular* in 2003 the Mexican government initiated to scale up UHC with the aim to reach 100% population coverage by 2010 (which was later extended to 2011). Affiliation was targeted towards the population previously not covered by social insurance. Official government sources declared 100% coverage in 2012 [13]. Seguro Popular seeks to provide health service coverage, through voluntary, public insurance for persons that are not affiliated to any social security institution. In 2014 it provided coverage for 275 medical interventions, described in the Universal Health Service Catalogue. *Seguro Popular* is operated at national level by the National Commission of Social Protection in Health (CNPSS). At State level the State *Seguro Popular* Fund Holders (REPSS) are responsible to manage funds and purchase care. As the health system is decentralized, the national policies are implemented in a heterogeneous manner throughout the states [14].

Strategies to promote cost-effective medicines use

For the four programs studied –NCMS, NHIS, Jamkesmas and Seguro Popular- strategies to select medicines were well documented in the literature. In contrast, purchasing, contracting and utilization were less well documented. Table 2 presents a comparison between the four programs.

The following strategies to promote cost-effective medicines use were common to all the four insurance programs (in bold in Table 2):

- use of formularies (at various levels in the healthcare system),
- bulk procurement,
- use of standard treatment guidelines and
- separation of prescribing and dispensing.

Formularies in the four cases were based on national essential medicines lists but each program adapting or modifying it for its specific needs. For instance, for the NCMS formularies, part of the medicines are selected from the national EML which in 2012 contained 520

Table 2 Overview of strategies used to promote cost-effective use of medicines in the four medicines benefit programs

Type of strategies	Strategies Medicines	NCMS (China)	National Health Insurance (Ghana)	Jamkesmas (Indonesia)	Seguro Popular (Mexico)
Selection	*Formulary*	✓	✓	✓	✓
	Cost sharing for medicines included in the formulary	✓	✗	✗	✗
	Generic substitution	✗	✓	✗	✗
Procurement	Medicines prices negotiation or rebates	✓	✗[c]	✓	(✓)
	Bulk procurement	✓	✓[a]	✓	✓
	Generic reference pricing	✗	✓	✗[a]	✓
Contracting	Fee for service for prescribers	✓			
	Fixed salary for prescribers[a]		✓	✓[a]	✓
	Fixed reimbursement rates for medicines	✓	✓	✗	✗
	Preferred provider network (accreditation)	✗	✓	✓	✓
Utilization	*Standard treatment guidelines*	(✓)	✓	✓	✓
	Payment for performance	(✓)	✗	✗	✗
	Separation of prescribing and dispensing	✓	✓	✓	✓
	Disease management programs	✓	No info	✓	✓
Monitoring and evaluation	User satisfaction monitoring	✗	✗	✗	✓
	Medicines purchasing monitoring	✓[b]		✓	✓
	Prescription monitoring	✗	✗	✗	✗

[a] = in the public sector; () = Limited use; [b] = information not publically available; [c] = healthcare facilities do their own negotiation with suppliers; italics = strategies common to all the four insurance programs

medicines, 317 Western and 203 Traditional. Since each province has their own EML (the National EML plus a provincial supplementary list), some medicines are taken from the provincial supplementary list. Programs made a distinction between medicines used at lower levels of care (e.g. primary care) versus those that should be available at high levels of care (second or tertiary care).

For all four programs the bulk procurement was done at regional level or national level (e.g. state or province). Systems to increase transparency of public procurement prices, volumes and bidding process were recently introduced in all of them [15–17]. Standard treatment guidelines had been developed in all four of them [18–21]. However, the extent to which they are implemented into clinical practice and linked to the selection of medicines for inclusion in the formulary varies. For instance, little information was found on the selection criteria of medicines included into the provincial formularies of NCMS and the establishment of evidence-based guidelines in contrast to experience-based care is a challenge in many settings [18]. In contrast, the formulary of Seguro Popular refers to clinical guidelines [22].

Furthermore, medicine price negotiation or rebates, generic reference pricing, fixed salaries for prescribers, accredited preferred provider network, disease management programs and monitoring of medicines purchases were implemented by three of the four schemes.

In Ghana, payment structures for public sector prescribers and dispensers is based on a policy which places all public service employees on a single vertical salary structure [23]. Thus prescribers are paid fixed salaries, irrespective of the quality and volume of services rendered. In Indonesia public health workers, including government physicians and pharmacists, receive a fixed salary independent of productivity or capitation [24]. In Mexico, prescribers in the public sector that provide services for Seguro Popular beneficiaries are paid by fixed salaries and do not receive any payment related to services provided (no financial incentives nor disincentives). Many physicians working in public health units also have their private consultancy offices [25].

In China, payment was linked to volume and type of dispensing services [15, 26, 27]. Whereas Indonesia [7] and Mexico (information provided by key informant) had fixed salaries for those filling prescriptions in the public sector, dispensing charges in China were included in the product reimbursements [27, 28]. There were no dispensing fees in Ghana [29].

There was a lack of information on payment for performance, monitoring user satisfaction and prescription monitoring.

Jamkesmas and Seguro Popular share many common strategies. In the case of Jamkesmas in Indonesia [7] and Seguro Popular in Mexico most providers (prescribers

and dispensers) are located in public clinics that operate under the provincial or state directed Ministry of Health [30]. Dispensing outlets and pharmacies are within the clinics. The decentralization of the health system in Indonesia and in Mexico results in variations in the pharmaceutical policy strategies implemented by provincial Jamkesmas administration [31] and state Seguro Popular Fundholders [32]. One important way in which Jamkesmas differs is in the variation in medicines procurement prices among provinces [33]. In Seguro Popular states are mandated to procure at a price that does not exceed a certain amount [34]. In addition to public and private hospitals and clinics, the NHIS in Ghana contracts private standalone pharmacies, and licensed chemical sellers to dispense medicines [29].

The rapid changes and large regional differences in the NCMS in China have made it difficult to describe the current general strategies to promote access and utilization via this insurance scheme. Users have to pay a deductible before the schemes start covering medicines [28, 35]. The coverage has a cap after a maximum insurance payment has been reached in a given time frame [28, 35, 36].

Reported impact of strategies of promote cost-effective use of medicines

With regard to China, in terms of the consequences of financing strategies on availability, access, and use of medicines, as well as on household and health system affordability, early cross-sectional appraisals of the health reforms found lower medicines prices in primary care facilities [37]. However, impacts of the health reform on generally low availability [38], total number of prescriptions [39, 40] or less-than-appropriate use [41] was not clear.

In Ghana, expenditures on medicines had increased after the introduction of NHIS [42, 43]. Supplier induced demand for medicines in private hospitals have also been documented [44]. Another study has shown that enrollment patterns did not match well with the medicines utilization changes and the authors have questioned whether the increased spending has improved equity in access and appropriate use [45].

In Ghana and Indonesia, key informants considered the claims-processing systems inefficient, which is often paper-based rather than electronic, and require resource-consuming reviews. Inefficient claims-review systems can lead to delays in payments to facilities, shortages of facility funds to purchase medicines, and medicines stock-outs [9].

In Mexico, no decrease in household expenditure on medicines was found 10 months after the introduction of the insurance scheme [46] or no statistically significant difference in household expenditure was found in comparison to households not insured by Seguro Popular [47].

Discussion

This study compares strategies to promote cost-effective use of medicines in insurance schemes targeting poor populations in middle-income countries. Whereas medicines policies to manage medicines in insurance schemes in high-income countries are well documented there is a lack of evidence from low- and middle-income countries [48, 49]. Transferability of evidence from high-income settings is limited and the creation of knowledge from low- and middle-income countries is relevant particularly given that many of them are making strides to move towards UHC. Our study contributes to the creation of evidence by analyzing four schemes operating in middle-income countries as case studies.

The results show that the identified country strategies aim to contain expenditure growth through budget caps on pharmaceutical expenditures (Mexico) and medicines price limits (all four countries). Moreover, all four schemes use strategies for cost containment through selection, bulk procurement and standard treatment guidelines. Price negotiation and rebates are also very common (China, Indonesia and Mexico). All these policies and practices including tendering are also commonly implemented in high-income settings [49].

However, the results show that there are a series of challenges in policies that aim to improve performance e.g. providers are mostly paid through fixed salaries, irrespective of the quality of their prescribing efficiency or the health outcomes actually achieved. On one hand, fixed salaries can protect against financial incentives to over-prescribe certain medicines for which prescribers receive a bonus [50]. On the other side, lack of incentives reinforcing good performance or sanctions to impede low quality can result in inadequate prescribing [51]. Policies to improve quality improvement are often more challenging to implement effectively; for instance, payment for performance requires advanced information systems to collect data on provider performance; the availability of such systems is usually limited in middle-income countries [52].

Three of the four schemes do not have cost sharing systems in place, in other words, beneficiaries receive the medicines included in the benefit package free of any co-payment. This protected individuals from financial hardship and out-of-pocket expenditure. An exception was China where there are many different kinds of cost-sharing schemes [53]. It is important to note that there is some evidence of cost-sharing in the Chinese NCMS reducing financial risk of the beneficiaries.

Of the four countries, only Ghana has generic substitution, an advantage in containing costs. Whether it is useful to introduce a generic substitution policy for cost containment depends very much on the context, such as architecture of the pharmaceutical supply and reimbursement system in place. Generic substitution policies are uncommon in systems where the same institution procures, distributes, and dispenses medicines. By design, these schemes procure generic medicines whenever available; originator or brand medicines are not available at the point of dispensing.

Finally, there was little information on any systematic monitoring and publishing performance metrics of medicines prescribing and expenditure by these insurance schemes. For instance, it was unclear how performance of prescribers was monitored, used for feedback or to inform future interventions to promote more appropriate use of medicines. The absence of information is not sufficient to say that schemes do not carry out these activities. In case these insurance schemes lack monitoring systems and performance metrics it will be challenging to implement the aforementioned policies efficiently, track their impact and adjust them if necessary.

The interpretation of the study results should take into consideration the following limitations: the analysis of strategies did not include an assessment of how well they were implemented. In addition, there is limited evidence to evaluate their impact on cost-effective use and access. Furthermore, rapid changes in strategies implemented by each of these insurance schemes make it difficult to keep track and accurately report the status quo. However, this is a limitation that applies to other policy analyses due to the nature of systems that are constantly changing. For certain types of strategies, it was easier to obtain information such as a selection of medicines (e.g. for instance, formularies were publiclly available). In contrast, strategies on procurement and reimbursement of providers were much harder to identify and report on. Hence, underreporting on these strategies is possible. However, we asked stakeholders specifically to provide us with information on documentation gaps to avoid publication bias.

Conclusions

Moving towards UHC requires countries to promote efficient use of financial resources in all areas of health services including medicines. Insurance schemes in middle-income countries have used a variety of strategies to ensure cost-effective use of medicines; there is no single strategy that will be suitable for all middle-income countries. There is an opportunity for insurance schemes to expand the type of strategies from cost-containment strategies towards those that incentivize quality use of medicines. To that end, we have identified a number of policy gaps that insurance schemes should address, in particular performance based payments and monitoring and performance metrics. Insurance schemes should pay closer attention to these policies.

Appendix

Table 3 Country profiles of four countries included in the case studies (2010)

	Indonesia	China	Ghana	Mexico
Demographics				
Number of inhabitants in 1,000 s	242,326	1,355,243	24,966	114.8
Life expectancy in years 2011				
Male	68	74	62	72
Female	71	77	65	78
Population distribution				
Median age	28	35	21	27
% population under 15	27	19	38	29
% population over 60	8	13	6	9
Economics and health systems financing				
Income group	Lower middle	Upper middle	Lower middle	Upper middle
% total health expenditure of GDP	2.8	5.0	5.2	6.3
% public expenditure of THE	36.1	54.3	58.2	49.0
% pharmaceutical expenditure of THE	1/3			
per capita total expenditure on health (PPP int. $)	123	373	85	962
Health indicators				
Age-standardized mortality rates by NCD (per 100,000 population) 2008	647	604	711	493
Prevalence of raised fasting blood glucose among adults aged ≥ 25 years] (%) 2008				
Male	6.6	9.6	9.9	13.2
Female	7.1	9.4	10.3	14.9
Prevalence of raised blood pressure among adults aged ≥ 25 years 2008				
Male	32.5	29.8	32.7	27.4
Female	29.3	25.6	31.6	21.5
Adults aged ≥20 years who are obese, 2008				
Male	2.5	4.6	4.4	26.7
Female	6.9	6.5	11.7	38.4
Prevalence of smoking any tobacco product among adults aged ≥15 years (%), 2009				
Male	61	51	11	24
Female	5	2	3	8
Alcohol consumption Among adults aged ≥15 years (litres of pure alcohol per person per year) 2008	0.6	5.6	3.1	8.6
Maternal mortality, 2011 Deaths per 100 000 live births	220	37	350	50
Under five mortality, 2011 Total number of such deaths per 1000 live births	151	15	78	16
Vaccination measles Immunization coverage among 1-year-olds (%) 2011	89	99	91	98
HIV prevalence HIV infections per 100 000 population per year	155	...	907	156
Health systems capacity				
Number of physicians per 10,000 inhabitants	2.0	14.6	0.9	19.6
Hospital beds (per 10,000 population)	6	39	9	17
Formal population coverage (% covered by insurance or tax-based arrangements)	40–60%			75–100%
Year of implementation UHC	2005			2003

Abbreviations

BPJS: Badan penyelenggara jaminan sosial; CNPSS: National commission of social protection in health; JKN: Jaminan kesehatan national; MSA: Medical savings account; NCMS: New rural cooperative medical scheme; NHIA: National health insurance authority; REPSS: State *Seguro Popular* fund holders; UE-BMI: Urban employees basic medical insurance; UHC: Universal health coverage; UR-BMI: Urban residents basic medical insurance; WHO: World Health Organization

Acknowledgements

We would like thank all the interviewees who participated in the study. In particular, we wish to acknowledge Maryam Bigdeli (World Health Organization), David H. Peters (Johns Hopkins Bloomberg School of Public Health) and Anita K. Wagner (Harvard Medical School and Harvard Pilgrim Health Care Institute) who originally proposed the idea of using the Faden et al. conceptual framework to analyze medicines in insurance schemes.

Funding

This paper is submitted as part of a special series that follows the publication of the Flagship Report on Access to Medicines from a Health Systems Perspective. The desk research in 2014 was funded by a grant of the Alliance for Health Policy and Systems Research. The Alliance for Health Policy and Systems Research provided input to the design of the study; data collection, analysis, and interpretation of data and in writing the manuscript were done independently.

Authors' contributions

VJW, PGA, WAK and MIB carried out data collection and analysis, and developed the first draft of the manuscript. VJW developed the first draft of the manuscript. All authors revised the manuscript, read and approved the final manuscript.

Competing interest

The authors declare that they have no competing interests.

Author details

[1]Department of Global Health, Boston University School of Public Health, Crosstown Center, Room CT-363, 801 Massachusetts Avenue, Boston, Massachusetts 02118, USA. [2]Pathfinder International, 9 Galen Street, Suite 217, Watertown 02472, Massachusetts, USA.

References

1. World Health Organization. Universal Health Coverage. Geneva: World Health Organization; 2015. Available at: http://www.who.int/mediacentre/factsheets/fs395/en/.
2. Bigdeli M, Jacobs B, Tomson G, Laing R, Ghaffar A, Dujardin B, Van Damme W. Access to medicines from the health system perspective. Health Policy Plan. 2013;28(7):692–704.
3. Yaghoubifard S, Rashidian A, Kebriaeezadeh A, Majdzadeh R, Hosseini SA, Akbari Sari A, Salamzadeh J. Developing a conceptual framework and a tool for measuring access to, and use of, medicines at household level (HH-ATM tool). Public Health. 2015;129(5):444–52.
4. Bigdeli M, Peters DH, Wagner AK. Medicines in Health Systems: advancing access, affordability and appropriate use. Geneva: Alliance for Health Systems and Policy Research/World Health Organization; 2013.
5. Faden L, Vialle-Valentin C, Ross-Degnan D, Wagner A. Active pharmaceutical management strategies of health insurance systems to improve cost-effective use of medicines in low- and middle-income countries: a systematic review of current evidence. Health Policy. 2011;100(2-3):134–43. http://dx.doi.org/10.1016/j.healthpol.2010.10.020.
6. Pan X-F, Xu J, Meng Q. Integrating social health insurance systems in China. Lancet. 2016;387:1274–5. http://www.thelancet.com/pdfs/journals/lancet/PIIS0140-6736(16)30021-6.pdf.
7. Harimurti P, Pambudi E, Pigazzini A, Tandon A. The nuts and bolts of Jamkesmas: Indonesia's government-financed health coverage programme. Washington (DC): World Bank; 2013.
8. Van Minh H, Pocock NS, Chaiyakunapruk N, Chhorvann C, Duc HA, Hanvoravongchai P, Lim J, Lucero-Prisno DE, Ng N, Phaholyothin N, Phonvisay A, Soe KM, Sychareun V. Progress toward universal health coverage in ASEAN. Glob Health Action. 2014; 7: doi: 10.3402/gha.v7.25856.
9. Apoya P, Marriott A. Achieving a Shared Goal: Free Universal Health Care in Ghana. Oxfam International, 2011. Avalable at http://www.oxfam.org/sites/www.oxfam.org/files/rr-achieving-shared-goal-healthcare-ghana-090311-en.pdf.
10. Saleh K. The health sector in Ghana, A comprehensive assessment. World Bank; 2013. Available at https://openknowledge.worldbank.org/handle/10986/12297.
11. Lakin JM. The End of Insurance? Mexico's Seguro Popular, 2001 - 2007. J Health Polit Policy Law. 2010.
12. Organization for Economic Cooperation and Development (OECD). Reviews of Health Systems: Mexico. Paris: OECD, 2016. http://www.oecd.org/publications/oecd-reviews-of-health-systems-mexico-2016-9789264230491-en.htm.
13. Presidencia de la Republica. Cobertura universal, un hito. Available at: http://calderon.presidencia.gob.mx/2012/11/cobertura-universal-de-salud-un-hito/. Accessed 23 June 2016.
14. Nigenda G, Wirtz VJ, González-Robledo LM, Reich MR. Evaluating the Implementation of Mexico's Health Reform: The Case of Seguro Popular. Health Syst Reform. 2015;1(3):217–28.
15. Tang S, Tao J, Bekedam H. Controlling cost escalation of healthcare: making universal health coverage sustainable in China. BMC Public Health. 2012;12 Suppl 1:S8. doi:10.1186/1471-2458-12-S1-S8.
16. Chunlin J, Wang L, Duan G, et al. Analysis and Suggestion on the current situation of the Essential Medicines Bidding and Procurement in China. Chinese Health Econ. 2013;32:80–1.
17. Public Procurement Authority (2003), Ghana. Manuals - Public Procurement Act, (Act 663) Available at: http://www.ppaghana.org/documents/FINALMANUAL_PPB.pdf?story_id=23.
18. Cheng T-M. A Pilot Project Using Evidence-Based Clinical Pathways And Payment Reform In China's Rural Hospitals Shows Early Success. Health Affairs. 2013. doi: 10.1377/hlthaff.2012.0640 http://content.healthaffairs.org/content/early/2013/04/01/hlthaff.2012.0640.full.html.
19. Zhang X-l, Yang X-w, Guo C-c, et al. Research on the variation of income and expenditure of County Public medical Institution in Shaanxi by Zero-Profit Drug Policy. Chinese Health Econ. 2009;9(1):20. http://en.cnki.com.cn/Article_en/CJFDTOTAL-WEIJ201211025.htm.
20. China clinical pathway network: pilot hospitals (2015), Available at: http://www.ch-cp.org.cn/m.php?name=hospital&mo_order=9.
21. Ministry of Health (2010) Standard Treatment Guidelines, Ghana, 2010. Available at: http://apps.who.int/medicinedocs/documents/s18015en/s18015en.pdf.
22. Comisión Nacional para la Protección Social en Salud/Seguro Popular. Catalogo Universal de Servicios de Salud. 2012. México, DF: CNPSS, 2012. http://www.oecd.org/publications/oecd-reviews-of-health-systems-mexico-2016.
23. Antwi J, Phillips D. Wages and health worker retention in Ghana: evidence from public sector wage reforms. 2012; Available at: https://openknowledge.worldbank.org/bitstream/handle/10986/13581/691070WP00PUBL0GhanaMigrationSalary.pdf?sequence=1.
24. Law No. 7/1977- Rules for Civil Servant Salary. Republic of Indonesia.
25. Zurita B, Ramírez T. Desempeño del sector privado de la salud en México. In: Knaul FM, Nigenda G. Caleidoscopio de Salud. Mexico D.F.: Funsalud, 2003. Availibility: http://funsalud.org.mx/portal/wp-content/uploads/2013/08/10-Desempenio.pdf.
26. Yip WC-M, Hsiao W, Meng Q, et al. Realignment of incentives for health-care providers in China. Lancet. 2010;375:1120–30.
27. Barber SL, Yao L. Development and status of health insurance systems in China. Int J Health Plann Manag. 2011;26(4):339–56.
28. Yu B, Meng Q, Collins C, et al. How does the New Cooperative Medical Scheme influence health service utilization? A study in two provinces in rural China. BMC Health Serv Res. 2010;10:116. doi:10.1186/1472-6963-10-116.
29. Seiter A, Gyansa-Lutterodt M. Polity Note: The Pharmaceutical Sector in

30. World Bank Seguro Popular: Health Coverage For All in Mexico, Washington DC. 2015. Available at http://www.worldbank.org/en/results/2015/02/26/health-coverage-for-all-in-mexico.

31. World Bank. Pharmaceuticals: Polic Note Series: Why Reform is Needed. Jakarta, Indonesia: World Bank, Washington DC 2009. Available at http://documents.worldbank.org/curated/en/2009/03/13743569/pharmaceuticals-reform-needed.

32. Knaul FM, González-Pier E, Gómez-Dantés O, García-Junco D, Arreola-Ornelas H, Barraza-Lloréns M, Sandoval R, Caballero F, Hernández-Avila M, Juan M, Kershenobich D, Nigenda G, Ruelas E, Sepúlveda J, Tapia R, Soberón G, Chertorivski S, Frenk J. The quest for universal health coverage: achieving social protection for all in Mexico. Lancet. 2012;380(9849):1259–79.

33. Anggriani Y. Personal Communication: Indonesia's Electronic Procurement System for Medicines. 2013.

34. Diario Oficial de la Gobernacion. LINEAMIENTOS para la adquisición de medicamentos asociados al Catálogo Universal de Servicios de Salud. Available at: http://www.dof.gob.mx/nota_detalle.php?codigo=5443837&fecha=07/07/2016.

35. Lei X, Lin Y. The new cooperative medical scheme in rural China: Does more coverage mean more service and better health? Health Econ. 2009; 18(S2):S25–46.

36. Long Q. et al. Changes in health expenditures in China in 2000s: has the health system reform improved affordability International Journal for Equity in Health. 2013. 12:40 at https://www.ncbi.nlm.nih.gov/pmc/articles/PMC3686675/.

37. Li Y, Wu Q, Xu L, Legge D, Hao Y, Gao L, Ning N, Wan G. Factors affecting catastrophic health expenditure and impoverishment from medical expenses in China: policy implications of universal health insurance. Bull World Health Organ. 2012;90(9):664–71. http://dx.doi.org/10.2471/BLT.12.102178.

38. Fang Y, Wagner AK, Yang S, Jiang M, Zhang F, Ross-Degnan D. Access to affordable medicines after health reform: evidence from two cross-sectional surveys in Shaanxi Province, western China. Lancet Glob Health. 2013;1(4):e227–37. http://dx.doi.org/10.1016/S2214-109X(13)70072-X.

39. Cheng W, Fang Y, Fan D, et al. The effect of implementing "medicines zero mark-up policy" in Beijing community health facilities. Southern Med Review. 2012;5(1):53–6.

40. Li Y, Ying C, Sufang G, Brant P. Bin Li and Hipgrave D. 2013. Evaluation, in three provinces, of the introduction and impact of China's National Essential Medicines Scheme. Bull World Health Organ. 2013;91:184–94.

41. Xue-He G, van den Hof S, van der Werf MJ, et al. Inappropriate Tuberculosis Treatment Regimens in Chinese Tuberculosis Hospitals. Clin Infect Dis. 2011; 52(7):e153–6.

42. Witter S, Garshong B. Something old or something new? Social health insurance in Ghana. BMC Int Health Hum Rights. 2009;9:20. doi:10.1186/1472-698X-9-20.

43. Blanchet NJ, Fink G, Osei-Akoto I. The effect of Ghana's National Health Insurance Scheme on health care utilisation. Ghana Med J. 2012;46(2):76–84.

44. Amporfu E. Private hospital accreditation and inducement of care under the Ghanaian national insurance scheme. Health Econ Rev. 2011;1(1):13.

45. Mensah S., Acheampong OB. Analysis of Top 100 Drugs by Cost and Utilization: First Quarter 2009." National Health Insurance Authority, Accra. 2009 (unpublished document).

46. King G, Gakidou E, Imai K, Lakin J, Moore RT, Nall C, et al. Public policy for the poor? A randomised assessment of the Mexican universal health insurance programme. Lancet. 2009;373(9673):1447–54. http://dx.doi.org/10.1016/S0140-6736(09)60239-7.

47. Wirtz VJ, Santa-Ana-Tellez Y, Servan-Mori E, Avila-Burgos L. Heterogeneous effects of health insurance on out-of-pocket expenditure on medicines in Mexico. Value Health. 2012;15(5):593–603. doi:10.1016/j.jval.2012.01.006.

48. Gray AL, Suleman F. The relevance of systematic reviews on pharmaceutical policy to low- and middle-income countries. Int J Clin Pharm. 2015;37(5):717–25.

49. Nguyen TA, Knight R, Roughead EE, Brooks G, Mant A. Policy options for pharmaceutical pricing and purchasing: issues for low- and middle-income countries. Health Policy Plan. 2015;30:267–80.

50. Alsan M, Schoemaker L, Eggleston K, Kammili N, Kolli P, Bhattacharya J. Out-of-pocket health expenditures and antimicrobial resistance in low-income and middle-income countries: an economic analysis. Lancet Infect Dis. 2015; 15(10):1203–10.

51. Das A, Gopalan SS, Chandramohan D. I Effect of pay for performance to improve quality of maternal and child care in low- and middle-income countries: a systematic review. BMC Public Health. 2016;16(1):321.

52. Lagarde M, Wright M, Nossiter J, Mays N. Challenges of payment-for-performance in health care and other public services – design, implementation and evaluation. Policy Innovation Research Unit, LSHTM: London, UK; 2013.

53. Qingyue M, Liying J, Beibei Y. Cost-sharing mechanisms in health insurance schemes: A systematic review. Alliance for Health Policy and Systems Research. Geneva: WHO; 2014. http://www.who.int/alliance-hpsr/projects/alliancehpsr_chinasystematicreviewcostsharing.pdf.

13

The effectiveness of naltrexone combined with current smoking cessation medication to attenuate post smoking cessation weight gain

Raewyn Rees[1] and Ali Seyfoddin[1,2*]

Abstract

Background: Smoking is the number one cause of preventable morbidity and mortality globally and although many countries have invested heavily in smoking cessation programs, 21% of the global population still smoke. Post cessation weight gain has been identified as a barrier to attempting cessation and is implicated in the high rates of relapse. Naltrexone has been touted as a possible solution to address post smoking cessation weight gain.

Results: The results from seven original studies assessing the effectiveness of naltrexone in combination with existing smoking cessation medications to attenuate post smoking cessation weight gain were obtained and critically reviewed. Five returned positive results and two returned results that were statistically insignificant. The positive results were seen more often in those identified as more likely to exhibit hedonic eating behaviour for example women and participants who were categorised as overweight or obese.

Conclusion: The evidence suggests further investigation in to a combination of naltrexone and approved smoking cessation medications is warranted and could provide a solution to attenuate post smoking cessation weight gain especially in women and those classified as overweight or obese. This may provide the tool required to remove a perceived barrier to smoking cessation and improve global statistics.

Keywords: Naltrexone, Smoking cessation, Weight gain

Background

Tobacco smoking is the leading cause of preventable morbidity and mortality globally and is causally linked to over five million deaths per year [1, 2]. There is overwhelming evidence that indicates it is the primary cause of nine different cancers and it is also implicated as a risk factor for stroke, cardiovascular disease, and numerous respiratory disorders [3]. Smoking affects every organ in the body and the financial burden for already stretched healthcare systems is crippling. With guidance from the World Health Organisation's framework convention for tobacco control, many countries have invested in smoking cessation programs to try and reduce the scourge [4, 5]. New Zealand is regarded as a leader in tobacco control with bold initiatives including Smokefree 2025 (less than 5 % of the population smoking by 2025) paving the way [6]. However, although smoking rates have been steadily reducing there are still sectors within society that are overrepresented in the statistics. For example, according to the Ministry of Health, New Zealand Health Survey 2014/2015, 42 % of Maori women reported being current regular smokers, in comparison with 17 % of the total population [7]. Under article three of the Treaty of Waitangi, New Zealand's founding document, the Crown has an obligation to ensure Maori are afforded oritetanga (equity) with non-Maori so action is needed [8]. Initiatives to improve smoking cessation statistics have been employed in New Zealand and globally. Education relating

* Correspondence: ali.seyfoddin@aut.ac.nz
[1]School of Interprofessional Health Studies, Faculty of Health and Environmental Sciences, Auckland University of Technology, Auckland, New Zealand
[2]Drug Delivery Research Group, School of Science, Faculty of Health and Environmental Sciences, Auckland University of Technology, Auckland, New Zealand

to the health consequences of smoking tobacco is widespread and is accompanied by governmental policies to restrict the purchase and use, yet there are still too many individuals not embracing the opportunity to improve their health [9, 10]. A number of studies have been conducted to identify any perceived barriers deterring individuals from attempting cessation and furthermore investigating why some relapse. Several of these studies concluded a fear of weight gain was a common barrier for cessation and contributed to relapse [6, 11–14]. This information was the driver behind researchers initiating investigations into the effectiveness of pharmacological aids to attenuate weight gain post smoking cessation. The aim of this review is to assess the effectiveness of naltrexone combined with currently available smoking cessation medications to reduce post smoking cessation weight gain. The current literature will be reviewed with the objective being to investigate a possible solution that may remove a perceived barrier to smoking cessation and achieve the overall goal of a reduction in the number of smokers thus reducing the impact on individuals and health systems. A brief outline of the literature highlighting perceived barriers to smoking cessation and causes of relapse will be followed by an outline of the pharmacological aspects of naltrexone that support an investigation in to its use for weight control post smoking cessation. A summary of the current research obtained will be followed by a critical discussion on the findings and the conclusion will summarise these findings and identify any gaps in the research.

Despite global efforts to encourage smoking cessation and evidence of an overall decline in the number of smokers, 21 % of individuals aged over fifteen still smoke [1, 15]. Studies have revealed more than two thirds of current smokers wish to quit; however only half will attempt cessation and approximately two thirds of abstainers' relapse in the first year [12, 16, 17]. This highlights a need for advancements in cessation methods to reach those for whom the current initiatives are not working [6, 12, 13]. Although research has revealed evidence that the majority of smokers are aware of the harm smoking causes [18], it also highlights a fear of weight gain as being a prevalent deterrent for attempting cessation, and a contributing factor to relapse with both these factors underpinned by the belief that smoking tobacco helps control weight [13, 19, 20].

With the introduction of tobacco, tobacco companies marketed cigarettes as a weight control product targeting women and this ideological belief appears to still be present in a number of smokers today [14, 21–23]. It is also apparent from the literature women allude to the fear of weight gain as being a barrier to smoking cessation more often than men and are three to four times more likely to relapse due to weight gain; however, it is acknowledged that some men do admit to believing

smoking helps regulate their weight [12, 14, 22, 23]. Medical literature gives some substance to this notion of tobacco smoking physiologically regulating weight and impacting on eating behaviour. There is experimental evidence to suggest nicotine from tobacco smoking is associated with neuroadaptations that suppress reward driven eating and impact on resting metabolic rates whilst also increasing energy expenditure [13, 14, 19, 21, 23]. During smoking cessation and the subsequent withdrawal of nicotine, these anorectic effects are supressed and without action to control previously blunted eating behaviours weight gain is likely [14, 21, 24]. Studies have shown up to 80 % of smokers gain on average between two and five kilograms in the first year after cessation; however, some will gain in excess of ten kilograms and women are more likely than men to gain substantial weight [1, 21–23, 25]. It was also recognised the average number of cigarettes smoked daily had a direct correlation to the amount of post cessation weight gain, the more an individual smoked the more weight they tended to gain post cessation [1, 14, 21, 22, 24, 25]. In a prospective study performed in New Zealand it was noted that even though smokers who quit gained more weight than those who continued to smoke, in general the gain was no more than those of similar age, who had never smoked, gained over the same time [26]. Despite varying evidence that suggests cigarette smoking can be implicated in weight control, other evidence reveals a substantial number of current smokers are classed as obese [11, 14, 24, 27]. One must question which came first the obesity or the smoking and are these smokers trying to reduce the chance of further weight gain by smoking? Yu et al., (2014) [24] found that obese smokers were less likely to be prescribed smoking cessation medication and questioned whether this was due to the fear of further weight gain preventing them seeking help or whether health professionals fear of further weight gain stopped them prescribing. Furthermore, studies have shown any weight gain post smoking cessation can be attributed to an increase in the incidence of type two diabetes and contributes to an increase in the risk of hypertension by up to 30 % which surmounts to very high risk for those already obese [11, 13, 21, 22, 25]. In summary the literature supports the theory that post cessation weight gain is a warranted barrier to attempting cessation and increasing the risk of relapse especially in women. Therefore, offering a solution to decrease the risk of weight gain post cessation may encourage and help individuals still smoking to successfully and permanently quit. First it is important to ascertain if the currently available cessation medications have an effect on post cessation weight gain.

To date clinical trials testing various currently available smoking cessation medications capacity to attenuate post cessation weight gain alone have returned mixed results. The most commonly used cessation medications include nicotine replacement therapy in the form of patches, bupropion, and varenicline [10]. Yang et al., (2016) [28], found that although participants receiving bupropion appeared to gain less weight than participants using varenicline, once the results were adjusted for confounding factors they were deemed to be statistically insignificant. Alternately Schnoll et al., (2012) [20] found participants using nicotine patches for longer than the standard cessation period appeared to gain less weight than those using them for the standard time frame and adherence to patch use was greater in the longer term participants. However, a limitation of this study was that patch adherence was determined by self-reporting which may affect the validity of the results [29]. Bush et al., (2012) [22], trialled cognitive behavioural therapy as a combination with nicotine patches to attenuate post cessation weight gain with positive results; however, once again self-reporting and surveys were used to acquire results. The mixed results received from these studies warrant further investigation in to alternate therapies such as combination pharmacotherapies. Naltrexone combined with existing cessation medications has been touted as a possible pharmacological combination that may be successful in helping to achieve this [9, 17, 30–34].

Naltrexone

Naltrexone is a semi synthetic opioid that acts as an antagonist at the μ receptors in the endogenous opioid system in the brain and is currently approved to treat opioid addiction and alcohol dependence [35, 36]. It has also recently been approved as an adjunct treatment to assist weight loss in morbidly obese individuals in the United States [34–37]. The endogenous opioid system has been implicated in hedonic eating behaviours and evidence suggests there is interaction between the opioid and nicotinic system, which is implicated in smoking addiction [17, 19, 31, 34, 38]. As mentioned previously post cessation weight gain can be partly attributed to hedonic eating behaviours that were formerly blunted by nicotine from tobacco smoking. Other sources of nicotine have also been proven to decrease hedonic eating in non-smokers which further supports the theory that withdrawing nicotine can increase the likelihood of hedonic eating behaviour leading to weight gain [19,]. Naltrexone has been proven to reduce eating behaviour synonymous with the endogenous opioid pathway by stopping the rewarding effects and increasing aversion to palatable foods (those high in fat and sugar) [19, 35–38]. Murray et al., (2014) [38], conducted a study to test the efficacy of naltrexone to blunt the desire for palatable food, and found participants administered naltrexone displayed a decreased response in reward stimuli to palatable foods and an increased aversion to other foods when compared

with placebo. A systematic review and meta -analysis investigating the use of opioid antagonists including naltrexone as a monotherapy for smoking cessation completed by David et al., (2014) [39], concluded that there was no evidence of any benefit of naltrexone on its own as a therapy to aid smoking cessation. However, there is evidence that supports naltrexone being an effective tool to halt eating behaviour driven by effects of the opioid pathway which are perceived to be enhanced by smoking cessation. The possibility that it could be effective as a pharmacological combination with approved smoking cessation medications to reduce post smoking cessation weight gain warranted further investigation and a number of studies have been conducted.

Method

To procure the current relevant literature for review a thorough search of the Auckland University of Technology library including the databases, CINAHL, EBSCO Health, Google Scholar, Medline, ProQuest, Science Direct and Scopus was performed. Each source was individually searched using the keywords and phrases "naltrexone", "smoking cessation", "weight reduction", "opioid antagonists", "barriers to smoking cessation", "obesity and smoking cessation", and "tobacco control strategies". To access studies directly relating to the use of naltrexone for post smoking cessation weight reduction a combination of these phrases was used: "naltrexone" and "smoking cessation" and "weight reduction". Furthermore, to ensure the results returned were current and from credible sources further parameters were set. Primarily studies that were published in peer reviewed journals and had been conducted within the past ten years were included. With advancements in pharmacotherapy to aid smoking cessation the authors deemed it necessary to consider research applicable to currently available smoking cessation medications hence any studies pre-dating 2006 were excluded as were studies using monotherapy: however, these studies were utilised for background information.

Discussion

Effectiveness of naltrexone to attenuate post smoking cessation

Several studies have tested the effectiveness of naltrexone to attenuate post smoking cessation weight gain. Of the seven studies found, five were double blinded randomised placebo controlled trials (RCT), one was an open label study with a control group, and one was an open label study with no control group. The studies all measured outcomes within the fifty-two weeks immediately post cessation which is in line with evidence suggesting the greatest weight gain usually occurs in the first year post cessation [21]. Five out of seven studies returned positive results suggesting a naltrexone combination could be effective in reducing post smoking cessation weight gain while two found results that were statistically insignificant [9, 10, 17, 32, 33, 40, 41]. Four of the studies returning positive results used a combination of nicotine patches and naltrexone and the remaining one used bupropion combined with the naltrexone [10, 32, 33, 41]. One of the studies that revealed statistically insignificant results used the nicotine patch combination and the other the bupropion [9, 17]. Of note, there appears to be no current studies trialling a combination including the other most commonly prescribed smoking cessation medication, varenicline. In previous studies, the two medications that were trialled, nicotine patches and bupropion, although results were deemed statistically insignificant appeared to have more positive effect on reducing post cessation weight gain as a monotherapy than varenicline [28]. However, varenicline has returned the best long term abstinence rates and is generally considered the most effective smoking cessation medication [10, 28]. One must question why a combination of naltrexone and varenicline appears to have not been tested thus far when existing evidence suggests it may produce better abstinence rates. Furthermore, having reviewed the pharmacological datasheet on varenicline there does not appear to be any identified interactions between naltrexone and varenicline that could prevent a combination being prescribed [42]. Nevertheless, nicotine patches with naltrexone were the most common combination used in the studies, this could possibly be due to less reported side effects from nicotine patch use as a monotherapy compared with bupropion and varenicline [43]. It is important to acknowledge all of the studies included pertaining to the effectiveness of naltrexone combined with smoking cessation medication to attenuate post cessation weight gain were conducted in the United States of America and several researchers were involved in more than one of the studies. Upon analysis overall the available studies returned varying results. A number of common themes including the role of hedonic eating in post cessation weight gain and treatment implications, abstinence rates, and the tolerability of naltrexone, were apparent.

Sex specific effectiveness of naltrexone

King et al., (2012) [32] and King et al., (2013a) [33] initiated studies where the aim was to assess the effectiveness and ascertain if there were any sex specific results when using a combination of naltrexone, nicotine patches, and cognitive behavioural treatment (CBT) to attenuate post cessation weight gain. Both the studies found that the women in the studies showed significantly reduced weight gain compared with the placebo group whereas the men did not. However, the women in the placebo group had greater weight gain than the men in the placebo group. A possible explanation for these results as mentioned previously could be due to the fact that some women have been shown to have lower cognitive control of brain responses to food stimuli and are somewhat predisposed to hedonic eating behaviour which during smoking is blunted by the effects of nicotine. Once nicotine is withdrawn and hedonic behaviours are amplified weight gain is inevitable if control is not regained hence those taking naltrexone gained less weight [31]. On the other hand, the results of a study undertaken by Toll et al., (2010) [9], investigating the effects of naltrexone combined with nicotine patches and CBT in highly weight concerned smokers returned negative results and may further support the notion that the lack of cognitive control apparent in some women may be implicated in post cessation weight gain. Participants included in this study were recruited according to their score on a weight concern scale and as women scored the highest the study included more women than men. The results showed that there was no significant difference in weight gain between the treatment group (receiving naltrexone) and the placebo group. A suggested reason for this was participants already had cognitive control over their eating and although advised not to, may have dieted throughout treatment [9]. Dieting is regarded as counterproductive during smoking cessation as it is suggested those who restrain their eating habits because of fear of weight gain are more likely to relapse due to a sub conscious reinforcement of smoking as a weight control mechanism [9]. This may offer an explanation for the extraordinarily high dropout rate from this particular study [9, 19]. The evidence from these studies suggest that to some extent naltrexone may be more effective for women than men due to commonly perceived differences in physiological driven eating behaviours [9].

Use of naltrexone in obese patients

Wilcox et al., (2010) [10], tested the use of a naltrexone with bupropion combination and behavioural therapies in already overweight and obese smokers. On completion of the study it was found there was no significant change in the weight measurements of participants when compared with their baseline measures. Existing evidence supports the perception that overweight and obese individuals may have low conscious control over their eating habits and are also prone to display hedonic eating behaviour [11, 19, 34, 35]. The study results support the hypothesis that naltrexone may curb this behaviour leading to reduced weight gain post smoking cessation [10]. However, there was no control group in this study so there is no evidence to prove the effects were not produced by the bupropion or behavioural therapy. In fact, efficacy studies indicate that specialised behavioural therapy has been successful in suppressing weight gain over the short term during smoking cessation [22]. Whilst King et al., (2012) [32] also included individuals in their research that were classed as overweight and obese the results were not stratified by body mass index. It is hard to determine if the positive results were due to the inclusion of obese and overweight participants. However, if compared with the Toll et al., (2010) [9], study which only included highly weight concerned smokers who fitted in the normal weight category and returned negative results, assumptions may be made that suggest the results could have been positive due to the inclusion of overweight and obese participants who were more likely to exhibit hedonic eating behaviour. There is some suggestion that naltrexone may be effective in overweight or obese individuals to attenuate post cessation weight gain. Even though the aim of this review is to assess the effectiveness of naltrexone regarding weight gain it is also important to consider the effect of naltrexone on abstinence rates. It would be counterproductive to offer a weight reduction pharmacotherapy that negatively affects abstinence rates.

Effect of naltrexone on cessation rates
There are mixed results reported in the literature regarding the possible effect of naltrexone on cessation rates. In two studies that extrapolated sex specific results, the men from the treatment group returned better abstinence rates than the placebo group, and the women in the treatment group [32, 33]. In contrast Toll et al., (2010) [9], found in a similar RCT combining nicotine patches and CBT with naltrexone that abstinence rates were greater in the placebo group than the treatment group. However, when considering the results from the sex stratified studies the ratio of men to women in the Toll et al., 2010 [9] study placebo group may have impacted on the results and furthermore according to Walker et al., (2016) [15], evidence shows that men are more likely than women to achieve and maintain abstinence. Whilst King et al., (2013b) [17], Wilcox et al., (2010) [10] and Toll et al., (2010) [9] found naltrexone appeared to reduce the urge to smoke and the number of cigarettes smoked pre cessation, this could have been attributed to the cessation medications, nicotine patches and bupropion, as during an investigation by Rohsenow et al., (2007) [44] in to the effects of naltrexone on smoking cessation it was found naltrexone did not reduce the urge to smoke after ten hours of nicotine deprivation. In a small open label study conducted by Toll et al., (2008) [41] with the aim of testing what effect a combination of bupropion and naltrexone may have on weight gain post cessation, the participants receiving bupropion monotherapy maintained a better rate of abstinence post treatment than those taking the naltrexone combination. However, due the extremely small number

of participants in this study the results cannot be deemed as indicative of expected results in a larger population [29]. Whilst all previously mentioned studies trialled combinations that included either 25 mg or 50 mg doses of naltrexone O'Malley et al., (2006) [40], tested the effects of a combination including a 100 mg dose of naltrexone, nicotine patch and CBT and found that those receiving the highest dose of naltrexone, 100 mg, returned better abstinence rates during the treatment period than those in the lower dose groups and those receiving placebo but these results were not observed in a post treatment follow up. It appears that whilst naltrexone may have shown better results in abstinence in men in two of the studies overall the placebo groups appeared to sustain a higher rate of abstinence. An important factor that these studies appeared to neglect was the number of previous quit attempts participants had made. Although several excluded those individuals who had made recent quit attempts, evidence from large study by Chaiton et al., (2016) [45] highlights it may take a smoker on average thirty attempts to quit before being successful. This raises questions on the validity of results correlating abstinence to type of therapy used unless quit attempts have been included as a possible confounder [29]. Tolerability and adherence to therapies can also effect overall results but were well documented during the included studies analyses.

Side effects of naltrexone use in smoking cessation therapy
The most common side effects attributed to naltrexone throughout the studies were nausea and dizziness; however, these were generally reported to be mild and on the whole were said not to have had an effect on overall adherence rates [9, 10, 17, 32, 33, 41]. It is important to note that nausea and dizziness are also common side effects of nicotine patches and even though there appeared to be less incidence in the placebo groups there is no definitive evidence to surmise which pharmacotherapy caused these effects as every individual reacts differently and more in the treatment group may have reacted to the nicotine patch [20, 46]. There was one exception to the generally acceptable adherence rates, O'Malley et al., (2006) [40] found that participants receiving a naltrexone dose of 100 mg did not show as greater compliance rates as those receiving the lower doses of 25 mg or 50 mg due to the persistence of unpleasant side effects. At the 100 mg dose there were also four cases of increased liver function values deemed to be outside the safe threshold and once naltrexone was stopped they returned to normal [40]. Liver function tests from the lower dose participants in the O'Malley et al., (2006) [40] study and the Toll et al., (2010) [9] study were all normal and within the safe range throughout

the duration of treatment. Furthermore, in the O'Malley et al., (2006) [40] study participants in the 25 mg treatment group reported side effects that were no different to those experienced by participants in the placebo group. Overall evidence suggests that 25 mg and 50 mg naltrexone were well received with few side effects and generally good tolerability.

Conclusions

In conclusion the evidence suggests that naltrexone combined with existing approved smoking cessation medications may be an effective pharmacotherapy to attenuate post smoking cessation weight gain in individuals whom are more likely to display hedonic eating behaviours, for example some women and those individuals who are already overweight or obese. This is promising as the literature reiterates that women and obese individuals are more likely to not attempt cessation due to fear of weight gain and furthermore women are three to four times more likely than men to relapse because of weight gain. A noticeable gap in the research pertained to the apparent exclusion in trials of a naltrexone combination with varenicline which is deemed to be the cessation medication that produces the best long term abstinence rates. Further research trialling varenicline and stratifying results by gender and weight status is recommended to find the most effective combination. Whilst abstinence rates did not appear to be significantly affected by the use of naltrexone and although men appeared to maintain more favourable abstinence results whilst receiving treatment with a naltrexone combination, without further gender specific research there is not enough evidence to draw conclusions other than naltrexone does not appear to have any negative effects on abstinence rates. Overall the combinations including the 25 mg and 50 mg naltrexone components were well tolerated by study participants and adherence rates were satisfactory. With smoking still causing the greatest number of preventable deaths globally and weight gain being touted as a significant barrier to attempting cessation whilst also contributing to relapse, the evidence suggests the use of naltrexone to attenuate post cessation weight gain may provide a solution. In a New Zealand context although regarded as leaders in tobacco control there are still sectors of society that are grossly overrepresented in smoking statistics and need to be reached. Māori women are one such group and with the positive results seen in the trials for women a naltrexone combination may help reduce these numbers by removing an identified barrier to cessation. With further research to find the optimal combination naltrexone could provide the solution to removing this barrier thus helping increase global smoking cessation rates and relieving unnecessary burden on individuals and healthcare systems. It may provide the impetus New Zealand needs to reach the goal of Smokefree 2025.

Abbreviations
CBT: Cognitive behavioural treatment; RCT: Placebo controlled trials

Funding
Not applicable.

Authors' contributions
"RR carried out the literature review and drafted the manuscript. AS supervised RR and participated in its design and coordination and helped to draft the final manuscript. Both authors read and approved the final manuscript."

Competing interests
The authors declare that they have no competing interests.

References
1. Scherr A, Seifert B, Kuster M, Meyer A, Fagerstroem K, Tamm M, Stolz D. Predictors of marked weight gain in a population of health care and industrial workers following smoking cessation. BMC Public Health. 2015; doi:10.1186/s12889-015-1854-7.
2. World Health Organisation. Tobacco Fact Sheet 339.2015 Retrieved from http://www.who.int/mediacentre/factsheets/fs339/en. Accessed 20 Oct 2016.
3. Alberg A, Shopland D, Cummings K. The 2014 surgeon general's report: commemorating the 50th anniversary of the 1964 report of the advisory committee to the US surgeon general and updating the evidence of the health consequences of cigarette smoking. Am J Epidemiol. 2014; doi:10.1093/aje/kwt335.
4. Kozlowski L. Prospects for a nicotine-reduction strategy in the cigarette endgame: Alternative tobacco harm reduction scenarios. Int J Drug Policy. 2015; doi: 10.1016/j.drugpo.2015.02.001.
5. Tobias M, Cavana R, Bloomfield A. Application of a system dynamics model to inform investment in smoking cessation services in New Zealand. Am J Public Health. 2010; doi:10.2105/AJPH.2009.171165.
6. Glover M, Fraser T, Nosa V. Views of low socio-economic smokers: what will help them to quit? J Smoking Cessation.2012; doi:10.1017/jsc.2012.2.
7. Ministry of Health. Annual update of key results 2014/15. New Zealand health survey. Wellington: Ministry of Health. p. 2015.
8. Shaw S, White W, Deed B. Health, wellbeing and environment in Aoteroa, New Zealand. Victoria: Oxford University Press; 2013.
9. Toll B, White M, Wu R, Meandzija B, Jatlow P, Makuch R, O'Malley S. Low dose naltrexone augmentation of nicotine replacement for smoking cessation with reduced weight gain: A randomised trial. Drug Alcohol Depend. 2010; doi:10.1016/j.drugalcdep.2010.04.015.
10. Wilcox C, Oskooilar N, Erikson J, Billes S, Katx B, Tollefson G, Dunayevich E. An open- label study of naltrexone and bupropion combination therapy for smoking cessation in overweight and obese subjects. Addict Behaviours. 2010; doi: 10.1016/j.addbeh.2009.10.017.
11. Dare S, Mackay D, Pell J. Relationship between smoking and obesity: a cross sectional study of 499504 middle age adults in the UK general population. PLoS One. 2015; doi:10.1371/journal.pone.0123579.
12. Memon A, Barber J, Rumsby E, Parker S, Mohebati L, deVisser R, Sundin J. What factors are important in smoking cessation and relapse in women from deprived communities? A qualitative study in Southeast England. Public Health. 2016; doi:10.1016/j.puhe.2016.01.014.
13. Pieroni L, Minelli L, Salmasi L. Economic evaluation of the effect of quitting smoking on weight gains: evidence from the United Kingdom. Value in Health. 2015; doi:10.1016/j.jval.2015.06.008.
14. White M, McKee S, O'Malley S. Smoke and mirrors: magnified beliefs that cigarette smoking suppresses weight. Addictive Behaviours. 2007; doi:10.1016/j.addbeh.2007.02.011.
15. Walker N, van-Woerden H, Kiparoglou V, Yang Y, Robinson H, Croghan E. Gender difference and effect of pharmacotherapy: findings from a smoking cessation service. BMC Public Health. 2016; doi: 10.1186/s12889-016-3672-y.
16. Greener M. Uncovering the basis of nicotine addiction. Nurse Prescribing. 2012;10(2):80–4.
17. King A, Cao D, Zhang L, Rueger S. Effects of the opioid antagonist

naltrexone on smoking and related behaviours in smokers preparing to quit: A randomised controlled trial. Addiction. 2013; doi:10.1111/add.12261.

18. Popova L, Halper-Felsher B. A longitudinal study of adolescents' optimistic bias about risks and benefits of cigarette smoking. Am J Health Behav. 2016; doi:10.5993/AJHB.40.3.6.

19. Criscitelli K, Avena N. The neurobiological and behavioural overlaps of nicotine and food addiction. Preventative Medicine.2016; doi:10.1016/j.ypmed.2016.08.009.

20. Schnoll R, Wileyto E, Lerman C. Extended duration therapy with transdermal nicotine may attenuate weight gain following smoking cessation. Addictive Behaviours. 2012; doi:10.1016/j.addbeh.2011.12.009.

21. Audrain-McGovern J, Benowitz N. Cigarette smoking, nicotine and body weight. Clinical Pharmacology & Therapeutics. 2011; doi:10.1038/clpt.2011.105.

22. Bush T, Levine M, Beebe L, Cerutti B, Deprey M, McAfee T, … Zbikowski S. Addressing weight gain in smoking cessation treatment: A randomised controlled trial. Am J Health Promot. 2012; doi:10.4278/ajph.110603-QUAN-238.

23. Jiloha, R. Pharmacotherapy of smoking cessation. Indian J Psychiatry. 2014; doi:10.4103/0019-5545.124726.

24. Yu Y, Rajan S, Essein E, Yang M, Abughosh S. The relationship between obesity and prescription of smoking cessation medications. Population Health Management 2014; doi:10.1089/pop.2013.0059.

25. Lycett D, Munafo M, Johnstone E, Murphy M, Aveyard P. Associations between weight change over 8 years and baseline body mass index in a cohort of continuing and quitting smokers. Addiction. 2010; doi:10.1111/j.1360-0433.2010.03136.x.

26. Robertson L, McGee R, Hancox R. Smoking cessation and subsequent weight change. Nicotine Tob Res. 2014; doi:10.1093/ntr/ntt284.

27. Tobias M, Yeh L, Jackson G. Co-occurrence and clustering of tobacco use and obesity in New Zealand: cross sectional analysis. Aust N Z J Public Health. 2007; doi:10.1111/j.1753-6405.2007.00004.x.

28. Yang M, Chen H, Johnson M, Essien E, Peters R, Wang X, Abughosh S. Comparative effectiveness of smoking cessation medications to attenuate weight gain following cessation. Substance Use & Misuse. 2016; doi:10.3109/10826084.2015.1126744.

29. Neuman W. Understanding research. Pearson Education: Boston, MA; 2009.

30. Apovian C, Aronne L, Rubino D, Still C, Wyatt H, Burns C, et al. A randomized, phase 3 trial of naltrexone SR/ bupropion SR on weight and obesity-related risk factors. Obesity. 2013; doi:10.1002/oby.20309.

31. Billes S, Sinnayah P, Cowley M. Naltrexone/bupropion for obesity: an investigational combination pharmacotherapy for weight loss. Pharmacol Res. 2014; doi:10.1016/j.phrs.2014.4.04.004.

32. King A, Cao D, O'Malley S, Kranzler H, Cai X, de Wit H, … Stachoviak R. Effects of naltrexone on smoking cessation outcomes and weight gain in nicotine dependent men and women. J Clin Psychopharmacol. 2012; doi:10.1097/JCP.0b013e3182676956.

33. King A, Cao D, Zhang L, O'Malley S. Naltrexone reduction of long term smoking cessation in women but not men: a randomised controlled trial. Biol Psychiatry. 2013; doi:10.1016/j.biopsych.2012.09.930.

34. Mason A, Laraia B, Daubenmier J, Hecht F, Lustig R, Puterman E, Epel E. Putting the brakes on the "drive to eat": pilot effects of naltrexone and reward based eating on food cravings among obese women. Eating Behaviours. 2015; doi:10.1016/j.eatbeh.2015.06.008.

35. Greig S, Keating G. Naltrexone ER/ bupropion ER: a review in obesity management. Drugs. 2015; doi:10.1007/s40265-015-0427-5.

36. Sudakin D. Naltrexone: not just for opioids anymore. Journal of Medical Toxicology. 2016; doi:10.1007/s13181-015-0512-x.

37. Mason A, Lustig R, Brown R, Acree M, Bacchetti P, Moran P, Epel E. Acute responses to opioidergic blockade as a biomarker of hedonic eating among obese women enrolled in a mindfulness -based weight loss intervention trial. Appetite. 2015; doi:10.1016/j.appet.2015.04.062.

38. Murray E, Brouwer S, McCutcheon R, Harmer C, Cowen P, McCabe C. Opposing neural effects of naltrexone on food reward and aversion: implications for the treatment of obesity. Psychopharmacology. 2014; doi:10.1007/s00213-014-3573-7.

39. David S, Chu I, Lancaster T, Stead L, Evins A, Prochaska J. Systematic review and meta-analysis of opioid antagonists for smoking cessation. BMJ Open. 2014; doi:10.1136/bmjopen-2013-004393.

40. O'Malley S, Cooney J, Krishman-Sarin S, Dublin J, McKee S, Cooney N, et al. A controlled trial of naltrexone augmentation of nicotine replacement therapy for smoking cessation. Arch Intern Med. 2006;166:667–74.

41. Toll B, Leary V, Wu R, Salovey P, Meandzija B, O'Malley S. A preliminary investigation of naltrexone augmentation of bupropion to stop smoking with less weight gain. Addictive Behaviours. 2008; doi:10.1016/j.addbeh.2007.05.012.

42. Pfizer New Zealand Ltd. Data sheet CHAMPIX (varenicline as tartrate).2015 http://www.medsafe.govt.nz/profs/datasheet/c/champixtab.pdf. Accessed 20 Oct 2016.

43. Zhang B, Chaiton M, Diement L, Bondy S, Brown K, Ferrence R. Health professional advice, use of medications and smoking cessation: a population based prospective cohort study. Prev Med. 2016; doi:10.1016/j.ypmd.2016.07.027.

44. Rohsenow D, Monti P, Hutchinson K, Swift R, MacKinnon S, Sirota A, Kaplan G. High dose transdermal nicotine and naltrexone: effects on nicotine withdrawal, urges, smoking, and effects of smoking. Exp Clin Psychopharmacol. 2007; doi:10.1037/1064-1297.15.1.81.

45. Chaiton M, Diemert L, Cohen J, Bondy S, Selby P, Philipneri A, Schwartz R. Estimating the number of quit attempts it takes to quit smoking successfully in a longitudinal cohort of smokers. BMJ Open. 2016; doi:10.1136/bmjopen-2016-011045.

46. Novartis Consumer Health Australasia. New Zealand data sheet: Habitrol. 2012. http://www.medsafe.govt.nz/Profs/Datasheet/h/HabitrollTTS.pdf. Accessed 20 Oct 2016.

14

Branded prescription drug spending: a framework to evaluate policy options

Jeromie Ballreich[1,2*] (iD), G. Caleb Alexander[2,3,4], Mariana Socal[1,2,5], Taruja Karmarkar[1,2] and Gerard Anderson[1,2,4,5]

Abstract

Background: High drug spending is a concern for policy makers due to limits on access for patients. Numerous policies have been proposed to address high drug spending. The existence of multifarious proposals makes it difficult for policy makers to consider all the alternatives. We developed an approach to select the most viable options to present to policy makers.

Methods: We identified 41 different proposals in the peer-reviewed literature to reduce the level of spending or change the incentives for branded prescription drugs; ten of which we identified as promising proposals. Based on criterion used to assess various legislative proposals regarding branded pharmaceuticals we developed a framework to evaluate the ten promising proposals. We then used a modified Delphi technique to iteratively evaluate these ten proposals starting with the initial criterion. During each iteration, five researchers independently evaluated the ten policies based on available criterion and assessed how to modify the criterion to achieve consensus on what attributes the criterion were intended to measure. We highlight areas of disagreement to show where modifications to existing criterion are needed.

Results: We found general agreement for most policy-criterion combinations after three iterations. Areas with the greatest remaining disagreement include possible unintended consequences, the concept of value implied by many of the policies, and secondary effects by the pharmaceutical industry, insurers, and the FDA.

Conclusions: Our analysis provides an approach that can be applied to evaluate policy proposals. It also suggests factors that policy analysts and researchers should consider when they propose policy options and where additional research is needed to assess policy impacts. Developing an objective approach to compare alternatives may facilitate the adoption of policies for branded prescription drugs in the U.S. by allowing policy makers to focus on the most viable options.

Keywords: Drug pricing, Pharmaceutical pricing, Drug policy, Pharmaceutical policy

Background

High levels of spending for branded prescription drugs have once again captured the concern of U.S. patients, clinicians, payers and policy makers. According to a recent U.S. government study, spending on prescription drugs increased 12.2% in 2014 [1], straining public sector budgets and causing some private insurers to put an increasing percentage of branded drugs on high cost sharing tiers. Much of the growth in spending is driven primarily by high priced branded drugs [2]. There is growing concern that the high prices are restricting access to branded drugs that have the potential to save lives and reduce morbidity. Perhaps the best example of these newly introduced, highly effective, yet very expensive products are the Hepatitis C drugs [3]. A recent CDC study found that hepatitis C was the infectious disease with the highest mortality rate in spite of the availability of a drug that is nearly a complete cure for most patients [4].

In response to these concerns, policy analysts and researchers have developed a wide range of policy options to address drug spending. Policy options have emerged from academic literature (e.g. see Conti and Rosenthal

* Correspondence: jballre2@jhu.edu
[1]Department of Health Policy & Management, Johns Hopkins Bloomberg School of Public Health, 624 N. Broadway, Baltimore, MD 21205, USA
[2]Center for Drug Safety and Effectiveness, Johns Hopkins Bloomberg School of Public Health, Baltimore, MD, USA
Full list of author information is available at the end of the article

[5]), trade and professional associations (e.g. see The American Medical Associations drug pricing policy initiatives [6]), and proposed legislation (e.g. see Medicare Prescription Drug Price Negotiation Act of 2015 [7]). The suggested policies impact all aspects of the U.S. pharmaceutical market ranging from altering demand of pharmaceuticals via value-based insurance design to increasing supply with changes to the generic regulatory process.

Given the multitude of policy options available, policy makers should be able to choose and institute appropriate policy; however, there has been no major legislation targeting drug spending in the U.S since the Drug Price Competition and Patent Term Restoration Act of 1984 [8] (informally known as Hatch-Waxman of 1984). One reason may be the discordance of priorities across stakeholders which makes consensus building difficult [9]. Another potential reason behind the lack of policy is that there are too many different proposals for policy makers to compare and build consensus around. A meta-analytic review on individual choices has shown that when individuals are presented with multifarious choices, they find it difficult to choose or sometimes fail to even make a choice [10]. The lack of choice or consensus on a policy can be attributed to the difficulty in comparing the relative merits of any given proposed policy without some existing criterion. The challenge is to develop and then apply criterion that can identify the most promising alternatives for the policy maker to consider. This paper presents promising policies based on a literature review, a framework and criterion to evaluate these policies, and demonstrates how this framework can help policy makers build consensus around promising policies.

Methods
Policies under consideration
We conducted a structured literature review with expert opinion to identify 41 policy proposals appearing in the peer-reviewed literature that are designed to reduce branded drug spending in the U.S. (Additional file 1). The technical appendix contains the specific search terms, algorithm, and flow chart describing the search process. Articles identified by this process were reviewed by three researchers (MS, JB, TK) and screened based on their relevance as a policy to reduce branded drug spending. Relevant articles were independently reviewed by two readers and a list of policy options was developed. Reference lists of articles identified by the literature review were also examined for other pertinent articles. We identified 41 policies addressing prescription drug spending in the peer reviewed literature and clustered these policies into five groups: revising the patent (and exclusivity) system; encouraging research to increase development of new drugs; altering pharmaceutical regulation; decreasing market demand; and developing innovative pricing

strategies. The five categories were based loosely on the economic fundamentals of the U.S. pharmaceutical market. The category "revision of the patent system" relates to the market protections in place to incentivize an industry with high upfront costs and low production costs. The category "encouraging research" relates to the supply of drugs on the market. Altering pharmaceutical regulation addresses the attributes of the market that contribute to imperfect competition such as regulatory barriers to entry. Decreasing market demand categorizes policies directly affecting demand for drugs. Lastly, the "innovative pricing strategies" category includes strategies that suggests alternatives to the current pricing strategy in the U.S. Simply clustering the various proposals into the five groups could make it easier for policy makers to compare policy options. However, some policy makers may not have preconceived ideas on the best approach and may want to compare all 41 ideas or some subset of them.

Since it was not possible to evaluate all 41 proposals in a single manuscript, we used a consensus process to narrow the list to the ten proposals listed in Table 1. We wanted representation from all five groups since they demonstrate very different approaches and chose at least one option from each group. Within each group, we chose proposals based on our assessment of its ongoing presence in policy discourse. It is important to note that the exact proposals we selected are not crucial to assess the value of our analytic approach. A policy analyst could use this framework, including its criteria, to assess any or all of the remaining 31 proposals or any other proposals in the grey literature.

Criteria to evaluate policies
The criteria we initially developed were based on our reading of the peer-reviewed literature; the arguments that individuals have made to support their proposals in the literature; discussion in the lay press, trade, and Congressional testimony. For example, a peer-reviewed article discussed framework on assessing policies targeting research and patents [11] while another highlighted challenges for policies to reduce spending [12]. These articles provided suggestions as to areas where criteria should be sensitive enough to assess the pros and cons of proposed policies. From recent congressional hearings, a Chief Executive Officer of a branded pharmaceutical company emphasized the importance of Research & Development (R&D), the Administrator of the U.S. Food and Drug Administration (FDA) stressed the role of regulation, and an executive of a Pharmacy Benefit Manager (PBM) company discussed the market dynamics of the US drug market [13]. We incorporated the concerns of each of these stakeholders into our initial criterion.

Table 1 Ten policy options

Policy	Description	Assumptions
Use of value-based pricing as a means for setting a fair price of new drugs [28]	In this mechanism, the price of new drugs is set after their effectiveness is compared to other existing treatments for the same indication. Drugs that add significant therapeutic benefits (added value) would be entitled to a premium, where drugs that do not add significant value may be priced at the same levels as the similarly effective existing drugs	Assumes that the premiums for drugs with added value are not as high as to offset the savings from drugs with no added value, but no assumption was made on the level of value accepted in the US.
Strengthening criteria for issuing and protecting patents [29]	Patents are crucial for the drug industry to recoup the R&D investment by providing a drug both market and pricing power. However, the patent system can be manipulated with drug patents "evergreened" with minor reformulations or subtle changes to the technology. A policy that strengthens the criteria for issuing and protecting patents should reduce patent system manipulation by making it harder for company to receive a patent for a minor drug reformulation, thereby preventing a company perpetuating market protection and high drug prices.	Assumes that it would make it harder for drugs that do not add significant value (for example me-too drugs or "evergreening" drugs) to enter the market altogether, or that the patents (or market exclusivity) for the non-beneficial drugs would be shorter.
Shift towards earlier approval, separate regulatory bodies (lethal vs. non-lethal diseases), simplified administrative and application details [30]	The current regulatory system is designed to require drugs achieve high standards of safety and efficacy; however, these high standards come with a high cost associated with regulatory burden. This policy would take into consideration a drug's target health condition and early trial attributes when developing a roadmap to regulatory approval. For example, drugs that target a high severity condition with limited treatment options could be granted approval or conditional approval with fewer required clinical trials. By reducing the regulatory burden for some drugs, this policy would lower the cost of drug development.	Assumes the gains with expediting processes related to severe, life threatening treatments would be higher than the losses from delaying the approval processes for other non-severe, non-life threatening therapies.
Increasing regulatory thresholds so as to increase value of products upon market entry [31]	The current regulatory system does not consider a drug's comparative effectiveness in the approval process. A policy requiring consideration of a drug's comparative effectiveness in the approval process increases the regulatory thresholds for drug to achieve approval, but it also limit market entry of drugs that offer no improvements in clinical effects to current drugs on the market. Currently, some drugs enter the market at high prices while offering no improvement in effectiveness. [32] Ineffective drugs do nothing to better patients care and only drive up drug costs.	Assumes that it would make it harder for drugs that do not add significant value (for example me-too drugs or evergreening drugs) to enter the market altogether, or that the patents (or market exclusivity) for the non-beneficial drugs would be shorter.
Adopting episode-based payments for physician administered drugs in Medicare [15]	Medicare currently reimburses physician-administered drugs using the ASP plus 6%. This reimbursement structure incentivizes physicians to administer drugs with the highest ASP since there profits are linear to the drug's selling price. Researchers have advocated changing the reimbursement to episode-based payments, which incentive physicians to maximizing the clinical care within a set budget.	Assumes that physicians will respond to the modified incentives by reducing the utilization of highly- expensive drugs and favoring other lower cost alternatives. Assumes there will be lower cost alternatives that can be used in order to control the expenditures.
Adopting value based insurance designs that alter coverage based on price, effectiveness, safety and other parameters [33–36]	Recognizing the potential that a formulary has on influencing prescribing and utilization behavior, a policy many researchers have the forward is to encourage wider adoption of value-based insurance designs. Fundamentally, a value-based insurance design uses formulary structure including co-pay, coinsurance, and deductibles to steer patients into choosing drugs that offer to patients the most value.	Assumes that patients and providers will respond to the incentives by increasing the use of value drugs and decreasing the use of non-value drugs. It is possible that manufacturers may reduce prices in order to increase the value of their drugs.

Table 1 Ten policy options *(Continued)*

Implementing risk-sharing contracts to ensure upside to pharmaceutical innovators and to protect payers against payments that do not return value to patients [37, 38]	A justification for high drug prices is often a drug's clinical benefit; however, there has to be skepticism on a new drug's claimed clinical benefit since much of the clinical benefit data is sourced from phase 3 trials which have strict inclusion/exclusion criteria and do not consider a drug's tolerability or ease of use. To adjust for the risk of a drug's claimed clinical benefit, a proposed policy for is the use of a risk-sharing contract between a drug manufacturer and a payer that sets specified clinical outcome targets as required for payment. This protect payers against for paying for drugs that do not offer clinical value or whose clinical value is less than promised.	Assumes risk-sharing contracts will promote utilization of drugs with hypothesized large clinical benefit in lieu of both lower cost drugs and the counterfactual that drugs with large clinical benefits would be automatically covered.
Empowering federal government to negotiate prices for Medicare, Medicaid, VA, PHS, DOD at one price [39–41]	Researchers have attributed high drug prices in part due to the inability of some major payors to negotiate drug prices. Researchers have suggested changes, including legislative changes, to allow the government purchasers of drugs, representing millions of patients, the ability to collectively negotiate prices using, for example, collective negotiation across the five big government purchasers and pharmacy benefit management tactics such as formulary exclusivity.	Assumes manufacturers will respond to the price negotiations with lowering the prices of their products. It is possible that prices will have different levels of decline across the multiple government programs.
Allow drug coupons only for branded drugs with no generic competitor or require disclosure of costs of drugs or alternative treatments [42]	While pharmaceutical companies offering drug coupons to patients appears benign on the face, drug coupons break-down the existing economic incentives that steer patients to potentially lower-priced or higher value drugs. Drug coupons are provided to patients, essentially reimbursing the patient for any cost-sharing. However, cost-sharing is one of the few tools that insurers used to steer patients to lower-priced or higher value drugs.	Assumes that physicians and patients will be sensitive to the price information and will choose to reduce utilization of a more expensive drug if there is a cheaper, similarly effective alternative. Assumes that removing drug coupons from drugs with generic alternative will spur competition and reduce prices.
Incorporating price information into clinical workflow to increase clinician and patient cost sensitivity [29, 43]	Across all of healthcare, there are calls for increased price transparency. The US healthcare market is notoriously fragmented and the fragmentation allows for market distortions such as wide price variation for products or services even though the price of inputs is the same. Incorporating price information into clinical work flow is a way of improving price transparency, an improved price transparency has been suggested to lead to better healthcare decisions.	Assumes that patients and providers will be sensitive to the price information disclosed. Assumes that the disclosed price information will be reflective of the true price for that patient, will be updated with sufficient frequency and will be available across the multiple insurers and government programs.

However, the criterion that were proposed were worded differently and often had slightly different meanings. We used a Delphi technique to attempt to reconcile the differences and to define criterion with unambiguous meanings. We also set the status quo as a reference point such that our evaluation using the criterion would suggest how a policy changes the U.S. drug market-this approach results in our criterion being value-laden. The criterion evolved as we evaluated each of the ten options and attempted to reconcile our different assessments.

We first present the final nine criterion and then discuss how they were developed. Refer to Table 2 for criterion.

Our first criterion assesses the *potential effect of a policy on investment in pharmaceutical research and development (R&D)*. Policymakers recognize the inherent trade-off between technological progress and drug prices

[14]. This criterion is designed to reflect the strong support for pharmaceutical innovation.

The second criterion assesses *whether the policy encourages the development of innovative drugs*. Unlike the first criterion, which evaluates policies' influence on the number of drugs in development, this criterion assesses the level of innovation in drug development. Given the concerns that some new drugs do not offer substantial clinical benefits over existing therapies [15], this criterion evaluates the potential for a policy to encourage the development of more innovative products.

The third criterion evaluates *how well a policy promotes uptake of high value drugs*. During our iterative assessment process, we learned that incentivizing development of new drugs and incentivizing appropriate use of drugs are different aspects of the drug-to-market

Table 2 Nine proposed criteria to evaluate policy proposals addressing the high price of branded prescription drugs in the U.S

Criterion	Rationale
Incentivize drug companies to invest in research & development	We assume that policies that increase manufacturer revenues will increase levels of R&D.
Promote R&D and marketing of high value drugs	Certain drugs provide greater value than other drugs as measured by things incremental cost effectiveness ratios or quality adjusted life years.
Encourage uptake of high value products	Policies that encourage uptake of high value drugs by promoting value decision making by patients, physicians, and payer.
Reduce financial barriers to drugs	Policies that reduce drug prices can facilitate greater access to drugs by reducing the financial burden of drugs.
Lower the overall spending on drugs and medical care	Policies that lower drug prices; reduce drug utilization; or give providers the proper incentives to substitute drugs for other clinical services will lower spending overall and for drugs
Administrative burden	We assume that policies requiring the FDA or companies to perform additional tasks will add to the administrative burden.
Facilitate entry to generic market	Policies encouraging providers to choose the less expensive generic can increase demand of generics on the market
Requirement for legislation	We assume any additional legislative change will prove difficult and policies significantly impacting the pharmaceutical industry will be most difficult to enact.
Potential for unintended consequences	We assume that there will always some level of unanticipated economic or clinical consequences that result from policies that change the rules or alter stakeholder incentives.

process. We crafted this criterion to align with policy-makers concerns around the uptake of high-value health-care including drugs by providers, patients and payers [16]. We define "high value" in a cost-effectiveness context as a drug offering a compelling incremental cost-effectiveness ratio.

The fourth criterion evaluates *the potential impact a policy has on patients' financial barriers to accessing drugs*. Access has proven to be challenging for many patients especially for specialty drugs. This criterion assesses the ability of proposed policies to ensure a patients' access to needed medications [17].

The fifth criterion evaluates *a policy's effects on lowering overall drug and medical care spending*. Some prescription drugs have been demonstrated to be substitutes for other medical care thereby offsetting other, potentially avoidable, medical costs [18]. Policy makers may want to recognize the possibility of a trade-off between high drug spending and lower medical care spending.

The sixth criterion targets *a policy's role in facilitating generic drug utilization*. Branded (on-patent) drugs are typically priced much higher than generic (off-patent) drugs. Policymakers are interested in drug policies encour-aging the use of generics [19], thereby, lowering spending-and this criterion assesses policies in this domain.

The seventh criterion evaluates *administrative burden for manufacturers and the FDA*. There is widespread concern that the queues in the FDA evaluation process are restricting timely access to drugs and that drug man-ufacturers have to spend significant funds on R&D [20]. Mechanisms that facilitate the regulatory process are of great concern to policy makers as long as they do not compromise safety and efficacy.

The eighth criterion examines *whether a proposed pol-icy will require legislation*; legislation is a potentially major hurdle for policy enactment. Policies that require regulatory or administrative changes may be more feas-ible to enact than policies requiring legislation.

The ninth and last criterion assesses the *risk of unin-tended consequences*. Incremental policies or policies with larger bodies of supporting evidence tend to have lower risk, as opposed to larger untested reforms that have been shown to unravel once implemented [21]. Pol-icies that have not been implemented in other settings; whose research is limited; or those that radically change current policies and practices pose a higher risk of unin-tended consequences.

It is possible to weight the criterion, but we did not elect to do this. We expect that some policy makers will place greater weight on controlling drug spending while others may place a higher emphasis on innovation or ac-cess. Because we did not assign weights, we computed overall scores for the ten alternatives, and overall scores reflect predicted policy effect and is not representative of strength of evidence nor magnitude of effect.

Policy assessment and evaluation
We used a modified Delphi technique to analyze the ten proposals [22]. Our team represented different areas of academic expertise including clinical medi-cine, health economics, pharmacoepidemiology, and health policy. However, all of the participants are academicians at a single academic institution. Our approach could be replicated with a larger and more diverse group of stakeholders and perhaps other cri-terion would evolve.

Our approach required three iterations in order to reach near consensus. During each iteration, all five members of the team independently evaluated the ten policies. Following the evaluation, results were compared and discussed. Discussions focused on areas of disagreement, with the purpose of understanding the reasons for the differences and adjudicating differences. Some disagreements were the result of differing interpretations of criterion, in which case revisions of criterion were undertaken. Revisions were constructed to reduce the uncertainty around the scope of a criterion before proceeding with the next round of assessments.

For the first seven criteria, policies were scored either "worse than status quo", "status quo", or "better than status quo". The eighth criteria, examining the need for legislation, was evaluated as either "requiring legislation" or "not requiring legislation", while the last criterion, the potential for unintended consequences, was scored as or "low", "medium" or "high".

Results

Preliminary review of each policy

We began with seven criterion gleaned from a variety of sources. Figure 1 depicts the results of the first round of analysis that we conducted. White boxes reflect areas where high levels of agreement were present; grey boxes represent areas where there was moderate agreement; and black boxes represent areas where there was low agreement. The numerical scores within each cell reflect the cumulative scores across the 5 reviewers, with a score range of –1 to 1 for each reviewer. For example, the use of value-based pricing received a score of 3 for the criterion *incentivize drug company innovation*. Although not seen on the matrix, four reviewers scored the policy of using value-based pricing as "better than status quo" for this criterion, and one reviewer scored the policy "worse than status quo", with the final score being +4 for "better than status quo" and –1 for "worse than status quo" for a total score of 3. Through the Delphi process we attempted to understand the reasons for the disagreement and revised the criterion.

As depicted by Fig. 1, in the first round approximately one-fourth (27.1%) of the seventy policy-criterion combinations had total agreement, while the remainder reflected either general agreement (32.9%) or disagreement (40%). We focused on the reasons for disagreement.

Much of the disagreement during Round 1 was about the meaning and wording of certain criterion. This suggests areas where the criterion is most uncertain and could foster the most policy debate. For example, an

Policy	Incentivize drug company innovation	Promote access to drugs	Reduce spending on drugs	Low administrative burden	Facilitate entry into generic market	Does not require legislation	Low risk for unintended consequences
Use of value-based pricing as a means for setting a fair price of new drugs	3	5	4	-5	1	3	4
Strengthening criteria for issuing and protecting patents	-1	2	1	-3	3	-5	1
Shift towards earlier approval, separate regulatory bodies (lethal vs. non-lethal diseases), simplified administrative and application details	2	5	4	3	2	-1	-2
Increasing regulatory thresholds so as to increase value of products upon market entry	3	-1	1	-5	0	-1	1
Adopting episode-based payments for physician administered drugs in Medicare	1	2	5	-3	2	-1	5
Adopting value based insurance designs that alter coverage based on price, effectiveness, safety and other parameters	2	2	5	-5	4	3	4
Implementing risk-sharing contracts to ensure upside to pharmaceutical innovators and to protect payers against payments that do not return value to patients	3	4	4	-5	2	1	3
Empowering federal government to negotiate prices for Medicare, Medicaid, VA, PHS, DOD at one price	-2	5	5	1	1	-5	3
Eliminating direct to consumer advertising	-2	-1	5	2	2	-5	5
Incorporating price information into clinical workflow to increase clinician and patient cost sensitivity	-1	2	5	-3	3	5	5

White cells indicate unanimous agreement. Light gray indicates disagreement. Dark gray indicates major disagreement. For numerical values "5" indicates better than status quo; "-5" indicates worse than status quo; "0" indicates status quo.

Fig. 1 Results of first round evaluating policies to reduce spending of branded prescription drugs in the United States

initial criterion was whether a specific policy *incentivizes drug company innovation.* Some interpreted this criterion as whether a policy increases R&D, while others interpreted this criterion as whether the policy shifts focus to developing truly innovative drugs rather than "me-too" drugs or "low-value" drugs. As a result, this one criterion was broken into two in order to achieve greater consensus. Similarly, the criterion *Reduce drug spending* raised concerns about whether this criterion was too general and missed the reduction of offsetting medical care, an argument raised in the justification of high priced hepatitis C drugs [23]. As a result of this first analysis, we clarified the definitions of each criteria and expanded the number of criteria from seven to nine.

Intermediate review of each policy

Figure 2 depicts the results of our second round of analysis. In this round, approximately two-fifths (40%) of the policy-criterion combinations had total agreement, while 32.2% reflected general agreement and 27.8%

reflected disagreement. While disagreements in the first round focused primarily on the interpretation of the criterion, disagreements during the second round generally focused on the projected effects of each policy (e.g., "to what degree will changes in FDA regulatory processes towards earlier approvals encourage the uptake of high value products"?). Revising criteria addressed much of the first round disagreement, the nature of the second round disagreements could not be fully addressed with criterion revisions; rather we attempted to address disagreements by discussing anticipated policy effects.

Final review of each policy

Figure 3 depicts the results of our final analysis. Through discussion of each researcher's position and the current literature, we reconciled most disagreements observed during the second round. However, there was still disagreement in 7.8% of the policy-criterion combinations, driven primarily on disagreements over unintended consequences, the concept of value implied by many of the

Policy	Incentivizes drug companies to invest in R&D	Promotes R&D and marketing of high value drugs	Encourage uptake of high value products	Reduce financial barriers to drugs	Reduces spending on drugs and Medical care	Administrative burden for manufacturers and FDA	Facilitates generic use	Requires legislation	Risk of unintended consequences
Use of value-based pricing as a means for setting a fair price of new drugs	-3	5	4	3	5	-4	2	-3	5
Strengthening criteria for issuing and protecting patents	-3	4	4	2	1	-3	4	-5	3
Shift towards earlier approval, separate regulatory bodies (lethal vs. non-lethal diseases), simplified administrative and application details	5	1	0	4	3	3	-2	-5	-1
Increasing regulatory thresholds so as to increase value of products upon market entry	-5	5	5	-2	-2	-4	1	-3	3
Adopting episode-based payments for physician administered drugs in Medicare	-3	1	4	4	5	2	4	1	3
Adopting value based insurance designs that alter coverage based on price, effectiveness, safety and other parameters	-3	5	5	5	5	-3	3	5	1
Implementing risk-sharing contracts to ensure upside to pharmaceutical innovators and to protect payers against payments that do not return value to patients	-2	5	5	5	5	-3	0	3	-1
Empowering federal government to negotiate prices for Medicare, Medicaid, VA, PHS, DOD at one price	-5	0	2	5	5	1	1	-5	3
Allow drug coupons only for branded drugs with no generic competitor or require disclosure of costs of drugs or alternative treatments	-5	1	2	1	4	1	4	-5	5
Incorporating price information into clinical workflow to increase clinician and patient cost sensitivity	-5	5	5	4	5	0	5	5	5

White cells indicate unanimous agreement. Light gray indicates disagreement. Dark gray indicates major disagreement. For numerical values "5" indicates better than status quo; "-5" indicates worse than status quo; "0" indicates status quo.

Fig. 2 Results of second round evaluating policies to reduce spending of branded prescription drugs in the United States

Policy	Incentivizes drug companies to invest in R&D	Promotes R&D and marketing of high value drugs	Encourage uptake of high value products	Reduce financial barriers to drugs	Reduces spending on drugs and Medical care	Administrative burden for manufacturers and FDA	Facilitates generic use	Requires legislation	Risk of unintended consequences
Use of value-based pricing as a means for setting a fair price of new drugs	-3	5	5	3	5	-5	5	-5	5
Strengthening criteria for issuing and protecting patents	-5	5	5	2	5	-5	5	-5	5
Shift towards earlier approval, separate regulatory bodies (lethal vs. non-lethal diseases), simplified administrative and application details	5	5	0	5	5	5	-5	-5	-5
Increasing regulatory thresholds so as to increase value of products upon market entry	-5	5	5	-5	-5	-5	5	-5	5
Adopting episode-based payments for physician administered drugs in Medicare	-5	5	5	5	5	5	5	5	5
Adopting value based insurance designs that alter coverage based on price, effectiveness, safety and other parameters	-5	5	5	5	5	-5	5	5	5
Implementing risk-sharing contracts to ensure upside to pharmaceutical innovators and to protect payers against payments that do not return value to patients	-5	5	5	5	5	-5	0	5	-5
Empowering federal government to negotiate prices for Medicare, Medicaid, VA, PHS, DOD at one price	-5	-1	5	5	5	5	5	-5	5
Allow drug coupons only for branded drugs with no generic competitor or require disclosure of costs of drugs or alternative treatments	-5	5	5	3	5	5	5	-5	5
Incorporating price information into clinical workflow to increase clinician and patient cost sensitivity	*-5	5	5	5	5	0	5	5	5

White cells indicate unanimous agreement. Light gray indicates disagreement. Dark gray indicates major disagreement. For numerical values "5" indicates better than status quo; "-5" indicates worse than status quo; "0" indicates status quo.

Fig. 3 Results of final round evaluating policies to reduce spending of branded prescription drugs in the United States

policies, and secondary effects by the pharmaceutical industry, insurers, and the FDA. Based on overall, unweighted scores, the three highest scoring policies are: adopting episode based payments, adopting value-based insurance design, and incorporating price information in the workflow.

Discussion

Many proposals have been proposed to reduce branded drug spending in the U.S., and we focused on those in the peer-reviewed literature. Multifarious proposals make it difficult for policy makers and other stakeholders to take action. To help policy makers build consensus around promising policies, we developed an evaluation framework that allows policy makers to make such comparisons, and used a modified Delphi technique to apply this framework to a select sample of ten policies.

From the literature, we found little direct research on how policy makers should build consensus around promising policies to address branded drug spending in

the U.S. Some international studies have examined the priorities of key stakeholders and policy makers, and suggest consensus building based on alignment of values [9, 24]. Others have discussed specific policies and their pros and cons of these policies [25]. While both approaches have merits in identifying stakeholder preferences and individual policy trade-offs, neither approach lends itself for an objective evaluation across multiple policies.

Our analysis demonstrates that it is possible to use a Delphi technique to revise the criterion used to assess alternative policies to minimize areas of disagreement. A limitation of this approach is generalizability; it is clearly possible that a different group would develop different criterion. However, our initial list is based on the arguments made by various individuals to support their proposals; discussion in the media, and trade and Congressional testimony. Early disagreement during Round 1 and to a lesser degree, Round 2, regarding the explicit criterion to use and the wording gave way to disagreements in the later rounds regarding the long run implications of specific policies and secondary effects of policies. A major benefit of this approach is that it can identify where there is disagreement on the criterion used to evaluate various options and help researchers developing policy alternatives to consider each criterion when the develop policy alternatives. Many important issues are not discussed in many policy proposals.

One important area of disagreement was related to the concept of "value" both regarding value-based pricing policies and value-based insurance design. When the authors developed policies promoting value-based practice, it was assumed that a value-premium or value-threshold would exist, thereby demarcating high-value versus low-value. However, without knowing specific details of a policy implementation and how value is defined, i.e. from whose perspective, what level, etc., the concept of "value" was a source of considerable disagreement among the five academics. Researchers and policy analysts developing alternatives may want provide better definitions of value.

The ambiguity around "value" hindered consensus around the effect of policies such as value-based purchasing. One argument was whether value premiums would be set at levels similar to those observed in Europe and the lower drug prices paid in Europe are in part due to the different level of value premiums [26]. However, others argued that a combination of the strength of the pharmaceutical lobby and fragmented payor market would result in US value premiums being set higher than Europe, and drug prices would be set to the maximum threshold. There was also disagreement concerning whether certain policies would increase administrative burden for manufacturers and FDA. Consider, for example, how value-based insurance design would impact manufacturers and the FDA: would manufacturers be more inclined to conduct phase 4 or pragmatic clinical trials testing the effectiveness rather than efficacy in order to demonstrate value? These issues require more discussion in the policy proposals.

There was residual disagreement regarding the secondary effects of proposed policies, especially the response from the pharmaceutical industry. For example, authors disagreed over whether strengthening criteria for issuing patents would reduce the likelihood of "evergreening" of existing patented drugs by the drug companies [27], thereby, facilitating a more robust and lower cost generic market. Alternatively, strengthening criteria could limit "me-too" drugs that act as competitors, and the reduction of competition would ultimately drive up prices.

Further disagreement centered on the potential secondary effects of some of the policies on payers, and in turn, patients. For example, consider a policy such as value-based pricing. While there was general agreement

that this type of pricing would encourage the development of high-value, innovative drugs, there were differing opinions as to whether changes to cost-sharing structures and drug prices would result in price increases for patients. A net increase in price exposure would increase the financial barrier to drugs.

The last theme of disagreement was the uncertainty regarding potential unintended consequences. The problem is that for some of these policies it is difficult to develop a control group since it is an all or nothing policy change. For example, we could only speculate on the nature of unintended consequences, due to the difficult assessing policies in largely hypothetical scenarios. For example, would an unintended consequence of requiring comparative effectiveness information on newly approved drugs significantly increase development costs? Alternatively, what value premiums are acceptable in the US and how would adoption of specific value premiums affect aggregate drug spending, and the impact of value premiums on patient, prescriber, and payer behavior.

Considering the motivation of the study was to provide a framework to assess policies aimed at reducing branded drug spending and not to suggest specific policy solutions, our limitations focused on the methodology. There were three main areas of limitations: selection of criteria, evaluation of policies, and generalizability. First, we attempted to identify the best criterion for a national policy discussion, however, our criterion may reflect our perceptions as five members of an academic institution. Other policy analysts may have different priorities and by extension criterion. The second main limitation is the evaluation of each criterion-policy pair. For most policy proposals, researchers tended to keep the proposal vague, which makes it difficult to assess the effects. Case in point is the policy to allow the federal government to negotiate drug prices. The U.S. Congressional Budget Office suggests price negotiations a range of effects depending on the circumstances of the negotiation [24]. Knowing the details of a negotiation policy could improve the confidence of the effects of this policy. Another limitation related to policy evaluation is the single policy approach for the evaluation. It is possible policies are not substitutes but rather complements, thus the effect is dependent on which policies to include. It is also realistic to assume any national policy will include multiple policies and there could be trade-offs across policies. The last limitation is generalizability, which cuts across multiple aspects. As suggested earlier, our criterion may not be generalizable to non-academic institute policy analysts. Evidence for policies chosen may not be generalizable to the U.S. national policy. Lastly, our framework may not be applicable to other countries.

Conclusions

Policy makers have a difficult time when there are multifarious policy options that address different aspect of the policy debate with different approaches. This makes it less likely for them to take action. An approach that allows policy analysts to use explicit criterion to examine the alternatives to reduce the number of available option is needed. Whenever possible, a comparison based on explicit and objective criterion is needed. In order to accomplish this there needs to be agreement on how to assess the criterion.

In this analysis of policy options to reduce spending of branded prescription drugs in the U.S., we found general agreement for most policy-criterion combinations. It required three iterations to reach general agreement starting from criterion initially gleaned from Congressional testimony, our reading of the peer-reviewed literature; the arguments that individuals have made to support their proposals in the literature; discussion in the lay press, and trade press. However, after three iterations disagreement persisted and the areas of continued disagreement suggest topics of further research especially empirical data to improve our understanding and quantification of the potential real-world effects of these policies.

Our findings also underscore the importance of clear definitions of the policies and their components as well as the importance of considering the primary and secondary outcomes of policies. Researchers developing policies need to consider the criterion that policy makers may use to assess the alternatives such as a policy's effect on research and development and whether it drives innovative medicine development or "me-too" drug development. Even with consensus on the direction of effect for a policy, our analysis suggests that the overall net effect of policies may be difficult to estimate, in part because of differences of opinion in their short versus long-term implications. This suggests areas for additional research. While uncertainties could increase the likelihood that policy makers will choose the status quo, pressure for change is building and policy makers will be reviewing the available options. More analysis on the unintended consequences of various alternatives is necessary. For a problem with a multitude of potential policy solutions, an approach such as we propose that focuses on the criterion that will be used to evaluate the options may be helpful. At a minimum, it suggests criterion that policies should address and points out areas where there is the greatest uncertainty regarding policy change.

Abbreviations

CDC: Center for Disease Control; FDA: Food and Drug Administration; PBM: Pharmacy Benefit Manager; R&D: Research and Development

Acknowledgements

This work was supported by the Arnold Foundation. Mr. Ballreich was funded by the Jayne Koskinas Ted Giovanis Foundation for Health and Policy. Ms. Karmarkar was supported by a T32 NRSA Training Grant from the Agency for Healthcare Research and Quality. The funding sources had no role in the design and conduct of the study, analysis, or interpretation of the data; and preparation or final approval of the manuscript prior to publication.

Funding

This work was supported by the Laura and John Arnold Foundation. The funding sources had no role in the design and conduct of the study, analysis, or interpretation of the data; and preparation or final approval of the manuscript prior to publication.

Authors' contributions

All authors contributed to the manuscript. JB, GA, and CA contributed to the conceptualization of the study. TK, MS, and, JB contributed to the literature review for the identification of pharmaceutical policies. All five coauthors developed the criterion and assessed the policies. JB analyzed the results during the iterations. All five wrote, edited, and reviewed the discussion and implications section. All read and approved final manuscript.

Competing interests

Dr. Alexander is Chair of the FDA's Peripheral and Central Nervous System Advisory Committee; serves as a paid consultant to PainNavigator, a mobile startup to improve patients' pain management; serves as a paid consultant to IMS Health; and serves on an IMS Health scientific advisory board. This arrangement has been reviewed and approved by Johns Hopkins University in accordance with its conflict of interest policies. Jeromie Ballreich, Mariana Socal, Taruja Karmarkar and Gerard Anderson have no disclosures to report. The authors declare that they have no competing interest.

Author details

[1]Department of Health Policy & Management, Johns Hopkins Bloomberg School of Public Health, 624 N. Broadway, Baltimore, MD 21205, USA. [2]Center for Drug Safety and Effectiveness, Johns Hopkins Bloomberg School of Public Health, Baltimore, MD, USA. [3]Department of Epidemiology, Johns Hopkins Bloomberg School of Public Health, Baltimore, MD, USA. [4]Division of General Internal Medicine, Johns Hopkins Medicine, Baltimore, MD, USA. [5]Department of International Health, Johns Hopkins Bloomberg School of Public Health, Baltimore, MD, USA.

References

1. Martin AB, Hartman M, Benson J, Catlin A. National Health Expenditure Accounts Team. National health spending in 2014: faster growth driven by coverage expansion and prescription drug spending. Health Aff. 2016;35(1): 150–60.
2. Medicine use and spending in the U.S. — a review of 2015 and outlook to 2020. IMS Institute for Healthcare Informatics, 2016. https://www.imshealth.com/en/thought-leadership/ims-institute/reports/medicines-use-and-spending-in-the-us-a-review-of-2015-and-outlook-to-2020. Accessed 20 May 2016.
3. Barua S, Greenwald R, Grebely J, Dore GJ, Swan T, Taylor LE. Restrictions for Medicaid reimbursement of sofosbuvir for the treatment of hepatitis C virus infection in the United States. Ann Intern Med. 2015;163(3):215–23.
4. Ly KN, Hughes EM, Jiles RB, Holmberg SD. Rising mortality associated with hepatitis C virus in the United States, 2003–2013. Clin Infect Dis. 2016;62(10): 1287–8.

5. Conti RM, Rosenthal MB. Pharmaceutical policy reform—balancing affordability with incentives for innovation. N Engl J Med. 2016;374(8):703–6.

6. AMA Supports Changing the Fundamentals of Drug Pricing. https://www.ama-assn.org/ama-supports-changing-fundamentals-drug-pricing. Accessed 24 Feb 2017.

7. Klobuchar A. S.31—Medicare Prescription Drug Price Negotiation Act of 2015. 114th Congress (2015–2016) Jan 6, 2015. Available at: www.congress.gov/bill/114th-congress/senate-bill/31/text. Accessed 24 Feb 2017.

8. Competition DP. Patent term restoration act of 1984. Public Law. 1984;98(417):98.

9. Vogler S, Zimmermann N, Habimana K. Stakeholder preferences about policy objectives and measures of pharmaceutical pricing and reimbursement. Health Policy and Technology. 2016;5(3):213–25.

10. Scheibehenne B, Greifeneder R, Todd PM. Can there ever be too many options? A meta-analytic review of choice overload. Journal of Consumer Research. 2010;37(3):409–25.

11. Grabowski HG, DiMasi JA, Long G. The roles of patents and research and development incentives in biopharmaceutical innovation. Health Aff. 2015;34(2):302–10.

12. Lotvin AM, Shrank WH, Singh SC, Falit BP, Brennan TA. Specialty medications: traditional and novel tools can address rising spending on these costly drugs. Health Aff. 2014;33(10):1736–44.

13. Developments in the Prescription Drug Market: Oversight - United States House Committee on Oversight and Government Reform. 114th United States Congress; 2016 [cited 2016Jul12]. Available from: https://oversight.house.gov/hearing/developments-in-the-prescription-drug-market-oversight/.

14. Scherer FM. The pharmaceutical industry-prices and progress. N Engl J Med. 2004;351:927–32.

15. Howard DH, Bach PB, Berndt ER, Conti RM. Pricing in the market for anticancer drugs. J Econ Perspect. 2015;29(1):139–62.

16. Schwartz AL, Landon BE, Elshaug AG, Chernew ME, McWilliams JM. Measuring low-value care in Medicare. JAMA Intern Med. 2014;174(7):1067–76.

17. Kaiser Health Tracking Poll: August 2015. Available at: http://kff.org/health-costs/poll-finding/kaiser-health-tracking-poll-august-2015/. Accessed 4 Nov 2015.

18. Zhang Y, Donohue JM, Lave JR, O'Donnell G, Newhouse JP. The effect of Medicare part D on drug and medical spending. N Engl J Med. 2009;361(1):52–61.

19. Gottlieb, S. 2017. https://blogs.fda.gov/fdavoice/index.php/2017/06/fda-working-to-lift-barriers-to-generic-drug-competition/. Accessed 28 July 2017.

20. Sacks LV, Shamsuddin HH, Yasinskaya YI, Bouri K, Lanthier ML, Sherman RE. Scientific and regulatory reasons for delay and denial of FDA approval of initial applications for new drugs, 2000-2012. JAMA. 2014;311(4):378–84.

21. Oliver TR. The politics of public health policy. Annu Rev Public Health. 2006;27:195–233.

22. Hsu CC, Sandford BA. The Delphi technique: making sense of consensus. Practical assessment, research & evaluation. 2007;12(10):1–8.

23. Chhatwal J, Kanwal F, Roberts MS, Dunn MA. Cost-effectiveness and budget impact of hepatitis C virus treatment with sofosbuvir and ledipasvir in the United States. Ann Intern Med. 2015;162(6):397–406.

24. Tordrup D, Angelis A, Kanavos P. Preferences on policy options for ensuring the financial sustainability of health care services in the future: results of a stakeholder survey. Applied health economics and health policy. 2013;11(6):639–52.

25. Cubanski J, Neuman T. Searching for savings in Medicare drug price negotiations. In: Henry J Kaiser Family Foundation; 2016.

26. Cohen J, Malins A, Shahpurwala Z. Compared to US practice, evidence-based reviews in Europe appear to lead to lower prices for some drugs. Health Aff. 2013;32(4):762–70.

27. Vernaz N, Haller G, Girardin F, Huttner B, Combescure C, Dayer P, Muscionico D, Salomon JL, Bonnabry P. Patented drug extension strategies on healthcare spending: a cost-evaluation analysis. PLoS Med. 2013;10(6):e1001460.

28. Jayadev A, Stiglitz J. Two ideas to increase innovation and reduce pharmaceutical costs and prices. Health Aff. 2009;28(1):w165–8.

29. Gillick MR. Molecular medicine, the Medicare drug benefit, and the need for cost control. J Am Geriatr Soc. 2006;54(9):1442–6.

30. Stewart DJ, Batist G, Kantarjian HM, Bradford JP, Schiller JH, Kurzrock R. The urgent need for clinical research reform to permit faster, less expensive access to new therapies for lethal diseases. Clin Cancer Res. 2015;21(20):4561–8.

31. Alexander GC, Stafford RS. Does comparative effectiveness have a comparative edge? JAMA. 2009;301(23):2488–90.

32. Bach PB, Mirkin JN, Luke JJ. Episode-based payment for cancer care: a proposed pilot for Medicare. Health Aff. 2011;30(3):500–9.

33. Zafar SY. Financial toxicity of cancer care: it's time to intervene. Journal of the National Cancer Institute. 2016;108(5):djv370.

34. Buxbaum J, de Souza J, Fendrick AM. Using clinically nuanced cost sharing to enhance consumer access to specialty medications. Am J Manag Care. 2014;20(6):e242–4.

35. Outterson K, Kesselheim AS. How Medicare could get better prices on prescription drugs. Health Aff. 2009;28(5):w832–41.

36. Thomson S, Schang L, Chernew ME. Value-based cost sharing in the United States and elsewhere can increase patients' use of high-value goods and services. Health Aff. 2013;32(4):704–12.

37. Cook JP, Vernon JA, Manning R. Pharmaceutical risk-sharing agreements. PharmacoEconomics. 2008;26(7):551–6.

38. Antonanzas F, Juarez-Castello C, Rodriguez-Ibeas R. Should health authorities offer risk-sharing contracts to pharmaceutical firms? A theoretical approach. Health Economics, Policy and Law. 2011;6(3):391–403.

39. Medicare Prescription Drug Savings and Choice Act, S 330, 111th Cong., 1st Sess. 2009.

40. Brixner DI, Watkins JB. Can CER be an effective tool for change in the development and assessment of new drugs and technologies? J Manag Care Pharm. 2012;18(5 Supp A):S06–11.

41. Frank RG, Newhouse JP. Should drug prices be negotiated under part D of Medicare? And if so, how? Health Aff. 2008;27(1):33–43.

42. Mackey TK, Yagi N, Liang BA. Prescription drug coupons: evolution and need for regulation in direct-to-consumer advertising. Res Soc Adm Pharm. 2014;10(3):588–94.

43. Newcomer LN. Changing physician incentives for cancer care to reward better patient outcomes instead of use of more costly drugs. Health Aff. 2012;31(4):780–5.

15

Controlled Substance Agreements for Opioids in a Primary Care Practice

Lindsey M. Philpot[1], Priya Ramar[1], Muhamad Y. Elrashidi[1,2], Raphael Mwangi[1], Frederick North[2] and Jon O. Ebbert[1,2]*

Abstract

Background: Opioids are widely prescribed for chronic non cancer pain (CNCP). Controlled substance agreements (CSAs) are intended to increase adherence and mitigate risk with opioid prescribing. We evaluated the demographic characteristics of and opioid dosing for patients with CNCP enrolled in CSAs in a primary care practice.

Methods: We conducted a retrospective cohort study of 1066 patients enrolled in CSAs between May 9, 2013 and August 15, 2016 for CNCP in a Midwest primary care practice.

Results: Patients were prescribed an average of 40.8 (SD ± 57.0) morphine milligram equivalents per day (MME/day), and 21.5% of patients were receiving ≥50 MME/day and 9.7% were receiving ≥90 MME/day. Patients who were younger in age (≥ 65 vs. < 65 years, $P < 0.0001$), male gender ($P = 0.0001$), and used tobacco ($P = 0.0002$) received significantly higher MME/day. Patients with more co-morbidities (Charlson Comorbidity Index, CCI) received higher MME/day (CCI > 3 vs. CCI ≤ 3, $P = 0.03$), and reported higher average pain (CCI > 3 mean 5.8 [SD ± 2.1] vs. CCI ≤ 3 mean 5.3 [SD ± 2.0], $P = 0.0011$). Patients on an identified tapering plan (6.9%) had higher MME/day than patients not on a tapering plan ($P = 0.0002$).

Conclusions: CSAs present an opportunity to engage patients taking higher doses of opioids in discussions about opioid safety, appropriate dosing and tapering. CSAs could be leveraged to develop a population health management approach to the care of patients with CNCP.

Background

Pain is the one of the most common reasons that people seek medical care [1]. An estimated 14.6% of U.S. adults experience chronic (≥3 months) regional or widespread pain [2], and 25.3 million adults (11.2%) suffer chronic daily pain [3]. Up to one-third of patients in the primary care setting pain suffer from chronic non cancer pain (CNCP) [4]. Opioids are commonly prescribed for CNCP [5] in primary care despite their unproven long-term efficacy for this indication [6, 7].

Controlled substance agreements (CSAs) have been developed as a clinical risk mitigation strategy and are recommended by clinical practice guidelines [8, 9]. CSAs are documented agreements providing education and mutual consent between patients and providers informing patients of their responsibilities when using prescribed opioids [10]. CSAs have been associated with modest reductions in the misuse of prescribed opioids [11]. Despite their widespread use for patients receiving opioids, no consensus exists on the goals and compositions of CSAs [12].

Published studies have evaluated the content of CSAs [13], how frequently they are used [14–16], and how frequently enrolled patients abuse opioids [17]. Previous studies have described patient characteristics and indications for and types of opioids prescribed to patients with CNCP in primary care [4, 18, 19] and in specialty care pain clinics [20]. However, few published studies [19] have described the clinical characteristics of patients on CSAs for CNCP and the amount, type and dose of opioids they receive and the degree to which daily dosing exceeds recommendations in the recently released

* Correspondence: ebbert.jon@mayo.edu
[1]Robert D. and Patricia E. Kern Mayo Clinic Center for the Science of Health Care Delivery, Mayo Clinic College of Medicine, 200 1st Street SW, Rochester, MN 55905, USA
[2]Primary Care Internal Medicine, Mayo Clinic College of Medicine, Rochester, MN, USA

Centers for Disease Control and Prevention (CDC) clinical practice guideline [7]. Previous studies of patients on CSAs have not assessed the relationship between opioid dose and patient characteristics.

In the present study, we analyzed patients receiving opioids for CNCP enrolled in a CSA through a primary care practice in the Midwest United States. We report on the clinical characteristics of enrolled patients and the type and amount of opioids they received. We explore associations between total daily opioid doses received and demographics characteristics.

Methods

Study overview

We conducted a retrospective cohort study using patient data collected at CSA enrollment, administrative sources, and electronic health record (EHR) chart review and abstraction.

Study setting

The study took place at the Mayo Clinic, a tertiary care academic medical center with a multispecialty primary care practice serving patients in Rochester, Minnesota and the surrounding area. This multispecialty primary care practice includes the divisions of internal medicine, family medicine, and pediatric/adolescent medicine which are situated within five distinct practice sites and provide care to approximately 152,000 patients.

Study population

Individuals were included in our cohort if they were placed on a CSA for opioid therapy for CNCP between May 9, 2013 and August 15, 2016 within our primary care practice. The Mayo Institutional Review Board reviewed and approved this research. Patients were only included if they had provided research authorization.

CSA enrollment

Our institutional guidelines recommend enrolling patients in a CSA if they are expected to be on a DEA Schedule II, III, or IV medication for ≥3 months. Enrollment is not expected for hospice, nursing home, palliative care, or group home patients. Clinicians can exercise discretion on enrollment if patients are receiving less than ten pills per month. Upon CSA enrollment, nursing staff discuss CSA expectations with patients. Language on the CSA form includes direction on only having a single provider or health care team prescribe medications, safe medication storage, prohibitions on medication sharing and medication dose changes without clinician contact, urine drug testing requirements, follow-up appointment attendance, and requesting refills at least 1 week before renewal. Both the nursing staff member and patient sign the form which is scanned into the EHR.

After CSA enrollment is completed, the Minnesota Prescription Drug Monitoring Program is queried.

Data collection

CSA

Information collected at the time of CSA enrollment included patient demographics, the primary indication for chronic opioid therapy, and screening tests for depression and anxiety if the patient had a documented history of anxiety and/or depression. Patients with this history completed the Patient Health Questionnaire-9 Item Scale (PHQ-9) [21] to screen for depression and the Generalized Anxiety Disorder-7 Item Scale (GAD-7) [22] to screen for anxiety. Data were stored in a secured, intranet-based registry environment.

Administrative data

Data were extracted from administrative data feeds of patient provided information and billing data, and a data collection window of up to 1 year prior to program enrollment was used. Patient provided information included race, educational status, employment status, relationship status, and alcohol and/or tobacco use. This information is collected using a current visit information form completed yearly or as needed by patients at an outpatient clinic visit or inpatient hospitalization. Patient data is entered into discrete data fields upon completion and are extracted electronically. Due to decreased availability of these data elements for all patients across the study period, we provided the number of patients with this data available within all results tables. Administrative billing data 1 year prior to enrollment date were used in applying an institutional protocol to calculate age-weighted Charlson Comorbidity Index [23–25] (CCI) for each patient to serve as a measure of comorbidity burden.

EHR data

Chart abstraction was performed to determine details of opioid therapy at CSA initiation (opioid type, formulation, dose, and dose frequency), evidence of an opioid tapering plan, pain score (current pain, weekly average pain, weekly worst pain), and CSA status (active or terminated contract). Active status was defined as currently receiving an opioid prescription and terminated status was defined as opioid presciptions not currently being supplied. If the patient was taking more than one opioid at CSA initiation, the most potent opioid was listed first. If patients did not pick up their first prescription, they were not included in the cohort.

Statistical analyses

Morphine milligram equivalents per day (MME/day) were calculated in order to allow for comparisons across opioid types. Total opioid dose per day was calculated by multiplying the amount of opioid per dose by the maximum prescribed doses per day. MME/day was calculated by multiplying total opioid dose per day by a morphine equivalent conversion factor [26, 27]. Bivariate analyses were performed to understand differences between populations by demographic characteristics, CCI, contract status, total and reported average pain, and MME/day.

Each variable was treated as continuous and checked for normality using histogram plots, measures of skewedness and kurtosis, and the Shapiro-Wilk Test for Normality. MME/day were not normally distributed and comparisons were made using the Wilcoxon Two Sample Test. Reported average pain was normally distributed and differences between groups was ascertained using a Two Sample t-Test. Pooled t-statistics are provided where the Folded F Equality of Variance estimates were equal ($p > 0.05$) and Satterthwaite t-statistics where variances were unequal ($p \leq 0.05$). All data management and statistical analyses were performed using Statistical Analysis Software (SAS) Version 9.3 (Cary, North Carolina). In order to estimate the percentage of patients receiving opioid amounts above specific thresholds, we dichotomized opioid amounts above 50 MME/day and 90 MME/day.

Results

Demographics

We identified 1066 patients enrolled in a CSA with an average age of 63.6 years (standard deviation [SD] ± 15.1) of whom 65.7% were female (Table 1). More than one-half of patients had completed at least some college (54.9%). More than one-third of patients (37.3%) were retired, and 64.3% had a public payer as their primary insurer. Four percent of patients indicated a need to cut down on their alcohol consumption and 15.9% indicated that they use tobacco.

Significant differences were observed in MME/day by age (≥ 65 years mean 35.8 MME/day [SD ± 50.0] vs. < 65 years mean 45.0 MME/day [SD ± 62.0] Wilcoxon Two Sample Test, t Approximation, $P < 0.0001$), gender (females mean 35.2 MME/day [SD ± 42.4] vs. males mean 49.8 MME/day [SD ± 73.8]; Wilcoxon Two Sample Test, t Approximation, $P = 0.0001$), and tobacco use status (non tobacco user mean 39.5 MME/day [SD ± 61.1] vs. tobacco user mean 49.5 MME/day [SD ± 55.6]; Wilcoxon Two Sample Test, t Approximation, $P = 0.0002$). No significance differences in MME/day were observed between education (≤ high school vs. > high school, $P = 0.20$), patient living arrangements (living alone vs. all other, $P = 0.64$) or between reporting the need to cut down on alcohol consumption compared those who did not ($P = 0.27$).

No significant differences were observed between average pain scores by age, gender, living arrangement, tobacco use status, education, or reported need to cut down on alcohol consumption.

Table 1 Demographic Characteristics of 1066 Patients Enrolled in a Controlled Substance Agreement

Age (Mean (SD))	63.6 (15.1)
Gender (n (%))	
Female	700 (65.7)
Male	366 (34.3)
Race (n (%))	
Black	25 (2.3)
Other/Unknown	40 (3.8)
White	1001 (93.9)
Marital Status (n (%))	
Divorced	167 (15.7)
Married	607 (56.9)
Single	143 (13.4)
Widowed	149 (14.0)
What is the highest grade or level of school that you have completed? (n (%))	
High School or Less	260 (24.4)
Some College or 2 yr. Degree	351 (32.9)
4-year College Graduate	130 (12.2)
Graduate and Post Graduate Studies	105 (9.8)
Missing	220 (20.6)
What is your current employment status (check all that apply)? (n (%))	
Employed	237 (22.2)
Full Time Homemaker	25 (2.3)
Other	35 (3.3)
Retired	398 (37.3)
Self-Employed	29 (2.7)
Unemployed	43 (4.0)
Work Disabled	122 (11.4)
Missing	176 (16.5)
Insurance Information (n (%))	
Medicare	596 (55.9)
Other Government	90 (8.4)
Private	380 (35.7)
Felt the need to cut down on alcohol consumption (n (%))	
No	873 (81.9)
Yes	46 (4.3)
Missing	147 (13.8)
Current tobacco use (n (%))	
No	736 (69.0)
Yes	170 (15.9)
Missing	160 (15.0)

SD Standard Deviation

Opioids indication, pain scores and co-morbidity

Musculoskeletal pain (67.6%), chronic pain syndrome (14.6%), and neuropathy (8.5%) were the three leading indications among patients on opioid CSAs (Table 2). Patient reported current pain scores were a mean of 4.2 (SD ± 2.5) and worst pain scores were a mean of 7.6 (SD ± 2.1). Eight percent of patients had moderate to severe anxiety (GAD ≥10) and 11.4% had moderate to moderately severe depression (PHQ-9 ≥ 10). The overall population had an average age-weighted CCI of 3.9 (SD ± 3.1). Patients with higher CCI scores were taking significantly higher opioid doses (CCI > 3 mean 51.7 MME/day [SD ± 87.2] vs. CCI ≤ 3 mean 37.7 MME/day [SD ± 44.1] Wilcoxon Two Sample Test, t Approximation, $P = 0.03$). Patients with CCI ≤ 3 also reported lower average pain (CCI ≤ 3 mean 5.3 [SD ± 2.0] vs. CCI > 3 mean 5.8 [SD ± 2.1], Pooled Two Sample t-Test, $t = 3.27$, $P = 0.0011$).

Opioids and contract status

Eighty-nine percent of patients had only one type of opioid prescribed (Table 3). Tramadol (54.5%) and Oxycodone (23.5%) were the most commonly prescribed opioids. Patients were on an average of 40.8 (± 57.0 SD) MME/day. A minority of patients (21.5%) were receiving ≥50 MME/day and 9.7% were receiving ≥90 MME/day.

Contracts had been terminated in 18% of patients by the end of the study period, 66% of which ($N = 126$) were discontinued for contract violation or patient preference. No significant differences were observed in MME/day or in pain scores between patients having a contract end during the study and those who did not (MME/day $P = 0.26$; average pain, Pooled t-Test $t = 1.49$, $P = 0.37$). Only 6.9% of patients were on an opioid tapering plan. MME/day were significantly higher among patients with an opioid tapering plan (mean 58.3 MME/day [SD ± 60.6] vs. mean 39.5 MME/day [SD ± 56.5]; Wilcoxon Two Sample Test, t Approximation, $P = 0.0002$), while reported average pain scores did not differ (Pooled t-Test, $t = 0.3$; $P = 0.74$).

Table 2 Indication for Opioids, Pain Scores and Co-Morbid Medical and Psychiatric Diagnoses ($N = 1066$)

Condition (n (%))	
Musculoskeletal pain	721 (67.6)
Chronic pain syndrome	156 (14.6)
Neuropathy	91 (8.5)
Headache/Migraine	45 (4.2)
Abdominal pain	11 (1.0)
Cutaneous/subcutaneous	10 (0.9)
Colorectal disease	8 (0.8)
Autoimmune disease	7 (0.7)
Nephrolithiasis	3 (0.3)
Sleep disorder	3 (0.3)
Autonomic dysfunction	2 (0.2)
Multiple sclerosis	2 (0.2)
Sarcoidosis	2 (0.2)
Syringomyelia	2 (0.2)
Angina	1 (0.1)
Dyspnea	1 (0.1)
Lymphedema	1 (0.1)
Age-Weighted Charlson Index (Mean (SD))	3.9 (3.1)
Pain (Mean (SD), $N = 860$)	
Current	4.2 (2.5)
Average	5.4 (2.1)
Worst	7.6 (2.1)
Moderate to Severe Anxiety Diagnosis (GAD-7 ≥ 10), N (%), $N = 578$	83 (7.8)
Moderate to Moderately Severe Depression Diagnosis (PHQ-9 ≥ 10), N (%), $N = 785$	121 (11.4)

SD Standard Deviation

Table 3 Opioid Prescriptions and Agreement Status

Number of Opioids Prescribed, N (%)	
1	948 (88.9)
2	111 (10.4)
3	7 (0.7)
Opioid Prescribed, N (%)	
Tramadol	581 (54.5)
Oxycodone	250 (23.5)
Hydrocodone	113 (10.6)
Codeine	52 (4.9)
Morphine	31 (2.9)
Hydromorphone	17 (1.6)
Fentanyl	9 (0.8)
Methadone	10 (0.9)
Other	3 (0.3)
Morphine Milligram Equivalents Per Day	
Mean (SD)	40.8 (57.0)
Median (Q1, Q3)	25.0 (15.0, 45.0)
Mode	20
Range	2.5–743.0
Medication change (Dose Change, New Opioid), N (%)	144 (13.5)
Tapering Plan, N (%)	74 (6.9)
Agreement Termination Reason, N (%),	
Admission to hospice/palliative care	12 (1.1)
Death	20 (1.9)
Contract violation or patient preference	126 (11.8)
Contract termination	32 (3.0)

SD Standard Deviation

Discussion

In our cohort of primary care patients on CSAs for CNCP in a Midwest primary care practice, we observed that patients who were younger in age, male gender, and used tobacco received higher MME/day. Patients with more co-morbidities and higher reported average pain were receiving higher MME/day. Patients who were on an identified tapering plan had higher MME/day than patients not on a tapering plan and 18% of the CSAs were discontinued by the end of the study period.

Compared to previous studies in the primary care population [4, 18, 19] our study sample was older [4, 19] with more medical comorbidity. The leading indication for opioid use in our population was musculoskeletal pain which is consistent with other studies of opioid prescribing in primary care [4, 18, 19]. Comorbid anxiety and depression were significantly higher in previous studies of CNCP patients in the primary care setting. In a study of 209 patients receiving opioids for CNCP, 36% had depression and 21% of women and 9% of men had anxiety [18]. In a study of 48 patients receiving opioids for CNCP, 54% had depression and 21% had anxiety [4]. However, these previous studies assessed lifetime depression through chart review while we assessed for current anxiety and depression using the PHQ-9 and GAD-7 at CSA enrollment. We observed a prevalence of moderate to severe anxiety of 7.8% and moderate to moderately severe depression of 11.4%. Depression is a risk factor for medical non adherence [28]. Patients with comorbid chronic pain and anxiety and depression are more likely to continue opioids [29] and to develop opioid use disorder [30]. Clinical assessment tools such as the Opioid Risk Assessment Tool (ORT) have been designed to assess the probability of a patient displaying aberrant behaviors when prescribed opioids for CNCP. However, screening tools such as the ORT are not routinely employed in clinical practice. The CDC guideline on opioid prescribing for chronic pain suggested that clinicians should not overestimate the ability of these tools to rule out risks from long-term opioid therapy [7]. A need exists for the development of effective screening tools to risk-stratify patients initiating CSAs. Such tools could allow clinical practices to engage patients at higher risk for opioid use disorders in counseling or more frequent follow-up and monitoring as opposed to a "one size fits all" strategy which may currently pervade clinical practice.

The daily prescribed opioid dose in our population (mean 40.8 MME/day) is comparable to a mean of 50–60 MME/day observed in a previous study of patients on long-term opioids for CNCP enrolled in two health plans serving over 1% of the U.S. population [26]. Our observed MME/day is lower than that observed in a study of 889 patients on opioids for CNCP in primary care with a mean of 92 MME/day [28]. The observed MME/day in our study is significantly lower than the median 180 MME/day observed in a Canadian study of patients attending a specialty chronic pain clinic for CNCP [20]. Our results also differ from these studies with respect to the most commonly prescribed opioids. Our patients most commonly received tramadol compared to hydrocodone [26], hydromorphone [20], and oxycodone [28]. Differences in the type of opioid prescribed to patients likely reflect regional practice patterns or health benefit design as evidenced by the differences in oxycodone prescribing for long-term opioid use between Kaiser Permanente (3%), Group Health Collaborative in Washington State (21%) [26], our Midwest population (23%), and five Wisconsin healthcare systems (50%) [28]. Available data suggests oral oxycodone has an elevated abuse liability profile compared to oral morphine and hydrocodone [31]. Consideration could be given to placing recommendations into clinical practice guidelines relating to the order in which opioids are prescribed to patients with CNCP, reserving opioids with greater abuse liability for later steps in order to reduce the risk for the development of opioid use disorder.

The mean MME/day among most of our patients on a CSA was below the dose level recommended by the CDC clinical practice guideline for prescribing opioids for chronic pain [7]. This guideline was aimed at primary care clinicians prescribing opioids for chronic pain outside of active cancer treatment, palliative care, and end-of-life care [7]. The CDC guideline recommends that clinicians should "carefully reassess evidence of individual benefits and risks when considering increasing dosage to ≥50 morphine milligram equivalents (MME)/day, and should avoid increasing dosage to ≥90 MME/day or carefully justify a decision to titrate dosage to ≥90 MME/day." In our population, 21.5% were receiving ≥50 MME/day and 9.7% were receiving ≥90 MME/day. The likelihood of opioid abuse among patients differs by dose with estimated ranges from 0.7% with lower doses (≤36 MME/day) to 6.1% with higher doses (≥120 MME/day) as compared to 0.004% in patients not prescribed opioids [7]. CSAs are intended to increase adherence through "contingency contracting" which leverages written documents delineating expected behaviors and the consequences contingent upon these behaviors [32]. To the extent that they incorporate adherence monitoring (e.g., drug evaluation, urine drug screening, and pill counts), CSAs may reduce the risk for dose escalation and the development of opioid use disorders [17] although the data for this is limited [11].

Eighteen percent of our population had contracts terminated by the end of the study period. Twelve percent of our population had CSA discontinuation for violation or patient preference; however, we were not able to ascertain the type of violation warranting discontinuation.

Previous studies have observed that 17% of contracts were cancelled by the clinician [19]. The most common reason for this was a urine toxicology screen positive for marijuana or cocaine. Controversy exists regarding the proper corrective action when illicit drugs are discovered. Clinicians may discharge patients from a CSA for this discovery, but some experts recommend preserving the therapeutic alliance with patients and using it as an opportunity to educate or facilitate treatment for other drugs of addiction [33].

Only 6.9% of our population was on a clearly identified tapering plan. We observed a higher mean MME/day among patients with an opioid tapering plan compared to those without a tapering plan with no significant differences in pain scores. The CDC guideline recommends that patients on higher doses of opioids ($\geq$90 MME/day) should be informed of the risks of overdose and offered the opportunity to work toward tapering to safer dosages [7]. Significant barriers to engaging patients in opioid tapering exist including patient perception of low risk for overdose, increased pain with tapering, lack of effectiveness of non opioid pain treatment modalities, and opioid withdrawal [34]. However, available evidence suggests stable or improved pain after an opioid taper [35]. Opioid withdrawal can be avoided through gradual tapering, and the daily dose to prevent acute withdrawal is approximately 25% of the previous day's dose [36]. Maintaining a healthy therapeutic relationship with CNCP patients can enhance patient care [37] and facilitate tapering if deemed appropriate by the treating clinician [34]. CSAs should be leveraged as an opportunity to engage patients in discussions about the benefits of ongoing opioid use rather than an automatic renewal system and opioid maintenance program. The percentage of patients who should be tapering within a CSA program at any given time is unknown.

The major strength of our study is the size of the population on a CSA for CNCP. A limitation of our study includes our evaluation of a population in a single center in the Midwest through a convenience sampling frame with a low prevalence of minority populations which limits the generalizability to other primary care practices. Another limitation is that we could not ascertain the precise reasons for contract discontinuation due to inconsistent reporting in the EHR, and we did not assess for the prevalence of possible opioid use disorder.

Conclusions

CSAs have been proposed as contingency contracting, but their greatest strength may lie in providing clinicians an opportunity to take a population health management approach to manage patients with CNCP on opioids. EHR registries that could alert clinicians to opioid doses exceeding pre-determined thresholds, drug screens that

are positive for illicit substances, and patients at high risk for opioid use disorder may hold tremendous potential for mitigating risk for patients and providers and improve the overall care of patients on opioids for CNCP.

Abbreviations

CCI: Charlson Comorbidity Index; CDC: Centers for Disease Control and Prevention; CNCP: Chronic non cancer pain; CSA: Controlled substance agreement; EHR: Electronic health record; GAD-7: Generalized Anxiety Disorder-7 Item Scale; MME: Morphine milligram equivalents; ORT: Opioid Risk Assessment Tool; PHQ-9: Patient Health Questionnaire; SD: Standard deviation

Acknowledgements

Not applicable.

Funding

This study was funded by the Robert D. and Patricia E. Kern Center for the Science of Healthcare Delivery and the Mayo Clinic College of Medicine.

Authors' contributions

LMP and JOE participated in the conception and design of the work, data analysis and interpretation, drafting of the article, critical revision of the article, and final approval of the version to be published. PR participated in the conception and design of the work, data collection, data analysis and interpretation, critical revision of the article, and final approval of the version to be published. MYE and FN participated in the data analysis and interpretation, critical revision of the article and final approval of the version to be published. RW participated in the data collection and final approval of the version to be published.

Competing interests

The authors declare that they have no competing interests.

References

1. St Sauver JL, Warner DO, Yawn BP, et al. Why patients visit their doctors: assessing the most prevalent conditions in a defined American population. Mayo Clin Proc. 2013;88(1):56–67.
2. Hardt J, Jacobsen C, Goldberg J, Nickel R, Buchwald D. Prevalence of chronic pain in a representative sample in the United States. Pain Med. 2008;9(7):803–12.
3. Nahin RL. Estimates of pain prevalence and severity in adults: United States, 2012. J Pain Official J Am Pain Soc. 2015;16(8):769–80.
4. Reid MC, Engles-Horton LL, Weber MB, Kerns RD, Rogers EL, O'Connor PG. Use of opioid medications for chronic noncancer pain syndromes in primary care. J Gen Intern Med. 2002;17(3):173–9.
5. Zerzan JT, Morden NE, Soumerai S, et al. Trends and geographic variation of opiate medication use in state Medicaid fee-for-service programs, 1996 to 2002. Med Care. 2006;44(11):1005–10.
6. Martell BA, O'Connor PG, Kerns RD, et al. Systematic review: opioid treatment for chronic back pain: prevalence, efficacy, and association with addiction. Ann Intern Med. 2007;146(2):116–27.
7. Dowell D, Haegerich TM, Chou R. CDC guideline for prescribing Opioids for chronic pain–United States, 2016. JAMA. 2016;315(15):1624–45.
8. Manchikanti L, Abdi S, Atluri S, et al. American Society of Interventional Pain Physicians (ASIPP) guidelines for responsible opioid prescribing in chronic non-cancer pain: part 2–guidance. Pain Physician. 2012;15(3 Suppl):S67–116.
9. Chou R, Fanciullo GJ, Fine PG, et al. Clinical guidelines for the use of chronic opioid therapy in chronic noncancer pain. J Pain Official J Am Pain Soc. 2009;10(2):113–30.

10. Jamison RN, Serraillier J, Michna E. Assessment and treatment of abuse risk in opioid prescribing for chronic pain. Pain Res Treat. 2011;2011:941808.

11. Starrels JL, Becker WC, Alford DP, Kapoor A, Williams AR, Turner BJ. Systematic review: treatment agreements and urine drug testing to reduce opioid misuse in patients with chronic pain. Ann Intern Med. 2010;152(11):712–20.

12. Arnold RM, Han PK, Seltzer D. Opioid contracts in chronic nonmalignant pain management: objectives and uncertainties. Am J Med. 2006;119(4):292–6.

13. Collen M. Analysis of controlled substance agreements from private practice physicians. J Pain Palliat Care Pharmacother. 2009;23(4):357–64.

14. Watkins A, Wasmann S, Dodson L, Hayes M. An evaluation of the care provided to patients prescribed controlled substances for chronic nonmalignant pain at an academic family medicine center. Fam Med. 2004;36(7):487–9.

15. Penko J, Mattson J, Miaskowski C, Kushel M. Do patients know they are on pain medication agreements? Results from a sample of high-risk patients on chronic opioid therapy. Pain medicine (Malden, Mass). 2012;13(9):1174–80.

16. Khalid L, Liebschutz JM, Xuan Z, et al. Adherence to prescription opioid monitoring guidelines among residents and attending physicians in the primary care setting. Pain Med. 2015;16(3):480–7.

17. Manchikanti L, Manchukonda R, Damron KS, Brandon D, McManus CD, Cash K. Does adherence monitoring reduce controlled substance abuse in chronic pain patients? Pain Physician. 2006;9(1):57–60.

18. Adams NJ, Plane MB, Fleming MF, Mundt MP, Saunders LA, Stauffacher EA. Opioids and the treatment of chronic pain in a primary care sample. J Pain Symptom Manag. 2001;22(3):791–6.

19. Hariharan J, Lamb GC, Neuner JM. Long-term opioid contract use for chronic pain management in primary care practice. A five year experience. J Gen Intern Med. 2007;22(4):485–90.

20. Busse JW, Mahmood H, Maqbool B, et al. Characteristics of patients receiving long-term opioid therapy for chronic noncancer pain: a cross-sectional survey of patients attending the pain Management Centre at Hamilton General Hospital, Hamilton, Ontario. CMAJ Open. 2015;3(3):E324–30.

21. Kroenke K, Spitzer RL, Williams JB. The PHQ-9: validity of a brief depression severity measure. J Gen Intern Med. 2001;16(9):606–13.

22. Spitzer RL, Kroenke K, Williams JB, Lowe B. A brief measure for assessing generalized anxiety disorder: the GAD-7. Arch Intern Med. 2006;166(10):1092–7.

23. Charlson ME, Pompei P, Ales KL, MacKenzie CR. A new method of classifying prognostic comorbidity in longitudinal studies: development and validation. J Chronic Dis. 1987;40(5):373–83.

24. Deyo RA, Cherkin DC, Ciol MA. Adapting a clinical comorbidity index for use with ICD-9-CM administrative databases. J Clin Epidemiol. 1992;45(6):613–9.

25. Quan H, Sundararajan V, Halfon P, et al. Coding algorithms for defining comorbidities in ICD-9-CM and ICD-10 administrative data. Med Care. 2005;43(11): 1130–9.

26. Von Korff M, Saunders K, Thomas Ray G, et al. De facto long-term opioid therapy for noncancer pain. Clin J Pain. 2008;24(6):521–7.

27. Washington State Agency Medical Directors' Group (AMDG). Interagency Guideline on Prescribing Opioids for Pain. 2015; http://www.agencymeddirectors. wa.gov/Files/2015AMDGOpioidGuideline.pdf. Accessed 25 Feb 2017.

28. Brown RT, Zuelsdorff M, Fleming M. Adverse effects and cognitive function among primary care patients taking opioids for chronic nonmalignant pain. J Opioid Manag. 2006;2(3):137–46.

29. Sullivan MD, Edlund MJ, Zhang L, Unutzer J, Wells KB. Association between mental health disorders, problem drug use, and regular prescription opioid use. Arch Intern Med. 2006;166(19):2087–93.

30. Edlund MJ, Martin BC, Fan MY, Devries A, Braden JB, Sullivan MD. Risks for opioid abuse and dependence among recipients of chronic opioid therapy: results from the TROUP study. Drug Alcohol Depend. 2010;112(1–2):90–8.

31. Wightman R, Perrone J, Portelli I, Nelson L. Likeability and abuse liability of commonly prescribed opioids. J Med Toxicol Official J Am College Med Toxicol. 2012;8(4):335–40.

32. Kirkpatrick AF, Derasari M, Kovacs PL, Lamb BD, Miller R, Reading A. A protocol-contract for opioid use in patients with chronic pain not due to malignancy. J Clin Anesth. 1998;10(5):435–43.

33. New York State Office of Alcoholism and Substance Abuse Services. Clinical Practice Guidance Number 2012.3: Guidance on Urine Drug Testing. 2012; https://www.oasas.ny.gov/AdMed/recommend/guide3test.cfm. Accessed 3 Mar 2017.

34. Frank JW, Levy C, Matlock DD, et al. Patients' perspectives on tapering of chronic Opioid therapy: a qualitative study. Pain Med. 2016;17(10):1838–47.

35. Berna C, Kulich RJ, Rathmell JP. Tapering long-term Opioid therapy in chronic noncancer pain: evidence and recommendations for everyday practice. Mayo Clin Proc. 2015;90(6):828–42.

36. Fishbain DA, Rosomoff HL, Cutler R. Opiate detoxification protocols. A clinical manual. Ann Clin Psychiatry. 1993;5(1):53–65.

37. Upshur CC, Bacigalupe G, Luckmann R. "They don't want anything to do with you": patient views of primary care management of chronic pain. Pain Medicine. 2010;11(12):1791–8.

16

Evaluating the impact of Brexit on the pharmaceutical industry

Fawz Kazzazi[1,5,6*], Cleo Pollard[2,5†], Paul Tern[1,5], Alejandro Ayuso-Garcia[3], Jack Gillespie[3] and Inesa Thomsen[4,5†]

Abstract

Introduction: The UK Pharmaceutical Industry is arguably one of the most important industries to consider in the negotiations following the Brexit vote. Providing tens of thousands of jobs and billions in tax revenue and research investment, the importance of this industry cannot be understated. At stake is the global leadership in the sector, which produces some of the field's most influential basic science and translation work. However, interruptions and losses may occur at multiple levels, affecting patients, researchers, universities, companies and government.

Goals: By understanding the current state of pharmaceutical sector, the potential effect of leaving the European Union (EU) on this successful industry can be better understood. This paper aims to address the priorities for negotiations by collating the analyses of professionals in the field, leading companies and non-EU member states.

Research methods: A government healthcare policy advisor and Chief Science Officer (CSO) for a major pharmaceutical firm were consulted to scope the paper. In these discussions, five key areas were identified: contribution, legislative processes, regulatory processes, research and outcomes, commercial risk. Multiple search engines were utilised for selecting relevant material, predominantly PubMed and Google Scholar. To supplement this information, Government documents were located using the "GOV.UK" publications tool, and interviews and commentaries were found through the Google News search function.

Conclusion: With thorough investigation of the literature, we propose four foundations in the advancement of negotiations. These prioritise: negotiation of 'associated country' status, bilaterally favourable trade agreements, minimal interruption to regulatory bodies and special protection for the movement of workforce in the life sciences industry.

Keywords: Brexit, Pharma, Pharmaceutical, Industry, Impact of Brexit, Leaving EU, Drug manufacture, Employment, Workforce, Funding

Background

A glance at the stock market suggests that the UK's pharmaceutical sector has emerged largely unscathed from Brexit, performing comparatively stronger than other industries in the immediate economic uncertainty that followed the referendum result in June 2016. As industries such as banking and insurance grappled with the pound falling to its lowest level in thirty years [1], the pharmaceuticals sector appeared to buoy calmly above the volatility. The British pharmaceutical company, GlaxoSmithKline (GSK), headquartered in Brentford, UK, even saw its share price rise in the immediate aftermath of the vote, highlighting the robustness of the industry [2]. These results panned out promisingly, flouting widespread speculation that the sector would be one of the worst hit. Some in the industry, whilst acknowledging the potential negative impacts of Brexit, even hailed independence from the EU as an opportunity for the UK to leverage its life science sector [3]. Such short-term observations would make an optimistic evaluation of the impact on the industry a seemingly straightforward one to write. However, it would likely prove short-sighted. As negotiations for a post-Brexit world take shape, the UK's pharmaceutical industry, one of the country's most reputable sectors, has perhaps more at stake than any other industry owing

* Correspondence: fk276@cam.ac.uk
†Equal contributors
[1]University of Cambridge, School of Clinical Medicine, Cambridge, UK
[5]Polygeia (Global Health Student Think-Tank), Cambridge, UK

to the complex nature of its current regulatory, funding and research structures.

The gravity of the potential disruption to the industry is reflected in the fact that the UK government has outlined science and innovation as one of the 12 'negotiating priorities' of Brexit [4]. This is matched by the insistence of industry leaders that a solution be reached swiftly in order to prevent financial damage to the sector and possible risks to all those who depend on the research, products and services it delivers. For example, Steve Bates, BioIndustry Association CEO, has called for an early agreement on issues such as regulation of medicines and the ability of non-UK nationals to work in the UK life science ecosystem, whilst the European Federation of Pharmaceutical Industries and Associations has warned that "disruption could lead to delays in medicines reaching patients" [5].

The pharmaceutical industry is being afforded attention and a sense of immediacy in these early stages of negotiation, yet the details that will determine its future remain unclear. This report aims to inform on the possible options available to the UK pharmaceutical sector now that its relationship with the EU faces potentially drastic changes. It is impossible to predict whether this new affiliation will be one of continuing partnership, lukewarm cohabitation or absolute divorce in terms of the deals reached on regulation, clinical trials, and the movement of persons and drugs (amongst other factors). It is possible, however, to shed light on the intricacies of any one these options, drawing knowledge from the EU's current relationships with non-EU states. Combining this insight with an outlining of the current state of the UK pharmaceutical sector should provide clearer understanding of where the priorities lie for pharma in these crucial Brexit negotiations.

Methodology

The impact of Brexit on the pharmaceutical industry is a diverse subject that is placed at the conjunction of economics, politics and science. In order to adequately represent the depth of discussions, the study consulted experts for their guidance in scoping this project. Three experts were selected for their breadth of knowledge: a government public health consultant, a member of parliament (MP) and a Chief Science Officer (CSO) of a major pharmaceutical firm. Following this scoping phase, five key areas were identified for exploration:

- Contribution*
- Legislative processes
  o Consideration of post-Brexit models*
    ■ Swiss
    ■ Canadian
    ■ European Economic Area
  o Potential cost burden from additional regulatory and market entrance requirements

- Regulatory processes
  o European Medicines Agency*
  o Medicines and Healthcare Regulations Agency*
  o Movement of people*
  o Professional standards
  o Clinical Trials Directive and Clinical Trials framework*
  o The Customs Union
- Research and outcomes*
  o Horizon 2020
  o Other EU funded projects
  o Continued access to EU funding in science and technology
- Creation of reputational and commercial risk for pharmaceutical companies wishing to do business from within and outside the UK

To find relevant literature, composite and extended terms containing the roots "pharm*" and "drug*" were searched with terms relating to Brexit, such as "Brexit", "EU", "eur*" and "leave EU", in search engines Pubmed and Google Scholar. Additionally, the same terms were used to locate government documents via the "GOV.UK" publication search tool. Furthermore, reports and commentaries were found through regulatory body websites and pharmaceutical associations such as "European Medicines Agency", "Association of British Pharmaceuticals" and "UK Biotech Association". Articles and interviews were discovered through the use of internet search engines such as "Google News". Finally, specific numerical figures and anecdotes from notable individuals were sought directly using the aforementioned search tools.

The research framework is outlined in Fig. 1. The initial search found 252 documents, of which 79 were used to inform an extended report and 60 of those used for this manuscript (Fig. 1). The items labelled with an asterisk (*) were the focus of this manuscript. Limitations in available literature excluded topics relating to: customs union, future trade risk and new British professional standards.

Pre-Brexit figures

The pharmaceutical industry constitutes an important component of the UK economy. The UK life sciences sector contributed £30.4 billion in UK GDP, supported 482,000 jobs and contributed £8.6 billion in taxes in 2015 [6], a significant portion (over half) due to the pharmaceutical industry [7]. Two of the world's largest pharmaceutical companies, AstraZeneca and GSK, are headquartered in the UK and almost all notable multinational pharmaceutical companies maintain a presence in the country.

The UK's life sciences industry is viewed as one of the most dynamic in Europe and has received substantial foreign investment over the last ten years [8]. Multiple

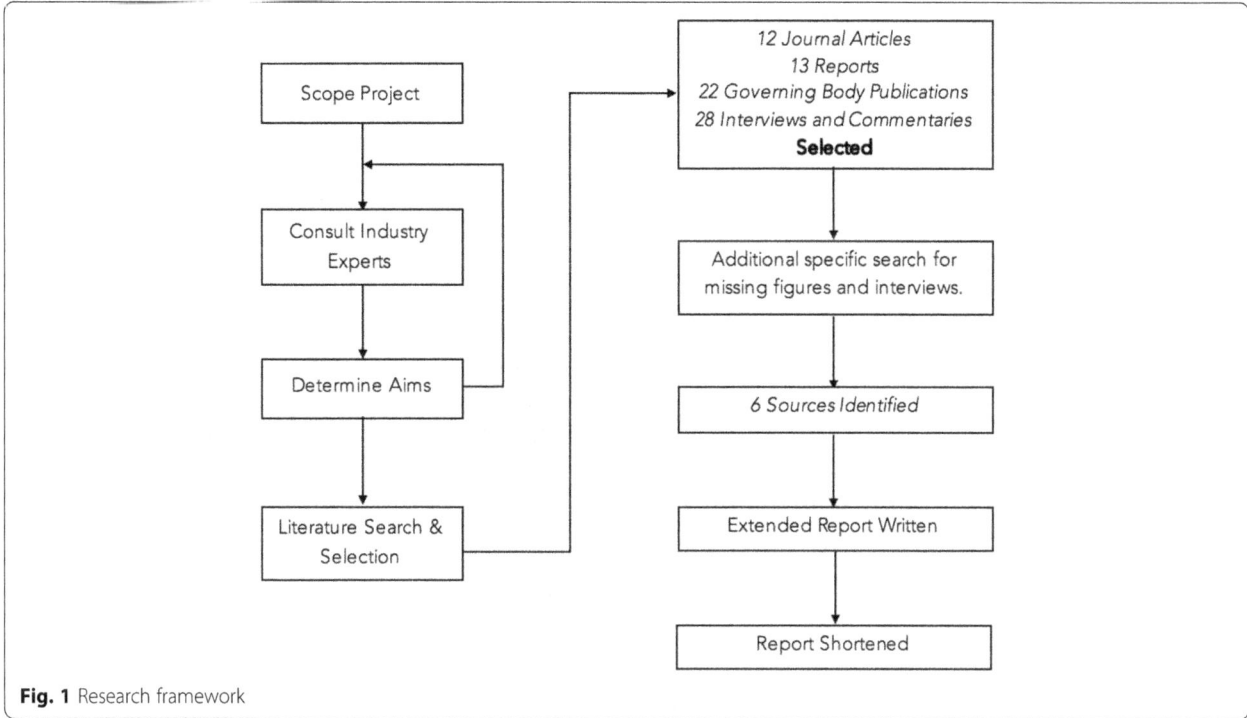

Fig. 1 Research framework

facets to the industry have allowed the UK to become a world leader in scientific research ahead of both China and the US, a feat which has ultimately benefitted the UK [9]. Investors appreciate the fairness and transparency of the UK's regulatory environment and have benefited from a collaborative government-industry relationship.

Industry overview

The pharmaceutical sector employs approximately 70,000 people in the UK [10] and provides jobs in a number of areas: manufacturing, distribution, clinical trials and R&D.

Pharmaceutical manufacturing is one of the few components of the UK's manufacturing sector to have experienced fairly consistent growth in output, productivity and employment over the last decade. Looking ahead, growth rates of 4–10% per annum had been forecast for the sector [11]. It is the most research intensive component of the UK economy and is responsible for around 25% of all commercial R&D conducted in the UK [12].

The UK is the main location in Europe for venture financing of pharmaceutical companies, accounting for over a third of the total Venture Capital (VC) raised in the pharmaceutical sector in Europe [13]. The London Stock Exchange, including its smaller sub-market, Alternative Investment Market (AIM), is an important source of funding for pharmaceutical companies, although it is not dominant within Europe [14] (Fig. 2).

Pharmaceutical manufacturing

The UK's reliable legal system and strong protection of intellectual property has helped to establish the country as a major centre for the manufacture of medical devices and pharmaceuticals. It is estimated that there are over 500 pharmaceutical manufacturers in the UK [15].

The UK's domestic market for pharmaceutical products is currently valued at ~£30 billion and demand for pharmaceutical products is expected to grow substantially due to the pressures of an ageing population [16]. Weak economic growth could reduce growth projections for the sector but, in general, demand for healthcare products has been resilient to economic downturns with the sector's growth remaining positive even during the 2008–09 crisis.

The EU remains the largest single export market for UK pharmaceutical companies. Exports to the EU have grown by around 30% over the last 10 years and further growth is expected. Germany is a crucial market due to its large and wealthy yet rapidly ageing population [15]. However, the EU now represents less than half of total UK pharmaceutical exports. Exports to outside the EU more than doubled over the last ten years. Key growth markets are Asia (especially China) and the US [15].

Drug pricing and reimbursement is an exclusive competency of EU member states. Consequently, third parties can purchase branded pharmaceuticals in EEA member states with lower prices and then resell them in other EU member states [17]. This process is known as parallel importation. Parallel imports of pharmaceutical products were prohibited in Sweden until it joined the

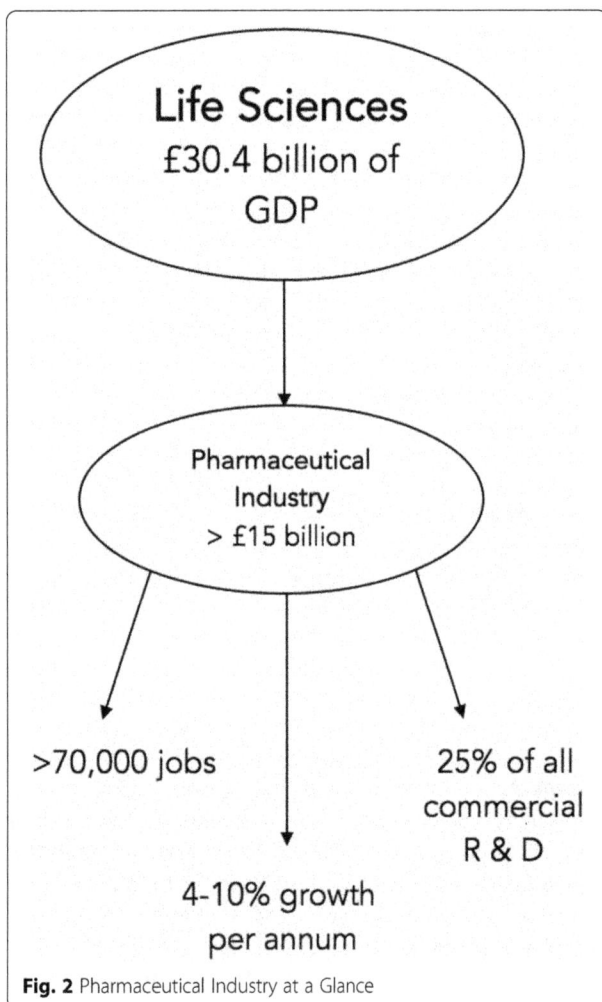

Fig. 2 Pharmaceutical Industry at a Glance

Life Sciences £30.4 billion of GDP

Pharmaceutical Industry > £15 billion

>70,000 jobs

25% of all commercial R & D

4-10% growth per annum

Since 2004, the UK has been party to the EU Clinical Trials Directive (CTD), 2001/20/EC EUCTD, which has received criticism for adding red tape, whilst bringing few tangible benefits and perhaps encouraging clinical trials to take place outside the EU. Sir Michael Rawlins, current chair of the Medicine and Healthcare Products Regulatory Agency (MHRA), referred to the original CTD as a "catastrophe" [21]. Nonetheless, with substantial changes to this directive due to be implemented in 2018, there is little support amongst the research community for leaving the EU-wide clinical trials network.

One key issue is the increased emphasis on rare diseases and genetic research. Both occur highly infrequently, making it impossible to generate a sufficiently large sample in any particular EU country [22]. This necessitates international longitudinal studies and it is feared that the UK will be unable to participate in such studies once outside the framework of the European CTD. That said, the UK is home to "The 100,000 Genomes Project", a national initiative aiming to sequence the DNA of 100,000 people. This is the largest project of its kind in the world [23].

Effect of Brexit on the pharmaceutical industry – Post-Brexit

Innovation
The pharmaceutical industry is one of the UK's main motors for innovation. Investing more in R&D than any other sector in the UK (£4 billion in 2014 [24]), the life sciences sector stimulates the creation of highly skilled jobs and the formation of partnerships and collaborations with academia and other sectors, which generates value for the UK.

The UK is a reference internationally in the life sciences industry, having discovered and developed 25 of the top 100 prescription medicines globally [15]. Nevertheless, to sustain the status of global leadership in the sector, it is essential to guarantee long-term funding, the brightest talent and the ability to collaborate at scale. Commercialisation of this research will require funding of small and medium enterprises (SMEs), from inception to sale, or Initial Public Offering (IPO).

The commercialisation and growth of SMEs rely heavily on the UK's VC, whilst also depending greatly on the European Investment Bank (EIB) and the European Investment Fund (EIF) funding; these constitute 25–40% of VC funds and attract further private investment [25]. If the European Investment Bank (EIB) funding pipeline is broken, UK SMEs will suffer and fewer start-ups will be created.

Diminished innovation
Framework Programmes (FPs) are the main EU funding mechanism for research, development and innovation, accounting for 78% of EU research funding received by

EU in 1995; evidence suggests that, since then, parallel imports have reduced pharmaceutical prices [18].

Biosimilar drugs are non-branded near-equivalents of branded biopharmaceutical products. It is possible that the government will also seek to encourage the use of biosimilars over the same period, although these drugs do not offer the same cost savings as generic drugs. The UK government has been focusing on cost reduction measures in recent years and this has included emphasising the use of generic drugs. Spending on generic drugs as a portion of total healthcare spending is expected to rise over the next decade [19].

Clinical trials
The UK's National Institute for Healthcare Research (NIHR) is the largest funder of clinical trial research in the EU [20]. Clinical trials provide important information for academics and R&D departments. The UK's status as a major location for clinical trials enhances its desirability as a location for pharmaceutical development.

the UK between 2007 and 2013 (FP7) [26] or 3% of UK's expenditure on R&D over the same period [27]. As a result of FPs and structural funds for research and innovation activities, the UK secured €8.8 billion in funding from the EU between 2007 and 2013 [28], earning €3.4 billion more than contributed [29].

Horizon 2020 is the current FP with a budget of €74.8 billion available for the period 2014 to 2020 [29]. This amount is distributed based on criteria of scientific excellence, alignment with a number of strategic objectives ('grand challenges'), geographical and disciplinary diversity, and potential for commercialisation.

The HM Treasury has committed to underwrite funding for approved Horizon 2020 projects applied for before the UK leaves the EU [30], providing short-term reassurance to applicants from the UK's research and innovation base. Access to EU funding beyond Horizon 2020 is still unknown, which is particularly worrying in the Life Sciences sector where projects can require extended periods of time. However, an individual of any country maintains the right to apply for funding from the European Research Council and the Marie Skłodowska-Curie funding.

Loss of global research leader status

Although 19% of the world's most cited life science academic publications in 2012 were produced by the UK [24], 60% of all internationally co-authored papers are with EU partners [31]. Cross-border collaborations between EU member states are becoming increasingly paramount in achieving the scale required to make breakthrough discoveries. Loss of EU membership presents a considerable obstacle in maintaining the UK at the forefront of global research. Furthermore, if non-EU countries see European scale as indispensable to meeting their objectives, it is likely that they will target partnerships outside of the UK.

Additionally, loss of alignment with the EU on data protection could further endanger the UK's leading position since the current UK Data Protection Act is insufficient to enable pan-European data sharing.

Falling R&D spending

There is a positive correlation between government spending on medical research and private R&D spending, a 1% increase in the former being associated with a 0.7% increase in the latter [32]. Any reductions in public funding could result in a decline in private R&D spending from pharmaceutical companies who, in 2014, spent 16% of their European R&D budget in the UK [33].

The benefit of increased government expenditure on research quality is demonstrated through Singapore's Agency for Science, Technology and Research (A*STAR), which was established in 1991. This body is credited with improving Singapore's output to the biotechnology sector by attracting top researchers from around the globe. Its success is believed to be rooted in the lack of stringent regime and control of research targets; investing in the best researchers, not just the best research proposals, has led to an influx of researcher applications [34]. In 2016, it committed 19 billion Singaporean Dollars (~£11 billion) to fund R&D until 2020 [35].

Regulation

It is difficult to assess the extent to which the UK's pharmaceutical industry will continue to be regulated by EU laws once the UK leaves the EU. A large part of this depends on whether the UK will continue to be part of the European single market and support free movement of medicinal products, a decision for both the UK and remaining EU member states to reach. The most likely outcome is that companies seeking to launch new products will have to apply separately for regulatory approval in the UK and in the EU. This will introduce delays to the system and may be detrimental to drug launches in the UK, as companies may prioritise applying for regulatory approval in the considerably larger EU market. As Japan's Ministry of Foreign Affairs states, the "appeal of London as an environment for the development of pharmaceuticals would be lost" if the EMA relocates, which would in turn drive negative impacts on R&D [36]. Not committing to the full implementation of the European Falsified Medicines Directive (FMD) would deprive the UK of the EU's efforts to prevent falsified medicines entering EU countries and thus reaching UK patients.

Furthermore, whilst the MHRA has released a statement announcing that it currently remains committed to playing a full and active role in European regulatory procedures for medicines and devices, its position beyond this interim period is not known. Rawlins has expressed the MHRA's preference for working closely with the EMA and maintaining the current regulatory system to the extent of even contributing to the deliberations of the Scientific Advisory Committee. Ultimately, however, the extent to which the MHRA will continue to engage with the EMA will be determined by Parliament's Scientific Advisory Body [37]. Regardless of the UK's path in terms of EU market access, there will be an increased authorisation burden for the UK, as drugs that have already been centrally approved by the EMA would need additional authorisation in the UK.

The EMA has already forecast potentially significant disruptions to its operations following Brexit but it remains unclear as to whether a relocation will take place or what other changes will emerge in terms of the UK's relationship with the EMA [38].

However, these problems could be circumvented by various administrative streamlining measures such as those used by EFTA states. For example, Liechtenstein uses processes that automatically approve medicines authorised by the EMA, whilst Norway and Iceland remain under the EMA's umbrella.

In April 2014, a new Clinical Trials Regulation (CTR), Regulation EU No. 536/2014, was adopted by the EU with the aim of full implementation by 2018 [25]. This CTR focuses on the simplification of current rules, streamlining applications for the conduction of clinical trials and their authorisation, and aiming to increase the transparency of the data produced [39]. Should the UK not adhere to Regulation EU No. 536/2014, innovation could be hindered as opportunities for doctors and academics to conduct clinical trials will be restricted and companies will begin to look elsewhere to carry out theirs.

Regulation of medical devices

Medical devices are regulated by the EMA and the MHRA. The Medical Devices Directive (MDD) similarly attempts to apply EU-wide standards to medical devices. This means that, at present, devices licensed in one EU country can be sold throughout the EU. This 'lowest common denominator' system allows manufacturers to deliberately register their products in countries with lower standards.

With Brexit, the MHRA is likely to impose tighter standards on medical devices, putting in place regulations that the EMA failed to install due to resistance from member states. This will benefit larger pharmaceutical companies with more sophisticated R&D and manufacturing infrastructure for ensuring products are of a high quality. Simultaneously, these regulations may create barriers to entry for new start-ups lacking the capital to produce high quality products to meet the more stringent regulations.

An end to cooperation with the EU on matters of European pharmacovigilance (PV) and future medical device databases (EUDAMED) will diminish the ability of the UK to detect side effects and respond to safety issues. In addition, loss of access to the European Centre for Disease Prevention and Control (ECDC) could hinder the UK's ability to produce medicines that fight pandemics, and may delay the manufacture and supply of vaccines.

Loss of certainty and scale

The Association of the British Pharmaceutical Industry (ABPI) supports.

the current regulatory system, which is regarded as highly effective, but has expressed concern about the potential additional bureaucracy that a new independent UK regulatory system would create [25].

If separate regulatory processes exist for the UK, companies seeking to launch new products will have to apply for regulatory approval in the UK and EU regions, which would cause delays. This could be detrimental to drug launches in the UK, as companies are likely to prioritize applying for regulatory approval in the considerably larger (500 million) EU market; the UK only constitutes 3% of the world's market for new medicines (60 million). As Rawlins stated: "One of the biggest worries I have about Brexit and standing alone as a regulator is that we are only 3% of the world market for new drugs and, if we are not careful, we are going to be at the back of the queue" [37]. David Jeffreys, spokesperson for the Association of British Pharmaceutical Industries and Vice-President of Eisai, a Japanese pharmaceutical firm, says, "The early innovative medicines will be applied for in the USA, in Japan and through the European system and the UK will be in the second, or indeed the third, wave - so UK patients may be getting medicines, 12, 18, 24 months later than they would if we remained in the European system." [40].

Conversely, some scientists take a more positive view, arguing that Brexit provides an opportunity for more liberal regulatory rules that will permit drugs to be launched more quickly in the UK [41]. Rawlins has also suggested the possibility of launching a system giving provisional licenses to new medicines whilst more real-world data is being collected, which would make the UK market more attractive for pharmaceutical companies.

Influence

The MHRA has a wide range of international links and is respected worldwide as one of the leading regulatory authorities for medicines and medical devices. The MHRA has shared its regulatory expertise with Malta, Latvia and the Czech Republic in a bid to help countries that have recently joined the EU to develop the systems necessary to playing an active part in European regulation [42]. The MHRA was:

- lead regulator in granting licensing to 7 out of 10 European medical products in 2007 [43];
- a rapporteur in 15% of the procedures of the PV Risk Assessment Committee (PRAC) and the Committee for Medicinal Products for Human Use (CHMP) in 2015 [25];
- responsible for inspections that resulted in 25% of Good Manufacturing Practice (GMP) certificates issued in 2015 for sites outside the EU [25].

The UK's VMD has also played a notable role in regulation, acting as a Reference Member State in 43% of Mutual Recognition Procedures in 2015 [25]. The loss of influence in the European system could deter regulatory experts from living and working in the UK, and result in the future implementation of regulations that are less favourable to UK interests, damage that will worsen if the EMA relocates.

Talent
Leadership
Approximately 17% of Science, Technology, Engineering and Mathematics (STEM) academics in UK research institutions are non-UK EU nationals [44]. Facilitating movement across borders is essential to ensuring the supply of talent demanded in current and emerging skill gap areas such as bioinformatics, genomics or Advanced Therapy Medicinal Product (ATMP) manufacturing.

The UK's global reference status therefore depends on removing any barriers to attracting, developing and retaining talent. This includes the current state of uncertainty regarding the UK's future immigration policy and the unwelcoming image projected on foreign workers.

The government remains committed to ensuring researcher mobility is protected. The House of Lords concluded that researcher mobility was "of critical importance to the UK science community, including academia, business and charities" and that "researcher mobility must be protected if UK science and research is to remain world-leading" [45]. A parliament report on the implications and outcomes for science and research concluded by saying: "We understand that the Government is not yet able to offer firmer guarantees regarding future immigration rules for researchers but remind them that this is essential in order to continue to attract top-quality researchers to the UK... There is clear agreement that researcher mobility is a crucial component of the UK's successful research and science sector." [46].

Headquarters
London is home to the EMA, as well as the European headquarters of over a dozen global pharmaceutical companies, the global headquarters of GSK and AstraZeneca, and considerable R&D and manufacturing operations for Amgen and Pfizer. This has attracted and nurtured talent across the value chain in areas such as research, development, regulation, manufacturing and commerce. GSK and AstraZeneca, for example, will employ 15 and 50 university graduates respectively in 2017 [47, 48]. Outside of the EU, the UK may see its capacity to attract talent significantly reduced, which could result in the relocation of operations, causing losses in job, economic contributions and innovation capacity.

Consideration of post-Brexit models
Initial overview
There are three existing models that could provide a solution which would allow the UK to continue receiving EU funding and benefitting from its association with EU-driven scientific research actions (Fig. 3).

A further, and likely, route will be that the UK negotiates its own model with the EU as it seeks to protect its current and future research funding. It should be noted that, even if the UK were able to adopt an existing model, such as that of an 'associated country', additional negotiations will be inevitable [49].

Associated countries
These are non-EU member states that have stipulated an individual formal agreement on full or partial association with an EU research funding programme. To be involved in these programmes in the same manner as EU member states, these countries must pay a fee which is calculated based on their GDP and on further negotiations.

Nevertheless, whilst these countries can receive and benefit from EU research funding, they cannot influence the direction of these programmes as access does not grant them a voice in the European Council or European Parliament. This is the key difference between EU member states and 'associated countries'.

Since the referendum result, lobbying by Universities UK (UUK) has sought to put pressure on the UK government to push negotiations for 'associated country' status [49]. This would secure the UK's participation in Horizon 2020 in a similar manner to other 'associated countries' [49].

Non-associated third countries
These are non-EU member states, such as Afghanistan and Argentina, which are not formally associated with EU research funding programmes and considered as 'developing' or 'industrialised'. Nevertheless, organisations and participants from these countries can become partners with the programmes and receive funding.

The pharmaceutical industry
In considering the post-Brexit options for the UK pharmaceutical industry, there are three key variations to be discussed: EEA (specifically Norway), EFTA (specifically Switzerland) and World Trade Organisations (WTO) (Fig. 4).

EEA
The EEA, established in January 1994, currently includes Norway, Iceland and Liechtenstein. These countries implement EU legislation, such as free trade (except for agriculture and fisheries in most cases) and free movement, acknowledge EU administrative decisions, contribute to the EU to help level social and economic disparities across member states, and pay custom taxes and other administrative costs. However, they cannot vote in the European Parliament and have no says in its laws.

Norway.
The EEA model can be considered a poor deal for Norway since it is so similar to that of EU member states. However, Norway has retained some autonomy

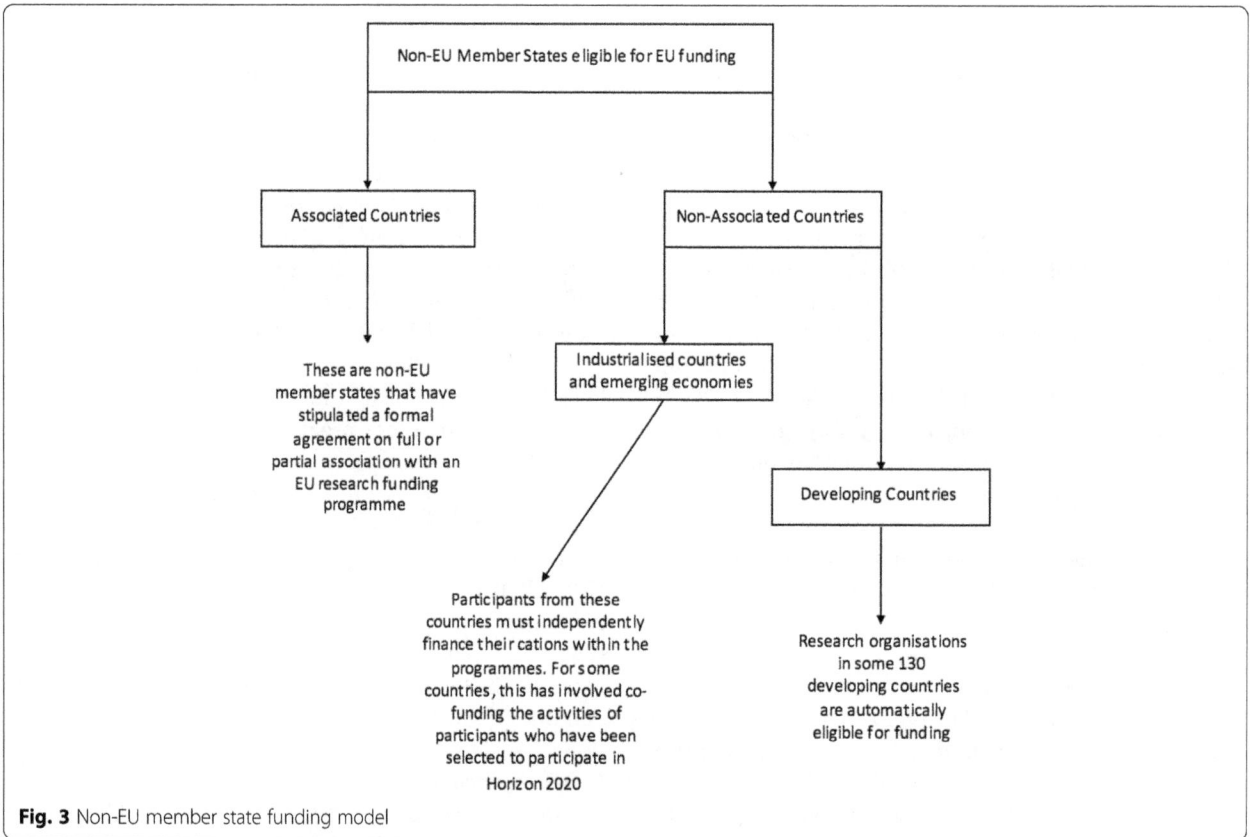

Fig. 3 Non-EU member state funding model

over its pharmaceutical sector. It has its own Medicines Agency (Statens legemiddelverk), which is a subsidiary to its national healthcare organisation. This is not so different to the UK where there is the NHS and the MHRA responsible for marketing medicines.

Although being part of the EEA means that Norway must adhere to EU regulations regarding marketing authorisations, its own Medicines Agency can influence the work of the EMA as EU member states can [50]. In addition, Norway has control over its own pricing and reimbursement, which is different for out- and inpatients, unlike for the rest of the EU [50].

There are therefore subtle differences in how Norway operates compared to that of EU member states, which could make it easier to sell this as a solution to the majority who voted for Brexit. In addition, considering that the UK's existing framework is similar to Norway's, it is feasible to envisage the UK transitioning to this model.

Advantages of the EEA model for the UK [51].

The EEA model would likely be the easiest option for the UK pharmaceutical industry, allowing for a transition to a legal framework only slightly different to the current model, whilst incentivising pharmaceutical companies to remain in the UK. An analysis of Norway suggests that the EEA model can succeed in maintaining

and even attracting key players in the pharmaceutical industry; as of 2015, all major pharmaceutical companies were present in Norway with 9 having production facilities there [50].

Adopting an EEA model would therefore protect the status quo, allowing for continued organisation and efficiency between the UK and the rest of the EU in terms of R&D, clinical trials, manufacturing, marketing, distribution etc. This model would also enable pharmaceutical companies that are only based in the UK to benefit from the new reform starting in 2018 which will introduce a single EU portal for clinical trials. This will ensure a harmonised process for approval of clinical trials across the EU and enable participating nations to access and share clinical trial information on an EU database [52].

If the UK attains membership to the EEA, it effectively retains its status within the EU. This incentivises those EU pharmaceutical companies with registered offices or manufacturing sites in the UK, as well as those that conduct clinical trials in the UK, to continue their activities in much the same manner. Without this security net, these companies will have to demonstrate that their work complies with EU standards, which could prove time-consuming and expensive, possibly resulting in these companies leaving the UK.

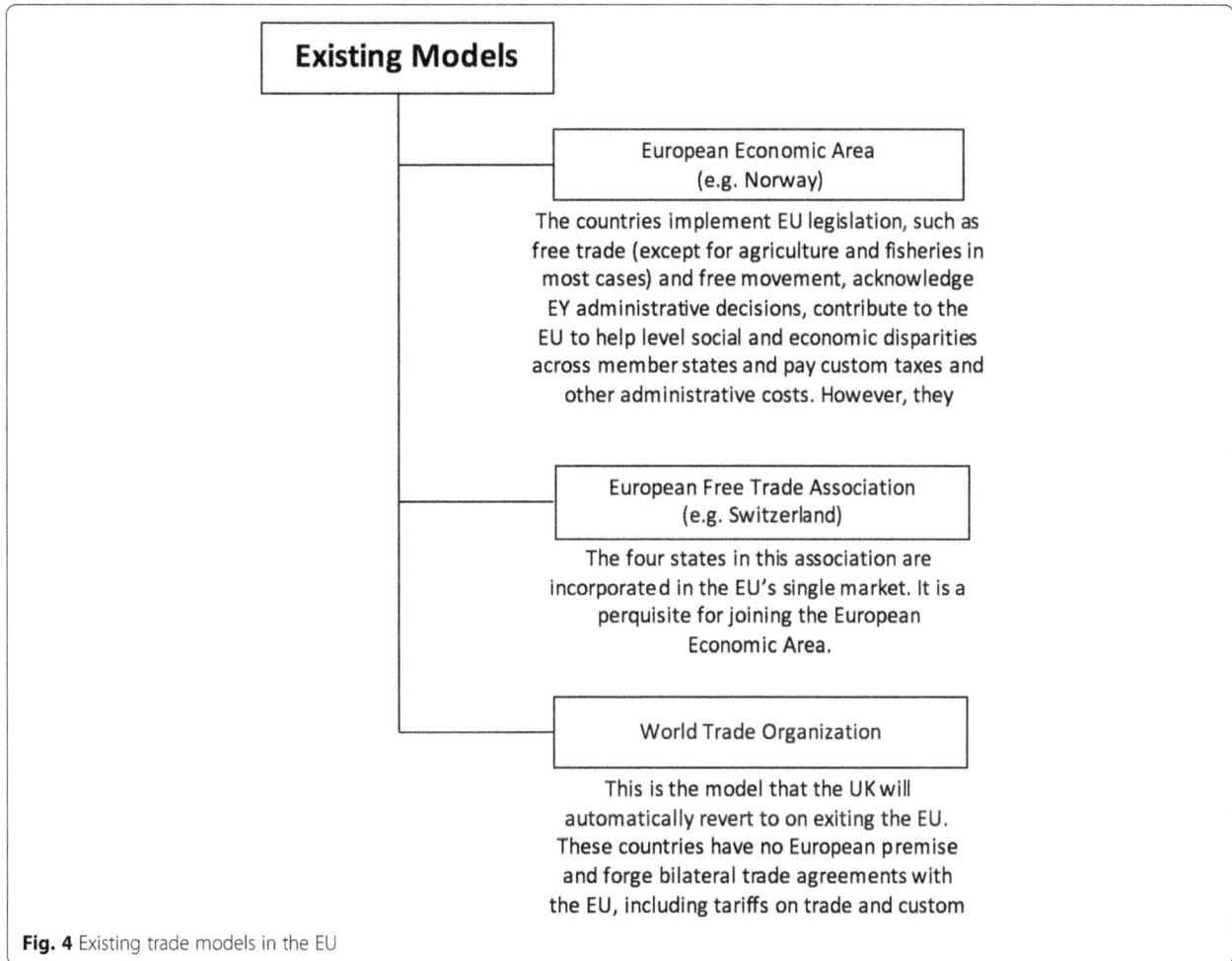

Fig. 4 Existing trade models in the EU

This is especially relevant to those EU pharmaceutical companies that have no offices or manufacturing plants outside of the UK. Unless the UK joins the EEA, these companies will likely relocate to EU or EEA countries in the pursuit of operational ease and business security, as it will be disruptive and time-consuming to establish new legislative practices within a changing business environment to boot. Joining the EEA should therefore protect the UK pharmaceutical industry from the organisational chaos and economic detriment of pharmaceutical companies leaving the UK.

EFTA
The EFTA was formed in 1960 and, today, comprises Switzerland, Norway, Iceland and Liechtenstein. It allows for these four states to be incorporated into the EU's single market. The EFTA is a prerequisite for joining the EEA.

As Switzerland is not also a member of the EEA (the Swiss rejected the idea in 1992), it has its own bilateral agreements with the EU, which took two years to finalise and cover all areas from trade to transport. The complexities of applying a similar model to the UK would therefore engender momentous negotiations.

Switzerland's model.
'Switzerland may guard its political and cultural independence fiercely, but its scientific sector has a strongly international flavour' [53].

Switzerland is a rich country and that is partly thanks to its pharmaceutical industry, which is geared towards high value exports and supported by expert research. Switzerland is home to some of the world's most successful pharmaceutical companies, such as Novartis and Roche, and noted for its scientific and academic institutions.

Despite not being an EU member state, Switzerland has also benefitted from EU FPs, such as Horizon 2020, which offer grants for research. The UK also has a strong reputation in the areas of science and research, and has received proportionately high funds through these programme (£67 billion alone through Horizon 2020). In fact, the UK receives more funding from the European Research Council than any other EU country and has priority access to scientific facilities across Europe, putting it at risk of losing a predicted £8.5 billion over the next four years [54].

Industry similarities and Switzerland's economic success outside of the EU makes it unsurprising that many leave campaigners are championing a Swiss-inspired model as Brexit negotiations take shape. However, it seems highly unlikely that the EU will facilitate furthering these aspirations; in 2010, it was already referring to a relationship with Switzerland "which has become complex and unwieldy to manage and has clearly reached its limits" [55].

In addition, leave campaigners are motivated by what they view as Switzerland's privileged position in terms of its unique relationship with the EU, yet many of them overlook the fact that the Swiss model aligns with many EU structures, laws and values. For example, in 1999, Switzerland accepted free movement of persons. Recently, Switzerland did indeed act to reinstate quotas on foreign workers. However, it was effectively punished by the EU which froze its Horizon 2020 grants and stalled its Erasmus + student mobility scheme [56]. This is a strong indication of the likelihood of failure if the UK attempts to negotiate entirely on its own terms.

WTO

Debate on this subject points to a third solution for the UK post-Brexit, that of the WTO, which is in fact the model that the UK will automatically revert to on exiting the EU [52]. This would be the most drastic option whereby the UK would abandon its European premise and use the established trade rules and norms of the WTO to forge bilateral trade agreements with the EU, resulting in a model similar to the rest of the world (that includes tariffs on trade with the EU, customs taxes etc.) [57].

This option could potentially offer the UK flexibility and the clean slate that leave campaigners rooted for, but it is the most ambiguous at this stage and would likely take many years to implement. For example, the UK could theoretically follow Canada which, after seven years of negotiations, signed the EU-Canada Comprehensive Economic and Trade Agreement (CETA) in 2013 and now profits from 98% tariff-free trade with the EU. Vicky Ford (Conservative MEP and Chair of the European Parliament Committee for the Internal Market and Consumer Protection) has stated that it is "much more important to look at the so called 'non-tariff barriers' which reflect the bureaucratic red tape faced by companies exporting into other markets and to recognise that the level of ease British companies currently have when selling into other EU markets is much, much

greater than that which is now offered to Canada in CETA" [58].

Final considerations

It should also be asked: is it really appropriate to compare the UK to Norway and Switzerland when demographically and economically these are very different nations? The former has a population of 5.1 million, the latter's is 8.2 million. The UK has a population of 64.7 million and a GDP of $2.678 trillion compared to that of Norway and Switzerland at $512.6 billion and $685.4 billion respectively. The economic impact of having to be a 'rule taker' as opposed to a 'rule maker' on issues such as free movement is therefore likely to be far greater for the UK than for Norway or Switzerland [57].

There is also the historical and societal context. Switzerland and Norway never voted to leave the EU because they were never member states in the first place; Switzerland rejected joining the EU in 2001 with a vote of 76.8% and Norway likewise turned down the idea on smaller margins in referendums in 1972 and 1994.

Moving forward

In 2011, the UK economy benefited by around £30 billion from pharmaceutical and chemical exports to the EU [59], which is just one of many figures serving to underpin the importance of investigating the impact of Brexit on this industry. The research conducted has yielded several policy recommendations and priorities based on their potential to maintain the UK's attractiveness as a pharmaceutical hub post-Brexit.

Negotiate an 'associated country' status in the EU's research funding programmes

This will guarantee access to the EU FPs and enable the UK to maintain its current dominance in the life sciences R&D sector. It will also sustain and encourage further collaborations between UK and European scientists, alleviating concerns over the uncertainty involved in working with UK-based partners. If the UK is to remain at the forefront of scientific innovation, it must work to preserve international collaborations.

Negotiate bilaterally favourable trade agreements for drugs and medical devices with the EU

The EU is an essential market for pharmaceutical companies in the UK. To prevent the exodus of pharmaceuticals companies currently based in the UK, the government must renegotiate trade conditions with the EU that are comparable to those pre-Brexit. This calls for a new streamlined customs system for UK-EU trade with low fee and administrative burden. This will also be important in preventing a sharp rise in the costs of drugs imported from the EU.

Mirroring the medicines regulatory approval process with the EMA, whilst retaining the MHRA's capacity to intervene

This would bypass the need for pharmaceutical companies to seek separate product approvals in the UK. By opting to follow the EMA's guidance, albeit with MHRA discretion for specific regulatory matters, the UK would incentivise pharmaceutical companies to remain in the country and prevent a delay in drugs reaching the UK market.

Assurance of free movement of high skilled professionals across UK-EU boarders

This will maintain the high skill level of the workforce in UK universities and the industry as a whole, whilst providing British nationals with the freedom to work, study and gain experience across the EU.

This option will appeal to multinational pharmaceutical companies who wish to quickly and easily relocate staff across international facilities. Free movement of professionals will therefore encourage foreign pharmaceutical companies to preserve their UK-based facilities. This will alleviate concerns regarding their EU staff members and their ability to attract and recruit the best in the field. Finally, such an agreement should encourage further foreign investment in the UK.

Abbreviations
ABPI: Association of the British Pharmaceutical Industry; ATMP: Advanced Therapy Medicinal Product; CETA: Comprehensive Economic and Trade Agreement; CHMP: Committee for Medicinal Products for Human Use; CTD: Clinical Trials Directive; CTR: Clinical Trials Regulation; ECDC: European Centre for Disease Prevention and Control; EEA: European Economic Area; EFTA: European Free Trade Association; EU: European Union; FMD: Falsified Medicines Directive; FP: Framework Programme; GMP: Good Manufacturing Practice; GSK: GlaxoSmithKline; IPO: Initial Public Offering; MDD: Medical Devices Directive; MHRA: Medicine and Healthcare Products Regulatory Agency; NHS: National Health Service; NIHR: National Institute for Healthcare Research; PRAC: PV Risk Assessment Committee; SME: Small and Medium Enterprises; STEM: Sciences, Technology, Engineering and Mathematics; UUK: Universities UK; VMD: Veterinary Medicines Directive

Funding
There was no funding for this work.

Authors' contributions
PT, AAG, and JG contributed research and wrote one section of this paper. FK edited the paper and contributed research and writing to multiple sections. CP researched and wrote two sections of the paper and edited the overall paper. IR researched and wrote one section of the paper and contributed to editing. All authors read and approved the final manuscript.

Competing interests
The authors declare that they have no competing interests.

Author details
[1]University of Cambridge, School of Clinical Medicine, Cambridge, UK. [2]King's College London, London, UK. [3]University of Cambridge, Cambridge, UK. [4]Imperial College London, MRC London Institute of Medical Sciences, London, UK. [5]Polygeia (Global Health Student Think-Tank), Cambridge, UK. [6]Leckhampton House, 37 Grange Road, Cambridge CB3 9BJ, UK.

References
1. Blitz R, Lewis L. Pound tumbles to 30-year low as Britain votes Brexit. Financial Times. 2016; https://www.ft.com/content/8d8a100e-38c2-11e6-a780-b48ed7b6126f. Accessed 1 Apr 2017
2. Nicholls A. SmartViews: Brexit - What's next for pharma? 2016. http://www.pharmatimes.com/magazine/2016/july_2016/smartviews_brexit_-_whats_next_for_pharma. Accessed 1 Apr 2017.
3. Surviving Brexit. 2016. http://www.pmlive.com/pharma_news/surviving_brexit_1136772. Accessed 1 Apr 2017.
4. The government's negotiating objectives for exiting the EU: PM speech - GOV.UK. GOV.UK. 2017. https://www.gov.uk/government/speeches/the-governments-negotiating-objectives-for-exiting-the-eu-pm-speech. Accessed 1 Apr 2017.
5. UK pharma strikes optimistic note as Brexit process begins. 2017. https://www.pmlive.com/pharma_news/uk_pharma_strikes_optimistic_note_as_brexit_process_begins_1190435. Accessed 1 Apr 2017.
6. Thompson M, Williams D-A, Ellingworth P, Bates S. The economic contribution of the UK Life Sciences Industry. 2017.
7. Anekwe L. Pharma contributes £32 billion to UK economy. Pharmafile. 2015;
8. Ward A. UK life sciences hit 7-year high. Financial Times. 2014; https://www.ft.com/content/6d0c13d6-4d55-11e4-bf60-00144feab7de. Accessed 17 Mar 2017
9. Galsworthy M, Davidson R. Debunking the myths about British science after an EU exit. LSE Blogs. 2015. http://blogs.lse.ac.uk/brexit/2015/12/05/debunking-the-myths-about-british-science-after-an-eu-exit/.
10. The Association of British Pharmaceutical Industry. Did you know? Facts and figures about the pharmaceutical industry in the UK. 2011. http://www.abpi.org.uk/our-work/library/industry/Documents/Did%20you%20know_Jan11.pdf. Accessed 28 Mar 2017.
11. Department for Business Innovation & Skill. Growth Dashboard. 2015. https://www.gov.uk/government/uploads/system/uploads/attachment_data/file/396740/bis-15-4-growth-dashboard.pdf. Accessed 17 Mar 2017.
12. Hirschler B. Brexit spells upheaval for EU and UK drug regulation | Reuters. Reuters. 2016; http://www.reuters.com/article/us-britain-eu-corporates-pharmaceuticals-idUSKCN0ZA26J. Accessed 17 Mar 2017
13. Bates S. UK biotech financing and deals in 2015/16. 2016.
14. Bradshaw J. UK biotech is surging but more support is needed, industry warns. Telegraph. 2016; http://www.telegraph.co.uk/business/2016/06/15/uk-biotech-is-surging-but-more-support-is-needed-industry-warns/. Accessed 17 Mar 2017
15. Business Monitor International. Pharmaceuticals & Healthcare Q416 Round-Up. 2016. http://store.bmiresearch.com/pharmaceuticals-healthcare-q416-round-up.html?ito=638&itq=bf6559e0-3ad7-495c-8cbd-223a6d16a0ae&itx%5Bidio%5D=4118473.
16. Hammett S. 2015 Life Sciences Outlook: United Kingdom 2014. https://www2.deloitte.com/content/dam/Deloitte/global/Documents/Life-Sciences-Health-Care/gx-lshc-2015-life-sciences-report-united-kingdom.pdf. Accessed 17 Mar 2017.
17. Norton Rose Fulbright. Impact of Brexit on life sciences and healthcare. 2016. http://www.nortonrosefulbright.com/knowledge/publications/136982/impact-of-brexit-on-life-sciences-and-healthcare. Accessed 17 Mar 2017.
18. Ganslandt M, Maskus K. Parallel Imports of Pharmaceutical Products in the European Union. 2001. http://apps.who.int/medicinedocs/documents/s17518en/s17518en.pdf. Accessed 17 Mar 2017.
19. King's Fund. Better value in the NHS The role of changes in clinical practice. 2015. https://www.kingsfund.org.uk/sites/default/files/field/field_document/better-value-nhs-summary-July-2015.pdf. Accessed 21 Aug 2017.
20. Davies SC, Walley T, Smye S, Cotterill L, Whitty CJ. The NIHR at 10: transforming clinical research. Clin Med. 2016;16:501–2. doi:10.7861/clinmedicine.16-6-501.
21. Cressey D. Overhaul complete for EU clinical trials. Nature. 2014; doi:10.1038/nature.2014.15339.
22. Science and Technologies Committee. EU regulation of the life sciences. 2016. https://www.publications.parliament.uk/pa/cm201617/cmselect/cmsctech/158/158.pdf. Accessed 17 Mar 2017.
23. Genomics England. The 100,000 Genomes Project | Genomics England.

2017. https://www.genomicsengland.co.uk/the-100000-genomes-project/. Accessed 17 Mar 2017.

24. Office for Life Sciences. Life Sciences Competitiveness Indicators. 2016.

25. Bates S, Thompson M. It is hard to think of an industry of greater strategic importance to Britain than its pharmaceutical industry &quot. In: Maintaining and growing the UK's world leading Life Sciences sector in the context of leaving the EU " 2016. http://www.abpi.org.uk/our-work/library/industry/Documents/UK-EU-Steering-Group-Report.pdf. Accessed 17 Mar 2017.

26. European Commission. Seventh FP7 Monitoring Report 2013. 2015.

27. Office for National Statistics. UK Gross Domestic Expenditure on Research and Development. 2015.

28. European Commission. EU Expenditure and Revenue 2007–2013. 2015.

29. Frenk C, Hunt T, Partiridge L, Thornton J, Wyatt T. UK research and the European Union: The role of the EU in funding UK research. R Soc. 2015; https://royalsociety.org/~/media/policy/projects/eu-uk-funding/uk-membership-of-eu.pdf. Accessed 17 Mar 2017

30. Clark G, Johnson J. Safeguarding Funding for Research and Innovation -. 2016. https://www.gov.uk/government/news/safeguarding-funding-for-research-and-innovation. Accessed 17 Mar 2017.

31. Frenk C, Hunt T, Partiridge L, Thornton J, Wyatt T. UK research and the European Union: The role of the EU in international research collaboration and research mobility. 2016. https://royalsociety.org/~/media/policy/projects/eu-uk-funding/phase-2/EU-role-in-international-research-collaboration-and-researcher-mobility.pdf. Accessed 17 Mar 2017.

32. The Policy Institute [King's College London]. Public medical research drives private R&D investment. 2016. https://www.kcl.ac.uk/sspp/policy-institute/publications/SpilloversFINAL.pdf. Accessed 17 Mar 2017.

33. European Federation of Pharmaceutical Industries and Associations. The Pharmaceutical Industry in Figures. 2016. http://www.efpia.eu/uploads/Modules/Documents/the-pharmaceutical-industry-in-figures-2016.pdf. Accessed 17 Mar 2017.

34. Singapore's salad days are over. Nature. 2010;468:731–731. doi:https://doi.org/10.1038/468731a.

35. Fai LK, Kek X. Govt commits S$19b to new 5-year plan for R&D initiatives RIE2020. Channel News Asia. http://www.channelnewsasia.com/news/business/singapore/govt-commits-s-19b-to-new/2409426.html. Accessed 28 Mar 2017

36. Brennan Z. Japan's Ministry of Foreign Affairs: Don't Move EMA Headquarters From London | RAPS. Regulatory Affairs Professionals Society. 2016; http://www.raps.org/Regulatory-Focus/News/2016/09/06/25773/Japan's-Ministry-of-Foreign-Affairs-Don't-Move-EMA-Headquarters-From-London/. Accessed 17 Mar 2017.

37. BBC World Service. BBC World Service - World Update: Daily Commute, Brexit Watch: Public Health After Brexit. 2017. http://www.bbc.co.uk/programmes/p04tmcp0#play, first aired 22 Feb 2017. Accessed 1 Apr 2017.

38. Benstetter M. EMA Management Board: Highlights of December. 2016. http://www.ema.europa.eu/docs/en_GB/document_library/Press_release/2016/12/WC500218416.pdf. Accessed 17 Mar 2017.

39. Office Journal of the European Union. REGULATION (EU) No 536/2014 OF THE EUROPEAN PARLIAMENT AND OF THE COUNCIL of 16 April 2014 on clinical trials on medicinal products for human use, and repealing Directive 2001/20/EC. 2014. http://eur-lex.europa.eu/legal-content/EN/TXT/?uri=celex:32014R0536. Accessed 17 Mar 2017.

40. Merrick R. Brexit will put UK patients at "back of queue" for vital new drugs, health experts warn. The Independent. 2017;

41. Boxall M. Brexit and the Pharmaceutical Industry. Investors Chronicle. 2016; http://www.investorschronicle.co.uk/2016/11/10/shares/sectors/brexit-and-the-pharmaceutical-industry-oZwUvT2tqnPDPCpgRBa8vl/article.html

42. Medicines and Health Regulatory Authority. Safeguarding public health through the effective regulation of medicines and medical devices. 2008. http://www.mhra.gov.uk/home/groups/comms-ic/documents/websiteresources/con2031677.pdf. Accessed 28 Mar 2017.

43. The Pharmaceutical Journal. MHRA/EMEA: rivalry or partnership? Pharm J. 2007;279:226. http://www.pharmaceutical-journal.com/news-and-analysis/mhra/emea-rivalry-or-partnership/10004834.article. Accessed 17 Mar 2017.

44. Campaign for Science and Engineering. Immigration: Keeping the UK at the heart of global science and engineering. 2016. http://www.sciencecampaign.org.uk/resource/caseimmigrationreport2016.html. Accessed 17 Mar 2017.

45. House of Lords Science and Technology Select Committee. EU membership and UK science. https://www.publications.parliament.uk/pa/ld201516/ldselect/ldsctech/127/127.pdf. Accessed 1 Apr 2017.

46. Blackman R, Blackwood N. Leaving the EU: implications and opportunities for science and research Seventh Report of Session 2016–17. Labour. 2016; https://www.publications.parliament.uk/pa/cm201617/cmselect/cmsctech/502/502.pdf. Accessed 1 Apr 2017

47. GlaxoSmithKline. GSK Graduate Jobs. 2017. https://www.graduate-jobs.com/scheme/gsk. Accessed 17 Mar 2017.

48. AstraZeneca. Graduate Jobs & Schemes. 2016. https://www.graduate-jobs.com/scheme/astrazeneca. Accessed 17 Mar 2017.

49. Morgan J. Brexit: could UK join EU research system as "associated country"? | THE News. Times Higher Education. 2016;

50. Festøy H, Ognøy AH. PPRI Pharma Profile. 2015. https://legemiddelverket.no/Documents/English/Price%20and%20reimbursement/PPRI_Pharma_Profile_Norway_20150626_final.pdf. Accessed 17 Mar 2017.

51. Salvatore V. The impact of Brexit on the pharmaceutical industry: some preliminary considerations | Pharmafile. Pharmafile. 2016; http://www.pharmafile.com/news/505928/impact-brexit-pharmaceutical-industry-some-preliminary-considerations. Accessed 17 Mar 2017

52. Privolnev Y. Brexit's Impact On The Global Pharmaceutical Industry Future Access To The EU Common Market. Pharm Online. 2016; https://www.pharmaceuticalonline.com/doc/brexit-s-impact-on-the-global-pharmaceutical-industry-future-access-to-the-eu-common-market-0001. Accessed 17 Mar 2017

53. Whelan J. Switzerland's thriving pharmaceutical industry. New Scientist. 2006;

54. Taylor K. What would Brexit mean for the pharma industry? - Health Solutions. Deloitte Health Solutions. 2016; http://blogs.deloitte.co.uk/health/2016/02/what-would-brexit-mean-for-the-pharma-industry.html. Accessed 17 Mar 2017

55. General Affairs Council Meeting. Council Conclusions on Eu Relations with EFTA. Brussels; 2010. https://eeas.europa.eu/sites/eeas/files/council_iceland.pdf. Accessed 17 Mar 2017

56. Wintour P. EU tells Swiss no single market access if no free movement of citizens. The Guardian. 2016;

57. HM Treasury. HM Treasury analysis: the long-term economic impact of EU membership and the alternatives. 2016. https://www.gov.uk/government/uploads/system/uploads/attachment_data/file/517154/treasury_analysis_economic_impact_of_eu_membership_print.pdf. Accessed 17 Mar 2017.

58. Ford V. Vicky Ford: The Canada deal is not the model Brexit negotiations should follow. 2017. http://www.conservativehome.com/platform/2017/02/vicky-ford-the-canada-deal-is-not-the-model-brexit-negotiations-should-follow.html. Accessed 28 Mar 2017

59. Edwards M. The Pink Book. 2012:2012. http://webarchive.nationalarchives.gov.uk/20160105160709/http://www.ons.gov.uk/ons/rel/bop/united-kingdom-balance-of-payments/2012/bod-the-pink-book-2012.pdf. Accessed 17 Mar 2017

17

Availability, prices and affordability of UN Commission's lifesaving medicines for reproductive and maternal health in Uganda

Denis Kibira[1,2*], Freddy Eric Kitutu[3,4], Gemma Buckland Merrett[5] and Aukje K. Mantel-Teeuwisse[6]

Abstract

Background: Uganda was one of seven countries in which the United Nations Commission on Life Saving Commodities (UNCoLSC) initiative was implemented starting from 2013. A nationwide survey was conducted in 2015 to determine availability, prices and affordability of essential UNCoLSC maternal and reproductive health (MRH) commodities.

Methods: The survey at health facilities in Uganda was conducted using an adapted version of the standardized methodology co-developed by World Health Organisation (WHO) and Health Action International (HAI). In this study, six maternal and reproductive health commodities, that were part of the UNCoLSC initiative, were studied in the public, private and mission health sectors. Median price ratios were calculated with Management Sciences for Health International Drug Price Indicator prices as reference. Maternal and reproductive health commodity stocks were reviewed from stock cards for their availability for a period of 6 months preceding the survey. Affordability was measured using wages of the lowest paid government worker.

Results: Overall none of the six maternal and reproductive commodities was found in the surveyed health facilities. Public sector had the highest availability (52%), followed by mission sector (36%) and then private sector had the least (30%). Stock outs ranged from 7 to 21 days in public sector; 2 to 23 days in private sector and 3 to 27 days in mission sector. During the survey, maternal health commodities were more available and had less number of stock out days than reproductive health commodities. Median price ratios (MPR) indicated that medicines and commodities were more expensive in Uganda compared to international reference prices. Furthermore, MRH medicines and commodities were more expensive and less affordable in private sector compared to mission sector.

Conclusion: Access to MRH commodities is inadequate in Uganda. Maternal health commodities were more available, cheaper and thus more affordable than reproductive health commodities in the current study. Efforts should be undertaken by the Ministry of Health and stakeholders to improve availability, prices and affordability of MRH commodities in Uganda to ensure that sustainable Development Goals are met.

* Correspondence: dkibira@gmail.com; dkibira@heps.or.ug
[1]WHO Collaborating Centre for Pharmaceutical Policy and Regulation, Utrecht Institute for Pharmaceutical Sciences (UIPS), Utrecht University, Universiteitsweg 99, 3584 CG Utrecht, the Netherlands
[2]Coalition for Health Promotion and Social Development (HEPS-Uganda), Plot 351A, Balintuma Road, Namirembe Hill, Kampala, Uganda
Full list of author information is available at the end of the article

Background

Maternal mortality is a major public health concern in Uganda. In 2016, Uganda's maternal mortality was estimated at 336deaths per 100,000 live births [1]. Judged against the Millennium Development Goal 5, Uganda did not achieve the 75% reduction in maternal mortality from the 1990 levels by 2015. [2]. Most of these maternal deaths are associated with events directly related to pregnancy and child birth, such as unsafe abortion and obstetric complications, severe bleeding, infections, pre-eclampsia and obstructed labour, and the proportion of deaths among women of reproductive age that are due to maternal causes is 13.4% [3]. Additionally, pregnancy increases the risk of maternal death from causes of malaria, diabetes, hepatitis, anaemia and HIV/AIDS. Indeed, 3.1% percentage of HIV/AIDS deaths is related indirectly to maternal causes [4]. Studies have shown that these deaths could have been averted if there was adequate access to maternal and reproductive health services [5–7].

The state of sexual reproductive health remains poor in Uganda with a high fertility rate of 5.8 children per woman of child bearing age [1], high rates of teenage pregnancies (24%) [8] and unsafe abortions accounting for 11% of maternal deaths annually [8]. In addition, there is limited demand for, and uptake of, reproductive health services, with only 20.4% of Ugandan women using a modern contraceptive method. The Contraceptive Prevalence Rate (CPR) stands at 30% and the unmet family planning need stands at 28% [9]. This situation is exacerbated by supply chain bottlenecks that impair the last mile delivery [10].

In 2010 the UN General Secretary launched the Every Woman Every Child (EWEC) movement to address challenges and bottlenecks to reduction of maternal and child mortality. The preceding review to the EWEC movement had identified unavailability and inadequate access to proven life-saving low-cost medicines and commodities. Therefore, the UN Commission on Life Saving Commodities (UNCoLSC) identified and highlighted 13 underused, low-cost and high impact medicines and medical devices for reproductive, maternal, new-born and child health with the greatest potential to reduce preventable deaths [11]. It also proposed mechanisms to increase the availability, adequate access and rational use of the 13 identified life-saving commodities.

Given the poor progress towards achieving MDG goal 5, Uganda received technical and financial support to conduct a reproductive, maternal, new born and child health (RMNCH) situation analysis to inform the development of an evidence-based country specific implementation plan [8]. Following a two-year implementation period, a nationwide survey was conducted to determine the availability and prices of the six maternal and reproductive health commodities from among the UNCoLSC commodities within the public, private and mission sectors. Additionally, this study also determined the stock out duration for the same basket of commodities to provide information on how fast the system responds to stock outs.

Methods

A survey measuring the availability, price and affordability of maternal and reproductive health (MRH) commodities at health facilities in Uganda was conducted in September 2015, using an adapted World Health Organisation (WHO) and Health Action International (HAI) standardized methodology [12]. This method was validated [13] and used by others [14–16]. It is based on quantitative techniques to analyse availability and prices of health commodities in the public, private and mission health sectors.

Public, private and mission sector health centres of level III or higher participated in the survey.

MRH commodity availability on day of survey and in 6 months preceding the survey was assessed and prices paid by patient were collected.

Selection of outlets

The central region which is the largest in the country and has the capital city was selected first. Three regions of Eastern, Western and Northern Uganda within 1 day's travel from the central region were then selected to provide a realistic representation of the diverse epidemiological, geographical and medicine supply chain characteristics in Uganda. Health facilities from both urban and rural areas were included in the study sample.

In each region, the main regional referral hospitals were selected with guidance of the Uganda Ministry of Health list of health facilities; public health centres level III or higher were randomly selected. Then private and mission sector health facilities that were within a three-hour drive radius from the enrolled regional referral hospitals were selected, respectively. Consecutive sampling was done with an intention of having 10 health facilities per sector in each region coming up to a total sample frame of 120 facilities. This was done to ensure that each sector had a minimum representation of 30 health facilities in the survey [12]. Health Centres level III are the lowest level of care at which MRH commodities are delivered according to the Ministry of Health (MoH) scheduling of basic of health services in Uganda [17].

Selection of medicines and commodities

The medicines and commodities surveyed included the six reproductive and maternal health medicines and commodities, which are required either to prevent or manage pregnancy as specified by the "United Nations Commission on Life Saving Commodities for Women and

Children" (UNCoLSC). UNCoLSC prioritized a core list of 13 life-saving commodities and medicines for reproductive, maternal, newborn and child health, and it specified their formulation or presentation. All countries, Uganda inclusive, were encouraged to grant marketing authorization to these medicines and commodities. The final list of products measured is shown in Table 1 below.

Data collection and analysis

Eight data collectors with previous experience of conducting medicine surveys worked in pairs of a pharmacist and a social scientist under close supervision of a qualified survey manager. Prior to data collection, these pairs were trained on the WHO/HAI methodology of monitoring medicine availability and prices. Data collectors used a semi-structured questionnaire to interview facility managers while ascertaining physical count and stock card records of surveyed medicines. Availability was measured by the physical presence of a product in the outlet at the time of the survey. For each medicine surveyed, data collectors recorded the stated product name for both the highest and lowest priced medicines available, the manufacturer, unit price of the product and number of stock-out days in the previous 6 months. In the public sector where medicines are free of charge to the care seekers, only availability and stock out days were recorded.

Once data collection was complete, survey data was entered centrally into the pre-programmed Microsoft Excel Workbook provided as part of the WHO/HAI methodology. Data input was independently checked for errors. Additional quality control measures were executed at various stages throughout the study. An advisory team provided the overall quality assurance by reviewing survey process, tools for data collection and validation of findings. The survey tools were pre-tested before the survey and prior to data collection. In addition, all survey personnel participated in training and field testing of the survey. Each regional/district team had a supervisor who cross checked the data on a daily basis for completeness, legibility and consistency and reported to the survey manager. A survey manager made field visits and follow-up telephone interviews to validate data in 10% of the sampled outlets. Prior to data entry all relayed data was checked for completeness and consistency.

The availability of individual medicines was calculated as the percentage of sampled medicine outlets where the medicine was found. Data were reported in aggregate as public, private or mission sector medicine outlets. Overall availability per sector was calculated as median of medicines surveyed. For stock data, facilities that had not stocked a particular medicine for 6 months preceding the survey were expressed as a percentage of total number of facilities. For those that reported to stock the medicine, a monthly average of stock-out days was calculated.

Patient prices were collected in Uganda Shillings and the median, minimum and maximum unit prices were estimated. To facilitate cross-country comparisons, medicine prices obtained during the survey were expressed as ratios relative to a standard set of international reference prices [18] by dividing the median local unit price by the international reference unit price. Medicine price ratios were calculated only for medicines with price data from at least four medicine outlets. The exchange rate used to calculate MPRs was 1$ = 3667.9 Uganda Shillings; this was the mid-rate (average of purchase and sale rate) taken from Bank Uganda website on the first day of data collection [19].

Affordability was calculated using the number of days it requires to pay for standard treatment or dose of treatment based on the daily income of the lowest-paid unskilled government employee [12]. The daily wage of the lowest paid government worker (attendants) is approximately UGX 6255 (USD 1.78) as per Uganda Ministry of Public Service salary structure [20]. Treatments that required more than 1 day's wages to purchase were considered unaffordable [12].

Table 1 List of medicines and commodities surveyed in Uganda, 2015, based on the standard World Health Organization/Health Action International Medicine Prices and Availability methodology

Medicine	Use
Reproductive Health	
1- Female condom (any brand)	Contraception
2- Contraceptive implants: a. Etonogestrel 68 mg/rod (Implanon) OR b. Levonorgestrel 0.75 mg/rod (Jadelle)	Contraception
3- Emergency contraceptive pill: a. Levonorgestrel (1.5 mg or 0.75 mg) tablet	Emergency contraception
Maternal Health	
4- Oxytocin injection 10 IU, 1 ml	Prevention and management of post-partum Haemorrhage
5- Misoprostol 200 µg tablet	Prevention and management of post-partum Haemorrhage
6- Magnesium sulphate 500 mg/ml injectable (2 ml, 5 ml, 10 ml ampoule)	Management of pre-eclampsia and eclampsia

Results

A sample of 114 facilities comprising of 37 public, 41 private and 36 mission sector health facilities participated in the study as is shown in Table 2 below.

Availability on the day of data collection

Availability of medicines on day of data collection is shown in Fig. 1. Overall none of the maternal and reproductive health commodities studied was found in all the surveyed health facilities. The public sector had the highest median (52%), followed by mission sector (36%) and then private sector had the least (30%). The most available commodity was oxytocin injection (86% in mission facilities and 84% in public facilities). The least available commodity was the female condom (in 5% of private facilities, 8% of mission facilities and 22% of facilities). In the public sector, three out of seven items were available in less than 50% of facilities. In the private sector, six of seven items were available in less than 50% of facilities whereas in mission sector five medicines were available in less than 50% of facilities.

Maternal health commodities were more available than reproductive health commodities. Among reproductive health commodities, the long term contraceptive etonogestrel implant (brand name Implanon) was most available at 76% in public facilities.

Medicine stock-out duration

During the review period, a large number of facilities (44% public facilities, 49% private facilities, 59% mission facilities on average) had not stocked MRH commodities in the 6 months preceding the survey; 38% public facilities had not stocked misoprostol, 19% private facilities had not stocked levonorgestrel tablets and 30% mission facilities had not stocked levonorgestrel implants (see Fig. 2).

For the facilities that had stocked the items in the previous 6 months preceding the survey, the stock out days ranged from 7 days to 20 days in the public sector; 2 days to 23 days in the private sector and 3 days to 27 days in the mission sector, respectively (see Fig. 3). Although ranges of stock out days were similar, pronounced differences existed between sectors for some commodities, e.g. for levonorgestrel tablets. Maternal health commodities had less stock out days in the 6 months preceding the survey than reproductive health commodities. Female condoms were the least stocked commodity across all sectors.

Table 2 Number and distribution of health facilities surveyed

Sector	Central	Eastern	Western	North	Total
Public	10	08	11	08	37
Private	13	09	09	10	41
Mission	11	07	09	09	36
Totals	34	24	29	27	114

Prices and affordability of commodities in private and mission sectors

Median price ratios (MPR) indicated that medicines and commodities were up to over four times more expensive in Uganda compared to international reference prices (Table 3). Also medicines and commodities were more expensive and less affordable in the private sector than the mission sector.

Discussion

Overall no MRH commodity was available in all the surveyed facilities. Commodities were available in just half of public facilities and in about one third of both mission and private sector facilities. Up to one in three facilities had not stocked many of the MRH commodities in a period of 6 months. Medicines and commodities were more expensive in Uganda than to the international reference prices and were less affordable in private sector than to mission sector.

A core obligation of state as regards the right to reproductive health is to ensure the availability, accessibility, acceptability and quality of services [21]. Essential commodity supplies are required to ensure that healthy reproductive care is made possible. Child bearing individuals have a right to choose, obtain and use contraceptives to avoid unintended pregnancies, to prevent and treat sexually transmitted infections (STIs), and to ensure healthy pregnancy and delivery. This concept is known as *Reproductive Health Commodity Security* (RHCS) and requires governments to ensure and maintain access to and availability of reproductive health commodities [22].

This survey found that universal access to medicines and commodities for reproductive and maternal health has not been achieved in Uganda. Availability was low, stock outs frequently occurred or medicines and commodities had not been stocked during the 6 months preceding the study and they were largely unaffordable because of high prices. This is similar to studies elsewhere; Silal et al. found access to obstetric services in South Africa was impeded by among others availability and affordability barriers and Adjei et al. found low availability of contraceptives in Ghana [5, 23].

Availability of maternal health commodities was better than availability for reproductive health commodities. Between 2012 and the current survey in 2015, availability of reproductive health commodities did not improve but there was an improvement in availability of maternal health commodities in the public sector. For example there was even a reduction in availability of emergency contraceptives from 61% to 24% in the public sector [24]. There was increase in availability of oxytocin in the public sector from 61% to 84% whereas it decreased slightly in the mission sector from 90% to 86% and in the private sector from 86% to 44%. Similarly availability

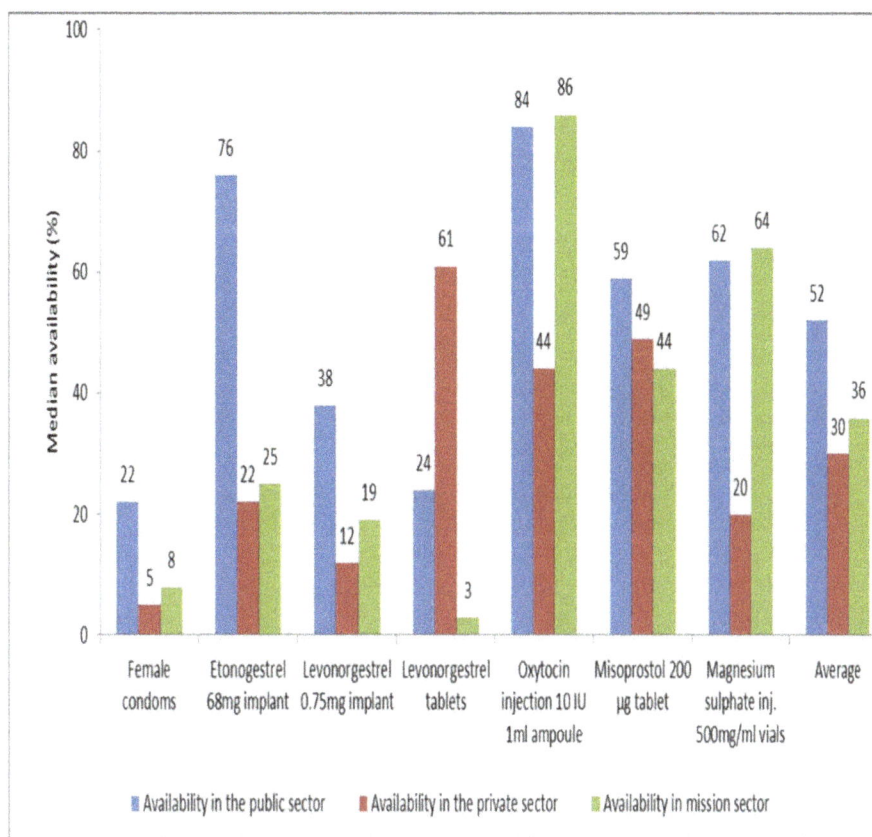

Fig. 1 Median availability of reproductive and maternal health medicines and commodities on day of data collection: Figure shows that overall no commodity was found in all facilities. The public sector had the highest availability, followed by mission sector and the private sector had the least availability

of magnesium sulphate in the public sector improved from 47% to 62% but reduced in mission facilities from 100% to 64%. Availability in the private sector remained minimal consistent with a previous survey [10]. This indicates that management of supplies for family planning programs remains a challenge. The improvement in the public sector may be related to the various government and civil society efforts to improve maternal health in this sector. These campaigns should also be targeted to the other sectors.

The results may indicate limited prioritisation of demand generation activities for reproductive and maternal health commodities by improving knowledge of providers and consumers of the commodities. Policy makers ought to emphasise among others provider skills and overcoming gender inequity and negative social norms to improve access to reproductive and maternal health commodities [25, 26].

Stock outs were high across all sectors but least prone in public sector; on average 63% of public facilities had a stock out in previous 6 months of survey, compared to 80% of mission facilities and 84% of private facilities. However, stock out duration per month was least in the

private sector. This implies that the private sector had the most readiness to respond to a stock-out.

Consumer prices for medicines and commodities were very high and unaffordable. For example the "emergency pill" levonorgestrel 0.75 mg had a median unit price of USD 1.52 per tablet and therefore the lowest government worker would have to spend 1.6 days' wages to afford two tablets required for a dose of treatment. This finding is consistent with many studies done in low and middle income countries which show that medicine prices are often high [27–29]. Efforts should be undertaken by the Ministry of Health and stakeholders like manufacturers, development partners and civil society to reduce commodity prices through measures such as price caps, subsidies, pooled purchasing mechanisms by all sectors and cost-effective strategies to increase the distribution coverage area of wholesalers [30, 31].

The WHO/HAI medicines Prices and Availability survey data can play an important role in analysing access, availability and affordability of essential medicines in low and middle-income countries. The major strength of this study is the use of a tested, reliable, standardized and

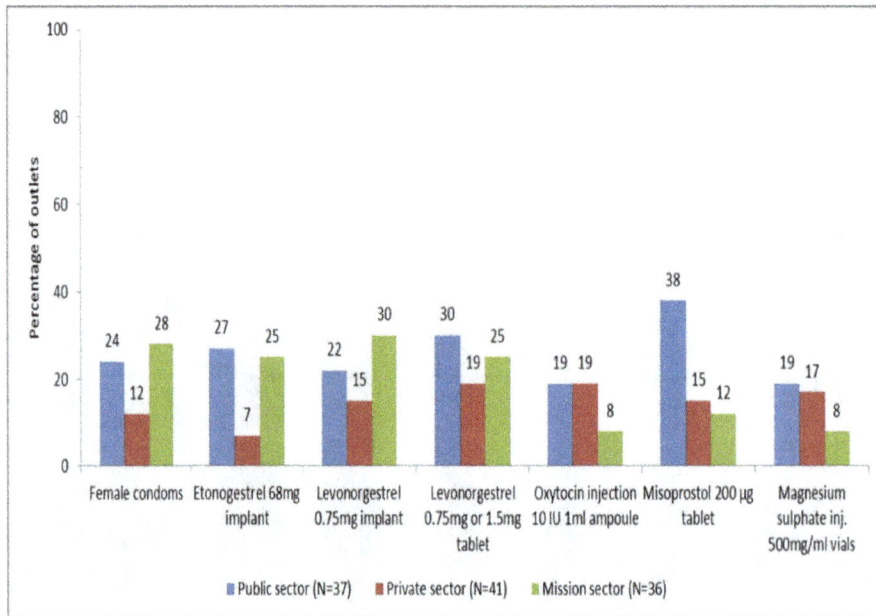

Fig. 2 Percentage of surveyed outlets that had not stocked the named reproductive or maternal medicine or commodity in 6 months preceding survey: a large number of facilities had not stocked many of the commodities

validated methodology which allows for the measurement of medicine prices and availability [13]. The study provides details on availability, cost, and affordability of individual medicines across three sectors (public, private and mission) and the methodology was adopted to incorporate stock-out rates for the various medicines and commodities and therefore provides a more reliable and accurate picture of availability over a longer period beyond the day of data collection. The study also explored alternative therapeutic alternatives, dosage forms

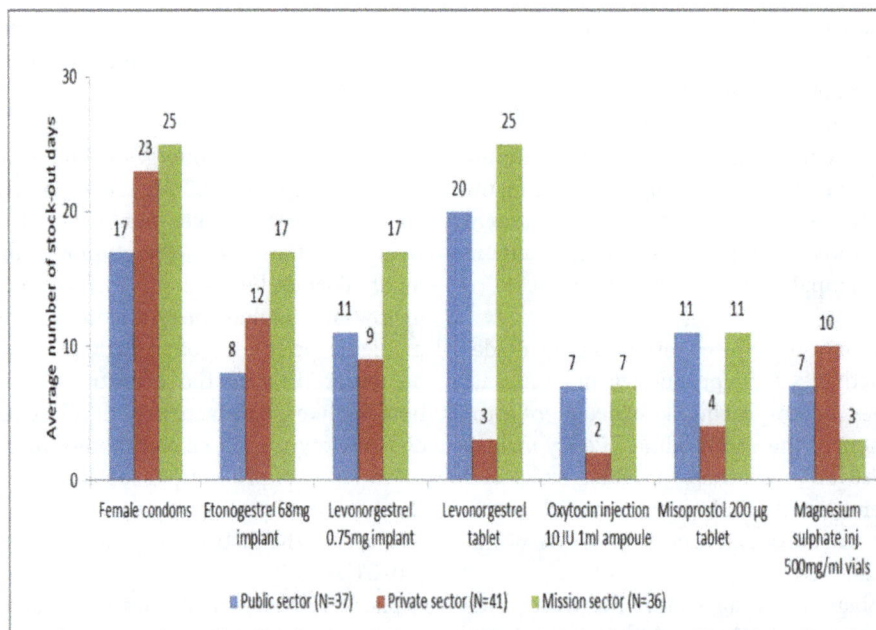

Fig. 3 Average number of stock-out days per month of each reproductive and maternal medicine or commodity at surveyed outlets in 6 months preceding survey: Stock out days per month ranged from 7 days to 20 days in the public sector; 2 days to 23 days in the private sector and 3 days to 27 days in the mission sector

Table 3 Prices and affordability of treatment

Medicine	Unit Price in USD (MPR)		Treatment unit	Affordability per treatment unit (in days)	
	Priv.	Mission		Private sector	Mission sector
Etonogestrel 68 mg/rod × 1 implant	3.03	–	1 implant	1.6	–
Levonorgestrel 0.75 mg tablet	1.52	–	2 tablets	1.6	–
Misoprostol 200 µg Tablet	1.52 (4.39)	0.91 (2.63)	I tablet	0.8	0.48
Oxytocin Injection 10 IU, 1 ml	0.61 (3.49)	0.61 (3.49)	1 ampoule	0.32	0.32
Magnesium sulfate Injection 500 mg/ml	2.04 (1.54)	1.52 (1.15)	1 ampoule	1.1	0.8

and strengths of the medicines and commodities. Findings in this study may not be generalizable to other countries with pharmaceutical markets and structures markedly different from Uganda's. However, such information can form an important component of advocacy efforts for rational pharmaceutical policies. In order to provide more useful information for effective policy intervention, and to counter the main limitations of this study, methods to elucidate factors influencing the differences in results between sectors, for example, should be incorporated.

Conclusions

Results indicate that access to medicines and commodities for reproductive and maternal health has not been achieved in Uganda. Access in terms of availability, prices and affordability was better for maternal health compared to reproductive medicines and commodities. The Ministry of Health therefore ought to emphasise among others, provider skills and overcoming gender inequity and negative social norms to improve access to reproductive and maternal health commodities. Efforts should be undertaken by the Ministry and stakeholders to reduce commodity prices for retailers and other measures such as subsidies, pooled purchasing mechanisms and cost-effective strategies to increase the distribution coverage area of wholesalers.

Abbreviations

HAI: Health Action International; MoH: Ministry of Health; MPR: Median price ratios; MRH: Maternal and reproductive health; RMNCH: Reproductive, maternal, new born and child health; UNCoLSC: United Nations Commission on Life saving Commodities; WHO: World Health Organisation

Acknowledgements

The authors recognize the contribution of HEPS-Uganda that availed the data used in this project.

Funding

This research used data that was publicly available from Coalition for Health Promotion and Social Development (HEPS-Uganda) and received no funding.

Authors' contributions

DK conceptualized the project, undertook data analysis and wrote the first draft of the manuscript; FEK and GBM revised the manuscript and critically reviewed its contents. FEK contributed to data analysis. AKMT critically reviewed the manuscript, provided comments and guidance on all drafts of manuscript. All authors read and approved the final manuscript.

Competing interests

The authors declare that they have no competing interests.

Author details

[1]WHO Collaborating Centre for Pharmaceutical Policy and Regulation, Utrecht Institute for Pharmaceutical Sciences (UIPS), Utrecht University, Universiteitsweg 99, 3584 CG Utrecht, the Netherlands. [2]Coalition for Health Promotion and Social Development (HEPS-Uganda), Plot 351A, Balintuma Road, Namirembe Hill, Kampala, Uganda. [3]Makerere University, School of Public Health and Pharmacy Department, College of Health Sciences, PO Box 7072, Kampala, Uganda. [4]Uppsala University, Department of Women's and Children's Health, International Maternal and Child Health, SE-751 85 Uppsala, Sweden. [5]Health Action International, Overtoom 60 (2), 1054 HK Amsterdam, The Netherlands. [6]WHO Collaborating Centre for Pharmaceutical Policy and Regulation, Utrecht Institute for Pharmaceutical Sciences (UIPS), Utrecht University, Universiteitsweg 99, 3584 CG Utrecht, the Netherlands.

References

1. Uganda Bureau of Statistics (UBOS). The National Population and housing census 2014 - main report. Kampala, Uganda: UBOS; 2016.
2. Ministry of Health (Uganda). In: Ministry of Health, editor. Annual health sector performance report - financial year 2014/2015. Kampala: Government of Uganda; 2015.
3. UNICEF. Maternal health - Maternal mortality; current status and progress. 2016 [cited 2016 October 21st]; Available from: http://data.unicef.org/topic/maternal-health/maternal-mortality/.
4. Uganda Ministry of Health. Annual health sector performance report - financial year 2015/16. Kampala: Uganda Ministry of Health; 2016.
5. Silal SP, et al. Exploring inequalities in access to and use of maternal health services in South Africa. BMC Health Serv Res. 2012;12:120.
6. Bhutta ZA, Das JK, Bahl R, Lawn JE, Salam RA, Paul VK, Every Newborn, et al. Can available interventions end preventable deaths in mothers, newborn babies, and stillbirths, and at what cost? Lancet Glob Health. 2014;384(9940): 347–70.
7. Pronyk PM, et al. The UN Commission on life saving commodities 3 years on: global progress update and results of a multicountry assessment. Lancet Glob Health. 2016;4(4):e276–86.
8. Ministry of Health (Uganda), A promise renewed; reproductive maternal, newborn and child health sharpened plan for Uganda, Ministry of Health, Editor 2013a, Ministry of Health,: Kampala, Uganda.
9. Uganda Bureau of Statistics, Uganda demographic and health survey, in government report. Kampala: Uganda Bureau of Statistics; 2016.
10. TARSC & HEPS. Women's health and sexual and reproductive health in Uganda: a review of evidence. Harare, Zimbabwe: TARSC, HEPS, EQUINET; 2013.
11. United Nations, Every woman every child. UN Commission on life-saving commodities for women and children: commissioners' report September 2012, 2012, United Nations: New York.
12. WHO/HAI. Measuring medicine prices, availability, affordability and price components. 2nd ed. Geneva, Switzerland: World Health Organization; 2008.

13. Madden JM, et al. Measuring medicine prices in Peru: validation of key aspects of WHO/HAI survey methodology. Rev Panam Salud Publica. 2010; 27(4):291–9.

14. Cameron A, et al. Switching from originator brand medicines to generic equivalents in selected developing countries: how much could be saved? Value Health. 2012;15(5):664–73.

15. Anson A, et al. Availability, prices and affordability of the World Health Organization's essential medicines for children in Guatemala. Glob Health. 2012;8:22.

16. Cameron A, et al. Mapping the availability, price, and affordability of antiepileptic drugs in 46 countries. Epilepsia. 2012;53(6):962–9.

17. Ministry of Health. In: Ministry of Health, editor. Package of basic health Services for Uganda. Kampala, Uganda: Ministry of Health; 1997.

18. Management Sciences for Health. International Drug Price Indicator Guide. 2014 [cited 2016 May 5th]; Available from: http://erc.msh.org/mainpage. cfm?file=1.0.htm&module=DMP&language=English.

19. Bank of Uganda. Exchange Rates. 2016 [cited 2016 April 22nd]; Available from: https://www.bou.or.ug/bou/collateral/exchange_rates.html.

20. Uganda Ministry of Public Service. New salary scales for public servants for FY 2014/15. Kampala, Uganda: Uganda Ministry of Public Service; 2014.

21. World Health Organization. Framework for ensuring human rights in the provision of contraceptive information and services. Geneva, Switzerland: WHO Document Production Services; 2014.

22. UNFPA, RHCS. The global program to enhance reproductive health commodity security. Denmark: UNFPA; 2010.

23. Adjei KK, et al. A comparative study on the availability of modern contraceptives in public and private health facilities in a peri-urban community in Ghana. Reprod Health. 2015;12:68.

24. Ministry of Health, H.-U., Monitoring reproductive health supplies in Uganda. 2012.

25. Lawry L, Canteli C., Rabenzanahary T, Pramana W, A mixed methods assessment of barriers to maternal, newborn and child health in gogrial west, south Sudan. 2017.

26. Jayanna K, Mony P, Ramesh BM, Thomas A, Gaikwad A, Mohan HL, Blanchard JF, Moses S, Avery L. Assessment of facility readiness and provider preparedness for dealing with postpartum haemorrhage and pre-eclampsia/eclampsia in public and private health facilities of northern Karnataka, India: a cross-sectional study. BMC Health Serv Res. 2014;14:304.

27. Chahal HS, Fort NS, Bero L. Availability, prices and affordability of essential medicines in Haiti. J Glob Health. 2013;3(2):020405.

28. Jiang M, et al. Medicine prices, availability, and affordability in the Shaanxi Province in China: implications for the future. Int J Clin Pharm. 2015;37(1):12–7.

29. Suh GH. High medicine prices and poor affordability. Curr Opin Psychiatry. 2011;24(4):341–5.

30. Palafox B, et al. Prices and mark-ups on antimalarials: evidence from nationally representative studies in six malaria-endemic countries. Health Policy Plan. 2016;31(2):148–60.

31. Mhlanga BS, Suleman F. Price, availability and affordability of medicines. Afr J Prim Health Care Fam Med. 2014;6(1):E1–6.

18

To what extent do prescribing practices for hypertension in the private sector in Zimbabwe follow the national treatment guidelines? An analysis of insurance medical claims

Victor Basopo and Paschal N. Mujasi[*]

Abstract

Background: Hypertension is the most prevalent cardiovascular disease in Zimbabwe. The prevalence of Hypertension in the country is above 30% regardless of the cut off used. Currently, majority of patients in Zimbabwe seek health care from the private sector due to limited government funding for the public health sector. However, Standard treatment guidelines for hypertension are only available in the public sector and are optional in the private sector. This study assesses compliance of private sector prescribing to Standard Treatment guidelines for hypertension.

Methods: We reviewed hypertension prescription claims to a private health insurance company in Zimbabwe for the period Jan 1-Dec 31 2015. We used the last prescription claimed in the year on the assumption that it represented the patient's current treatment. Prescription data was analyzed by comparing medicines prescribed to those recommended in the Zimbabwe 7th Essential Medicines List and Standard Treatment Guidelines 2015. We used Microsoft Excel© 2010 to conduct the analysis.

Results: A total of 1019 prescriptions were reviewed. Most patients were either on mono or dual therapy (76%). The mostly prescribed class of antihypertensive as first line were Angiotensin Converting Enzyme Inhibitors /Angiotensin Receptor Blockers. Regardless of whether they were being used as first, second or third line this class of antihypertensives emerged as the most prescribed (639 times). Only 358 (35%) prescriptions were compliant with standard treatment guidelines; the rest (661) did not meet several criteria. Areas of non-compliance included use of second line medicines as first line, failure to consider patient characteristics when prescribing, use of contraindicated medicines for certain patients, clinically significant interactions among prescribed medicines and illogical combinations that predispose patients to toxicity.

Conclusion: The poor compliance to standard treatment guidelines observed in our study indicates need to improve prescription practices for Hypertension in the private sector in Zimbabwe for its cost-effective management among the covered patients. However, further investigation is needed to understand the drivers of the prescribing habits and the non-compliance to the Essential Medicines List and Standard Treatment guidelines observed. This will enable design of appropriate educational, managerial and economic interventions to improve compliance.

Keywords: Compliance, Essential Medicines List, Hypertension, Insurance medical claims, Prescribing practices, Private sector, Zimbabwe, Standard treatment guidelines

* Correspondence: vbasopo@gmail.com
International Master in Health Economics & Pharmacoeconomics, Barcelona
School of Management, Universitat Pompeu Fabra, Balmes 132, 08001
Barcelona, Spain

Background

Globally, Cardiovascular disease is the leading cause of mortality, accounting for about a third of deaths [1]. Cardiovascular disease is a group of diseases comprising endocarditis, hypertension, cardiac failure, acute pulmonary oedema, angina pectoris and acute myocardial infarction. By 2014 deaths, from cardiovascular disease were ranked fourth among the top 10 causes of mortality in those over 5 years of age in Zimbabwe [2]. Hypertension is the most prevalent cardiovascular disease in Zimbabwe [3]. The prevalence of Hypertension in the country is 30% regardless of the cut off used [4–6]. There is also a 4% prevalence of severe undiagnosed hypertension in females and 3.7% in males [7, 8]. Thus, Hypertension, whose role in cardiovascular diseases is well established, is a growing medical problem in Zimbabwe.

The Zimbabwean government recognizes the growing importance of non-communicable diseases (NCDs) including Hypertension and has prioritized their management in the national health strategy [9]. The government, through the Ministry of Health has the largest network and infrastructure in the country to support health care activities in the form of hospitals (referral, provincial, district and rural hospitals) and clinics [2]. However, there is limited government funding for the provision of the required health care including the management of NCDs. The Ministry of Health and Child Care's 2016 budget allocation for example, was 8.3% of total government budget expenditure; this is less than the 15% agreed at the Abuja Declaration of 2000 and the Sub-Saharan average of 11.3% [10]. Given that 60.5% of government funding goes to employment costs, the basic health system in Zimbabwe is highly dependent on donor funding and individual patient payments, with the later reported to be 54.1% of total health expenditure at district hospitals by the end of 2015 [10]. Individual patient payments comprise direct payments to health care providers (out of pocket) and contributions to private health insurance or medical aid societies.

Due to the limited government funding for public sector health services in Zimbabwe, an increasing number of patients are forced to seek health care from the private sector. However, clinical practice guidelines are only available in the public sector. A multi-disciplinary team, the National Medicines Therapeutics Policy and Advisory Committee, is tasked by the Ministry of Health and Child Care to develop the Essential Medicines List and Standard Treatment Guidelines for Zimbabwe (EDLIZ) for the common diseases affecting the population. The Standard Treatment Guidelines outlined in EDLIZ are mandatory in the public sector but optional in the private sector. However, they are the only available clinical practice guidelines in the country and ideally should guide clinical practice in the private sector as well. Private health care providers tend to rely mainly on pharmaceutical company representatives as their source of prescribing information. This raises questions about the quality of care provided in the private sector, particularly whether private patients are being given the best possible care as intended by EDLIZ 2015.

Literature review

Recommendations for management of hypertension

Hypertension is defined as systolic blood pressure of 140 mmHg or higher or a diastolic blood pressure of 90 mmHg or higher [11]. High blood pressure is associated with an increased risk of stroke, myocardial infarction, heart failure, renal failure and cognitive impairment [11]. The complications of hypertension are related to either sustained elevations of blood pressure, with consequent changes in the vasculature and heart, or to the accompanying atherosclerosis that is accelerated by long-standing hypertension [1, 12].

The management of Hypertension involves a combination of life style interventions and the use of therapeutic agents [3, 12–19]. The goal of hypertension treatment using therapeutic agents is to keep the blood pressure under control and to manage all the identified risk factors for cardiovascular disease, including lipid disorders, glucose intolerance or diabetes, obesity and smoking [15].

Standard treatment guidelines as outlined in EDLIZ 2015 make the following recommendations in selecting medicines for high blood pressure for adults: start with first line medicine; start with the lowest recommended dose; if ineffective or not tolerated change the medicine or add a medicine from another class [3]. The therapeutic agents recommended in EDLIZ 2015 for management of Hypertension are in line with what is being used in other parts of the world [13], as presented in the Table 1 below.

Most patients will require more than one medicine to achieve control of their blood pressure [14, 16]. Patients of African origin respond well to treatment with calcium channel blockers and diuretics but have smaller blood pressure reductions with Angiotensin Converting Enzyme (ACE) inhibitors, Angiotensin Receptor Blockers (ARBs) and Beta blockers [3, 15, 16]. Beta blockers are not a preferred initial therapy for hypertension because clinical outcome benefits have not been as well established as with other agents [13, 15, 16]. Evidence linking Atenolol to higher rate of stroke among the elderly compared to other anti-hypertensives has led to its use in those over 60 years being discouraged unless there are compelling indications [15, 16].

The Zimbabwe clinical practice guidelines also provide an insight into what are considered logical combinations

Table 1 Recommendations for Management of Hypertension in Zimbabwe

Categorization	Therapeutic group	Recommended medicines	Dosage and Prescribing notes
First Line	Thiazide diuretic	• Hydrochlorothiazide	hydrochlorothiazide 12.5 – 25 mg once a day. Unwanted side effects include raised plasma glucose, uric acid, and cholesterol and reduced plasma potassium
	Calcium Channel blockers	• Nifedipine • Amlodipine	Nifedipine slow release 10- 40 mg once or twice a day or Amlodipine 5-10 mg once a day.
Second line	Angiotensin converting enzyme (ACE) inhibitors	• Enalapril • Lisinopril	Enalapril 5-40 mg once a day or Lisinopril 5-40 mg once a day. Unwanted side effects are reported as a persistent cough that might occur in 10–25% of the patients, angioedema, and postural hypotension. An additional warning is that all ACE inhibitors can cause excessive hypotension and renal failure is also listed. In the event of a cough developing, Angiotensin Receptors Blockers (ARBs) can be substituted for ACE inhibitors. Hyperkalaemia can develop with the concomitant administration of ACE inhibitors with potassium supplements or potassium retaining medicines and this should only be done with careful monitoring of serum potassium.
	Angiotensin receptor blockers (ARBs)	• Losartan	Losartan 25-100 mg once or twice a day.
	Beta blockers	• Atenolol	Atenolol 50 mg once a day. Unwanted side effects include precipitation or exacerbation of asthma, heart failure, impaired glucose control, fatigue and peripheral vascular disease.
	Alpha blockers	• Prazosin • Doxazosin	Prazosin 0.5 – 5 mg twice or three times a day; or Doxazosin 4- 16 mg once a day.

in the Zimbabwean context as shown in the Table 2 below.

According to the EDLIZ 2015, during selection of medicines for management of Hypertension, medicine interactions should always be considered such as in cases of concurrent use of nonsteroidal anti-inflammatory drugs (NSAIDs), aminophylline, corticosteroids etc. whenever cases of resistant hypertension are encountered [3]. Angiotensin converting enzyme inhibitors and ARBs should not be used in combination but rather ARBs should be used as an alternate to ACE inhibitors in patients who develop a persistent cough [15, 16]. Thiazides and beta blockers have been shown to be an effective combination for reducing blood pressure, but since both classes can cause hyperglycemia, the combination should be used with caution in patients at risk of developing diabetes [16].

Diabetes is one of the common co-morbidities with Hypertension and can influence the choice of medicines to manage Hypertension. Hydrochlorothiazide can impair glucose tolerance exacerbating hyperglycemia in Diabetes [3]. Further, beta blockers have a potential to mask symptoms of hypoglycemia in insulin dependent diabetics [3]. The use of low dose Thiazides in diabetics, is recommended if need dictates otherwise patients should be switched to an ACE inhibitor, calcium antagonist or alpha blocker if unwanted effects appear [3].

Table 2 Suggested combinations of Antihypertensive Medicines for Management of Hypertension in Zimbabwe

	Thiazide Diuretic	ACE inhibitor/ARB	Calcium channel blocker	Beta blocker	Alpha blocker
Thiazide Diuretic (Hydrochlorothiazide)		Yes		yes	Yes
ACE inhibitor/ARB (Enalapril/Losartan)	yes		Yes		Yes
Calcium channel blocker (Nifedipine SR/Amlodipine)		Yes		Yes*	Yes
Beta blocker (Atenolol)	yes		Yes*		Yes
Alpha blocker (Prazosin/Doxasosin)	yes	Yes	Yes	Yes	

Logical combinations * Verapamil, a calcium channel blockers and beta blockers are absolutely contraindicated. (Extract from EDLIZ 2015)

Rationale and significance of the study

The emergence of cardiovascular disease including Hypertension as the single most important cause of death in Zimbabwe after communicable diseases and the increasing number of patients seeking medical care in the private sector, make it necessary to study how hypertension patients are being managed in the private sector. This will help determine if patients are receiving proper care and if changes need to be made to current treatment practices.

The study uses prescription claims for hypertension medicines submitted to one medical aid society in Zimbabwe during 2015. Through an analysis of the claims data, the study compares the observed prescribing practices and medicines used with what is recommended in the 7th Essential Medicines List and Standard Treatment Guidelines for Zimbabwe, 2015 (EDLIZ 2015). The study demonstrates use of routinely available data through insurance claims to monitor adherence to guidelines and provides information which can be used to improve management of hypertension in the private sector in Zimbabwe. This would contribute to cost effective management of hypertension and reduction of the high mortality rates arising from diseases of the circulatory system. The study also adds to the body of knowledge on the management of Hypertension in Zimbabwe.

Aim and objectives

The aim of this study was to determine, through an analysis of insurance claims data, compliance of private medical practitioners' prescribing practices with the 7th Essential Medicines List and Standard Treatment Guidelines for Zimbabwe, 2015 (EDLIZ 2015) recommendations on the pharmacological management of hypertension.

The specific study objectives were to:

- Describe private medical practitioner's prescription practices for hypertension, specifically the extent of use of the medicines recommended in EDLIZ 2015 for management of hypertension
- Identify instances where the private medical practitioner's prescription practices do not comply with EDLIZ 2015 specifically existence of any clinically valid interactions between the prescribed medicines for the hypertensive patients in the study and use of combinations of medicines that are considered inappropriate per the standard treatment guidelines outlined in EDLIZ 2015

Methods

This was a retrospective descriptive cross sectional study using secondary data. The study focused on Hypertensive patients who were covered by the Medical Aid Society of

Central Africa (MASCA) and received treatment from private sector health facilities (hospitals and clinics) during the period 1 January 2015 to 31 December 2015. This included patients covered by all reimbursement schemes under the society receiving care from all levels of the health care system and from all types of prescribers. The MASCA remains one of the few viable medical insurance schemes in Zimbabwe hence the choice to study its members. MASCA has a membership of 15,000 spread across the country giving it a national character [20].

We obtained claims data submitted by patients in Zimbabwe to the Medical Aid Society of Central Africa (MASCA) during the period under study (1 January 2015 to 31 December 2015). Each claim related to a single prescription. The study was limited to medicine claims with medicines used for the management of hypertension. Thus, we extracted data on reimbursement claims containing hypertension medicines listed in EDLIZ 2015, filed with MASCA during the study period. Prescription data extracted from the MASCA database contained patient characteristics such as age, sex and race in addition to all the medicines reimbursed in the year. The information was provided in Excel format, from which hypertension prescription information was extracted manually, to create another Excel file that contained hypertension medicines only. The International Classification of Diseases, 10th Revision, Clinical Modification (ICD-10-CM) which physicians and other providers use to code all diagnoses, symptoms, and procedures recorded in hospitals and physician practices [21] is yet to be adopted so information captured by medical aids does not include diagnosis [20]. Hence, we used the prescribed medicines to identify hypertension patients. For these patients, we also collected data on other medicines for chronic conditions prescribed concurrently during the period to assess the appropriateness of combinations and clinically relevant drug interactions. We assumed that patients filed claims for all the chronic medications they acquired during the year through the scheme. The data collected represents a census of all active MASCA members and dependents suffering from hypertension who filed in claims during the 12-month study period.

The last prescription claimed by each patient during the 12-month period was used in the analysis, based on the assumption that it represented the patient's current treatment. Collection of data covering the 12-month period made it possible to capture prescribing information from lost patients due to inability to continue making contributions, death or exhaustion of allocated benefits for the year.

We conducted a descriptive and comparative analysis of the prescription data gathered using Microsoft Excel 2010. The basis for comparison of the observed prescription practices was the 7th Essential Medicines List and Standard Treatment Guidelines for Zimbabwe 2015 (EDLIZ 2015).

Results

Study sample

The study sample comprised of Hypertension prescriptions claims for 1019 patients that were submitted to MASCA in the period Jan 1-December 31, 2015. Majority of the prescription claims (58%) were for Male patients and the remaining 42% were for female patients.

Patients of European and Asian origin accounted for the bulk (65%) of the prescription claims and the majority (58%) of these claims were for patients over the age of 60 (Table 3).

Prescription practices

Number of prescribed hypertension medicines per patient

The number of prescriptions containing one medicine; Monotherapy (384; 38%) was found to be almost equal to that with two medicines; dual therapy (387; 38%). Overall, about three quarters (76%) of patients were either on mono or dual therapy for their hypertension. The number and proportion of prescriptions with three medicines; triple therapy (188, 18%) was greater than both those on four medicines; quad therapy (49; 5%) and those with five or more medicines (11; 1%) as illustrated in Fig. 1.

Prescription of anti-hypertensive first line therapy by therapeutic class

For patients who were on mono therapy, we considered the prescribed medicine as their first line therapy. For those who were on two or more medicines, if any of the medicines prescribed was in the first line therapeutic

class as recommended by the EDLIZ 2015 (as per Table 1) we considered that as their first line therapy. The assumption was that this was the initial medicine prescribed for them and the others having been added as required to achieve better hypertension control.

The most prescribed medicines as first line therapy were found to be ACE inhibitors/ARBs (29.6%), closely followed by thiazides (27.7%). Beta blockers, calcium channel blockers and other medicines contributed 19.3%, 17.9% and 5.5% of the first line therapy respectively (Fig. 2).

Commonly prescribed antihypertensive medicines by therapeutic classes

Figure 3 below shows the commonly prescribed therapeutic classes of Hypertension medicines regardless of whether they were being used as first, second or third line. Angiotensin converting enzyme inhibitors/Angiotensin Receptor Blockers emerged as the most prescribed (639 times) followed by Beta blockers (607), Thiazide diuretics (338), Calcium channel blockers (253) and Alpha blockers (72) in that order.

Other co-prescribed medicines

We reviewed the prescription data to establish the other medicines co-prescribed with Antihypertensives amongst the study sample. Figure 4 shows the other medicines that were commonly prescribed with antihypertensives. Anti-diabetic medicines were the other class of medicines most often prescribed for the hypertensive patients in our study followed by non-steroidal ant-inflammatory drugs (NSAIDs).

Metformin, Glibenclamide and Insulin are all indicated for the management of Diabetes [3]; Allopurinol for Gout; Isosorbide Dinitrate for Angina; Salbutamol for Asthma and Aspirin for the reduction of cardiovascular risk [3, 22]. Diabetes was the most common comorbidity (173 cases), while the existence of Angina required the administration of Isosorbide Dinitrate in 66 cases. Non-steroidal anti-inflammatory drugs were found in 142 prescriptions while aspirin and allopurinol were co-prescribed in 85 and 93 prescriptions respectively.

Prescription compliance with standard treatment guidelines

Almost two-thirds (65%) of the prescriptions were found not to be in line with EDLIZ 2015 recommendations. Compliance was referenced to correct use of first line medicines, prescribing to the appropriate population subgroups, administering medicines in the same therapeutic class to the same patient and avoidance of known drug interactions (Fig. 5).

Table 3 Sample Characteristics

		Number	Percentage
Gender	Male	423	42%
	Female	596	58%
Total		1019	100%
Race	White	538	53%
	Asian	123	12%
	Black	358	35%
Total		1019	100%
Age	Below 30 Years	6	1%
	31–40 Years	40	4%
	41–50 Years	128	12%
	51–60 Years	253	25%
	Over 61 Years	592	58%
Total		1019	100%

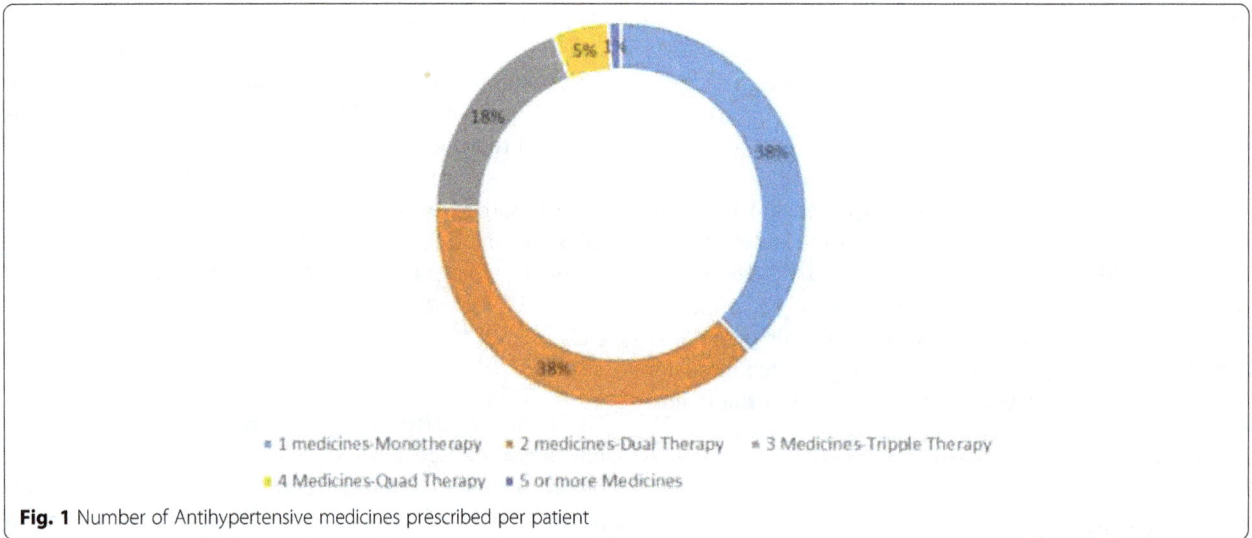

Fig. 1 Number of Antihypertensive medicines prescribed per patient

Reasons for non-compliance
Prescription of inappropriate medicines
Half of the non-compliant cases (52%) emanated from the inappropriate use of second line medicines to initiate therapy in patients. The balance of the noncompliance was accounted for by the prescribing atenolol to patients over 60 years of age (29%), use of beta blockers or ACE inhibitors/ARBs as monotherapy in people of African origin (10%), co-prescribing medicines in the same therapeutic class (4.7%), combining potassium sparing agents together (3%) and using beta blockers and ACE inhibitors as dual therapy in patients of African origin (Table 4).

Clinically significant interactions or contraindications
Clinical interactions can result in reduced effectiveness of medicines or an increase in side effects both to the disadvantage of the patient [6, 17, 18]. Potential interactions documented in the standard treatment guidelines

were identified in 406 prescriptions (about 40% of the prescriptions). Table 5 below shows the main interactions identified. The use of ineffective therapy in patients of African origin though not strictly an interaction was included here because of the impact it has on poor hypertension control.

Discussion
Calcium channel blockers (CCBs) and thiazide diuretics are the recommended first line medicines for Hypertension as per the EDLIZ 2015 guidelines [3]. However, from the survey, private practitioners seem to prescribe ACE/ARBs the most followed by Thiazides. This is at variance with EDLIZ 2015 that places ACE/ARBs as second line medicines that are only to be prescribed in the event of treatment failure or in situations where patients develop intolerance [3]. It is highly unlikely that the 30% of patients on ACE/ARBs had experienced treatment failure or intolerance suggesting doctor's preference to ACE/ARBs for initiating therapy.

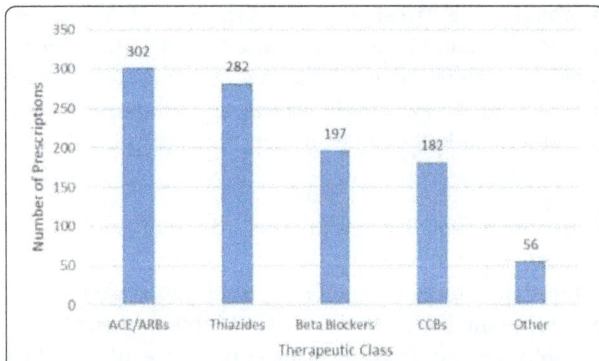

Fig. 2 Prescriptions of first line medicines by therapeutic class. ACE/ARBs - angiotensin converting enzyme inhibitors or angiotensin receptor blockers. CCBs - calcium channel blockers. Other - other anti-hypertensives

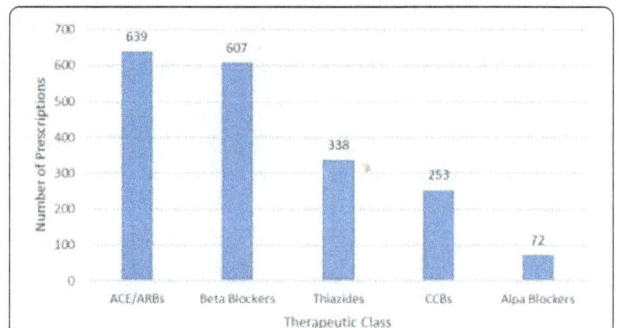

Fig. 3 Commonly prescribed Antihypertensives. ACE/ARBs – ACE inhibitors and angiotensin receptor blockers. CCBs-calcium channel blockers

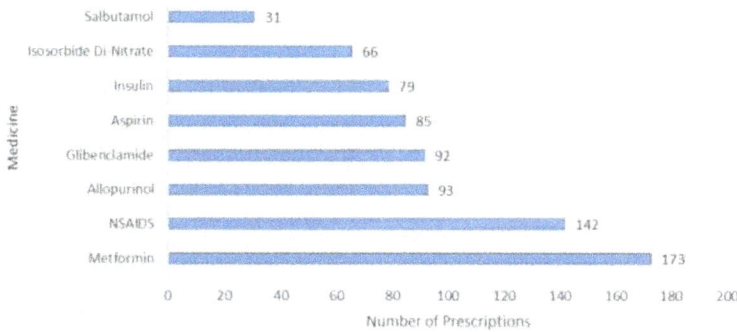

Fig. 4 Commonly co-prescribed medicines (Non-anti hypertensives). NSAIDs-Non-Steroidal Anti Inflammatory Drugs

Beta blockers and calcium channel blockers were used as initial therapy but to a lesser extent than thiazides and ACE/ARBs. The previous edition of EDLIZ 2015 had atenolol as a first line medicine therefore the continued use of the drug could reflect the slow pace at which doctors adjust to changes in guidelines. The same argument could be advanced for the lower than expected use of CCBs that only became first line in the current edition. Several guidelines [15–17] now discourage the routine use of beta blockers as first line because of poor health outcomes, therefore one can argue that their continued use as observed in this study disadvantages patients. Angiotensin receptor blockers and ACE inhibitors were used as first line possibly because of the influence of pharmaceutical promotion. A couple of studies suggest that promotion by pharmaceutical companies particularly through advertising contributed to adoption of newer hypertensive medicines in the United States [23–25]. It is also however possible that doctors in our study were following some international guidelines [16, 17] which recommend Angiotensin receptor blockers and ACE inhibitors as first line for white patients. As earlier indicated, about 53% of the prescriptions surveyed in our study were for white patients.

The recommended approach to the pharmacological management of hypertension is stepped care whereby if a single drug does not adequately control blood pressure, drugs with different modes of action can be combined to effectively lower blood pressure while minimizing toxicity. Rational drug prescribing in the circumstance is then defined as the use of the least number of drugs to obtain the best possible effect in the shortest period and at a reasonable cost [26]. The bulk of the patients (62%) in the study had their hypertension managed using two medicines or more, consistent with international best practice [16–18, 27]. A study of patients attending a cardiology clinic in India showed a similar trend with most of the patients on multiple therapies with two combined antihypertensive [28]. This pattern is encouraged by international guidelines which state that prescribing small doses of different classes of antihypertensive medicines is more beneficial than prescribing a high dose of one antihypertensive.

Given a sizeable proportion of severe undiagnosed hypertension (3–4%) in Zimbabwean population [5–7] it is possible that patients are presenting at health facilities late; this may explain the observation that most patients were on two or more anti-hypertensives since most guidelines recommend commencing treatment with two

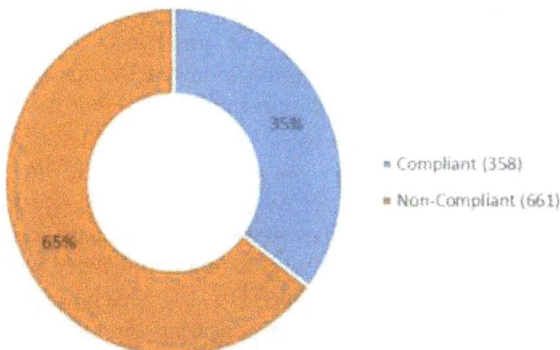

Fig. 5 Prescription compilance with Standard Treatment Guidelines, 2015

Table 4 Reasons for non-compliance

Compliance issue	Number of prescriptions	Percentage
Second line medicines being prescribed as first line	342	52%
Atenolol being prescribed to patients above the age of 60 years.	189	29%
Beta blocker or an ACE inhibitor being used as monotherapy in people of African origin	69	10%
Two medicines from the same therapeutic class being co-prescribed,	31	5%
ACE/ARBs inhibitors in combination with potassium sparing diuretics	19	3%
Combination of a beta blocker and an ACE inhibitor or ARB to treat people of African origin	11	2%
Total	661	100%

Table 5 Clinically significant interactions or contraindications

Interaction or contraindication	Number of prescriptions	Percentage
NSAIDs-non-steroidal anti-inflammatory drugs	142	35%
Beta blockers or ACE/ARBs used as monotherapy in patients of African origin,	69	17%
Atenolol administered to diabetics	53	13%
Thiazide-Amiloride combination containing hydrochlorothiazide 50 mg per tablet	45	11%
Medicines from the same therapeutic class being administered together	31	8%
Potassium sparing agents and ACE/ARBs administered together	19	5%
Hydrochlorothiazide prescribed to diabetics	17	4%
Hydrochlorothiazide prescribed to patients with gout	13	3%
Beta blockers and ACE/ARBs used as dual therapy in patients of African origin.	11	3%
Atenolol prescribed to asthmatics	6	1%
Total	406	100%

drugs whenever systolic blood pressure is above 160 mmHg [17, 18]. In such a scenario of severe undiagnosed hypertension in Zimbabwean population the relevance of monotherapy as observed in our study with 38% of patients being on monotherapy becomes questionable since it may not provide adequate control [25, 27]. Indeed, in a study by Al-Drabah et al. in which the majority of subjects were prescribed monotherapy, the researchers observed that target BP control was not achieved in most patients [29] which implies that monotherapy may not be sufficient for achieving adequate BP control in majority of patients [30].

Only 35% of the surveyed prescriptions were found to be following the Zimbabwe standard treatment guidelines and therefore can be considered compliant. Different studies have found different levels of compliance to treatment guidelines for hypertension in various contexts. Like this study, a study conducted in Malaysia observed that doctors poorly adhered to Malaysian Clinical Practice guidelines [30]. In another study in Malaysia as well, 85.3% of prescriptions at a Cardiac clinic were in accordance with guidelines [31]. In contrast to our study, findings from a study in Eritrea found that prescribing practice for hypertension followed the Eritrean National treatment guideline 2003 [32].

Several Studies have shown that application of guidelines to clinical practice improves treatment outcomes, especially better BP control [33–35]. Thus, the low level of adherence observed in our study is of concern. It is however important to note that guidelines are just to guide but physicians need to follow a patient-centric approach. Thus, it is not always surprising that inconsistencies exist between recommended and observed treatment approaches because clinicians sometimes individualize therapy based on specific patient characteristics and response to treatment. Several studies show that adherence to clinical guidelines and recommendations are not all uniform; they vary by time period and country, and by characteristics of patients and physicians [36–39].

We observed various areas of noncompliance in our study, ranging from failure to consider patient characteristics to using second line medicines as first line. Beta blockers and ACE/ARBs are known for being less effective as monotherapy in patients of African origin [3] yet these were prescribed to 22% of the surveyed African patients. Bearing in mind the Zimbabwean population is largely black, this is a huge concern. The use of second line medicines as first line was associated with beta blockers, ACE inhibitors or ARBs, all listed as second line in EDLIZ 2015. Possible explanations could be the effects of pharmaceutical promotion or doctors aligning themselves to guidelines that promote their use as such [15, 16, 18, 19]. Continued use of Atenolol as observed could be a sign of doctors reacting slowly to the new guidelines thus perpetuating old practices. Also, recent guidelines [13, 15, 16] discourage the use of Atenolol in elderly patients but doctors seem unaware because 32% (189 out of 592) of this age group was on Atenolol. Instances of prescribing medicines from the same therapeutic class as observed offers no advantages to the patients and instead a combination of medicines from different therapeutic classes is recommended in the event of treatment failure [3, 17, 25]. The combination of beta blockers and ACE/ARBs as observed in 3% of prescriptions has not been proven to have any synergistic hypotensive effects and is often discouraged [19].

The recommended chronology of adding antihypertensive medication is that of add-on i.e. in the event of treatment failure a new class of medicine is added onto the existing one unless there is intolerance which necessitates the withdrawal of the first medicine [3, 27]. It therefore follows that the most prescribed medicines should be the first line agents followed by the second line and so forth. It was interesting to note that the two most prescribed classes were ACE/ARBs (639) and beta blockers (607) yet these are considered second line in EDLIZ 2015. Popularity of ACE/ARBs could be two-fold namely the effect of pharmaceutical promotion or private sector doctors using international guidelines which recommend these as reference [16–18]. Ideally thiazides and CCBs should have been appearing on the bulk of the prescriptions but given that guidelines are recent, one may think that this was a transition period, with growing usage expected over time. However, thiazide-type diuretics have always been first line in previous editions perhaps indicating private sector prescribing is not aligned to EDLIZ 2015. The widespread use of atenolol observed in our study could be attributed to the previous edition that had placed it as first line and doctors were still to adjust to the new recommendations. The low usage of alpha blockers is in line with expectations as they are reserved for the resistant cases and men beyond 50 years with benign prostrate hypertrophy [3, 18].

Interactions between medicines or between medicine and patient characteristics can lead to poor hypertension control or an increase in toxicity [3, 16]. Non-steroidal anti-inflammatory drugs reverse the effects of antihypertensive medicines [3], predisposing patients to complications [12], but they were being routinely prescribed in 142 patients, about 14% of the study population. Regular use of the NSAIDs could be linked to joint problems often experienced by the elderly who constituted more than half the study population.

Insurance has been shown to increase access to antihypertensive drugs by patients [39–43]. Given the positive impact of Insurance on overall access to antihypertensive drugs, an important question is whether insurance also plays a role in shaping prescribing patterns of antihypertensive agents in line with treatment guidelines. Given the drive for efficiency and effectiveness by insurance companies, one would have expected to see a higher level of compliance to treatment guidelines in this cohort of antihypertensive patients who have private medical insurance through MASCA. This expectation is based on the popular view that health insurance companies in general are more likely to exercise management controls to encourage prescribing that is consistent with established national guidelines particularly if the recommended therapy also represents the lowest cost alternative. One possible explanation for the observed low compliance in our study despite coverage by health insurance is that the insurance society has relatively weak controls over prescribing.

Studies have shown that prescribing in the private for profit sector tends to be worse than in public sector as indicated by poorer compliance with Standard Treatment Guidelines (STGs), and lower use of Essential Medicines Lists (EML) and generic drugs [44]. However, it's important to note that the private sector in Zimbabwe is not bound to follow EDLIZ 2015 which is only mandatory in the public sector. Indeed, in many countries in Africa, the private sector is encouraged but not obliged to prescribe from EML as may be the case for public health centers [45]. In the absence of any binding guideline or effective regulations on prescribing behavior for clinicians, the current prescription pattern observed in this cohort of MASCA clients is probably a reflection of the mixed effect of the preferences of clinicians, the hypotensive efficacies of medications, and the tolerance levels of patients.

A methodological strength of our study is that it uses readily available claims data and demonstrates use of routinely available data to evaluate and monitor prescribing habits. This can help rapid identification of the necessary modifications to prescribing habits to achieve rational and cost effective treatment. Additionally, our analysis is based on observations of actual prescribing practices as recorded by clinicians rather than on reported practices which may be subject to recall bias. Since we used data for all clients covered by MASCA which has the largest coverage for private sector clients, we can be confident that our data provides a fair representation of hypertensive prescription habits in the private sector in Zimbabwe. Few studies have studied medicines use in the private sector [44]. The number of studies in the private-for profit sector is very small which precludes accurate comparison with other settings. This study contributes to the current knowledge and incipient knowledge on prescribing patterns in the private sector.

Findings from this study point to the need to improve prescription practices for Hypertension in the private sector in Zimbabwe. However, further investigation is needed to understand the drivers of the prescribing habits and the non-conformance to the EDLIZ 2015 observed in this study. Assuming that EDLIZ 2015 provides the most appropriate guidance for hypertensive treatment in Zimbabwe, our study indicates that there is room for significantly improving the cost effectiveness of hypertensive treatment among the covered patients. We recommend that the Association of Healthcare Funders of Zimbabwe (AHFoZ) through its membership actively encourages the use to EDLIZ 2015 by all private medical practitioners or instead develops its own clinical practice guidelines in consultation with all the stakeholders involved. Medical aids societies are encouraged to provide training and regular feedback to medical practitioners, through representative associations such as the Zimbabwe Medical Association or the College of Primary Care Physicians of Zimbabwe to improve their adherence to guidelines. A low percentage of medicines prescribed from an EML may highlight private sector prescriber's lack of knowledge on the role of the EML in cost-effectiveness optimization.

Study limitations and suggestions for future research

We did not have access to diagnosis or detailed clinical information for the patients in our study. Thus, we used the medicines as a surrogate for the diagnosis hypertension. We could also not distinguish between newly diagnosed or long standing hypertensive patients or even determine the severity of the hypertension. This lack of diagnosis and other clinical information (e.g. comprehensive data on co-morbidities over and above the few we concentrated on) made it difficult to accurately ascertain the appropriateness of prescribing especially when combined medicines were prescribed. Collecting this detailed information may provide different insights on the appropriateness of current prescribing and its adherence to guidelines.

The study was carried out soon after the updating of the guidelines. It is not clear to what extent poor dissemination or lack of knowledge about the guidelines could be responsible for the observed prescribing practices. Identifying which factors were at play was out of scope but an interesting area for further research. What determines the choice of antihypertensive therapies is a question of vital commercial, medical and public health importance. Thus, there is need to investigate factors that explain the observed practice. Also, there is need track trends in usage given the guidelines are new and see how this changes over time. A better understanding of the causes of the observed prescribing behavior could help target interventions to improve prescribing of hypertension for the covered patients. These would ideally involve a mix of educational components, managerial components and economic interventions depending on the identified causes.

This being a cross sectional study design considering the most recent prescription claim for each patient, any earlier switch of drug treatment could not be considered in the study design. Thus, we could not examine switches among antihypertensive drugs classes either due to non-response or side effects as this may explain the observed prescription patterns. Also, we did not have data about the prescribers-age, type of provider (Specialists or not) level of care (hospital or health center) etc. which might influence the prescribing patterns of antihypertensive drugs.

It would also be interesting to study the costs of care, clinical outcomes (was hypertension being controlled) and quality of life of the patients in the study and if this was affected by the prescribing practices observed. Such research may offer stronger grounds for use of the EDLIZ 2015 by MASCA since these are not currently mandatory.

Conclusion

The study uses prescription claims for hypertension medicines submitted to one medical aid society in Zimbabwe during 2015. It compares the observed prescribing practices and medicines used with what is recommended in the 7th Essential Medicines List and Standard Treatment Guidelines for Zimbabwe, 2015 (EDLIZ 2015). The poor compliance to standard treatment guidelines observed in

our study indicates need to improve prescription practices for Hypertension in the private sector in Zimbabwe for its cost-effective management among the covered patients. However, further research is needed to understand the drivers of the prescribing habits and the non-compliance to the Essential Medicines List and Standard Treatment guidelines observed. This will enable design of appropriate educational, managerial and economic interventions to improve compliance.

Abbreviations

ACE: Angiotensin converting enzyme; AIDS: Acquired immuno deficiency syndrome; ARB: Angiotensin receptor blockers; BP: Blood pressure; CCBs: Calcium channel blockers; EDLIZ 2015: 7th Essential medicines list and standard treatment guidelines for Zimbabwe; EML: Essential Medicines Lists; HIV: Human immunodeficiency virus; ICD-10-CM: International Classification of Diseases, 10th Revision, Clinical Modification; JNC: Joint National Committee; MASCA: Medical Aid Society of Central Africa; NCD: Non-communicable diseases; NSAIDs: Non-steroidal anti-inflammatory drugs; STGs: Standard treatment guidelines; WHO: World Health Organization

Acknowledgements

The authors would like to acknowledge the management of Medical Aid Society of Central Africa, Zimbabwe who provided the data on which this study is based.

Funding

The authors received no external funding for this study.

Authors' contributions

VB developed the proposal, collected and analyzed the data and prepared the first draft of the manuscript. PNM provided overall supervision for the process, in addition to critical review and finalization of the manuscript for publication. Both authors read and approved the final manuscript.

Competing interests

The authors declare that they have no competing interests.

References

1. Sawicka K, Syczyrek M, Jatrezbska I, Prasal M, Zwolak A, Daniluk J. Hypertension the silent killer. J Pre-Clin Clin Res. 2011;5(2):43–6.
2. Zimbabwe National Statistics Agency and the Ministry of Health and Child Care. Zimbabwe national health profile. 2014.
3. Ministry of Health and Child Care, Zimbabwe. The essential drug list and standard treatment guidelines. 7th ed; 2015.
4. Ibrahim HM, Damasceno A. Hypertension in developing countries. Lancet. 2012;380:611–9.
5. Mufunda J, Chatora F, Ndambakuwa Y, Nyarango P, Chifamba J, Kosia A, Sparks VH. Prevalence of non-communicable diseases in Zimbabwe: results from analysis of data from the national central registry and urban survey. Ethn Dis. 2006;16:718–22.
6. Mutowo MP, Mangwiro JC, Lorgelley P, Owen A, Renzaho A. Hypertension in Zimbabwe: a meta-analysis to quantify its burden and policy implications. World J Metaanal. 2014; 10.13105/wjma.v3.i1.54.
7. World Health Organization. Non-communicable diseases country profiles. 2014 apps.who.int/iris/bitstream/10665/128038/1/9789241507509_eng.pdf. Accessed on 29 Sept 2016.
8. World Health Organization. National health survey- Zimbabwe noncommunicable risk factors. 2005.

9. Ministry of Health and Child Welfare. The national health strategy for Zimbabwe (2009–2013). 2009.

10. Zimbabwe 2016 Health and Child Care Budget Brief. http://www.unicef.org/Zimbabwe. Accessed on 29 July 2016.

11. Sacks FM, Compos H. Dietary therapy in hypertension. N Engl J Med. 2010; 362:2102–12. Massachusetts Medical Society

12. Greene R, Harris ND. Pathology and therapeutics for pharmacists; a basis for clinical pharmacy practice. London: The pharmaceutical Press; 1998. p. 75–91.

13. National Institute of Clinical of Health and Clinical Excellence. Hypertension; the clinical management of hypertension in adults. August 2011.

14. Evidence based guideline for the management of high blood pressure in Adults. Report from the panel members appointed to the Eight Joint National Committee (JNC8). 2014.

15. Group Health Cooperative. Hypertension diagnosis and treatment guidelines. August 2014.

16. American Society of Hypertension and the International Society of hypertension. Clinical Practice guidelines for the management of hypertension in the community: A Statement by the American Society of Hypertension and the International Society of Hypertension. J Clin Hypertens. 2014;16(1):14–26.

17. National Heart Foundation of Australia. Guideline for the diagnosis and management of hypertension in adults-2016. Melbourne: National Heart Foundation of Australia; 2016.

18. European Society of Hypertension/European Society of Cardiology. Guidelines for the Management of Arterial Hypertension-2013. J Hypertens. 2013;31:1281–357.

19. Hypertension Canada. CHEP guidelines for blood pressure measurement, diagnosis, assessment of risk, prevention and treatment of hypertension. Can J Cardiol. 2016;32:569–88.

20. Oral communication with Mr. Josen Sigola, CEO of MASCA.

21. Association of Healthcare Funders of Zimbabwe. http://www.ahfoz.org. Accessed 29 July 2016.

22. World Health Organization: Prevention of cardiovascular disease- guidelines for assessment and management of cardiovascular risk. 2007.

23. Siegel D, Lopez J. Trends in antihypertensive drug use in the United states: do the JNC V recommendations affect prescribing? JAMA. 1997; 278:1745–8.

24. Soumerai SB, Mc Laughlin TJ, Spiegelman D, Hertzmark E, Thibault G, Goldman L. Adverse outcomes of underuse of beta-blockers in elderly survivors of acute myocardial infarction. JAMA. 1997;227:115–21.

25. Manolio TA, Cutler JA, Furberg CD, Psaty BM, Whelton PK, Applegate WB. Trends in pharmacological management of hypertension in the United States. Arch Intern Med. 1995;155:829–37.

26. Gross F. Drug utilization-theory and practice the present situation in the Federal Republic of Germany. Eur J Clin Pharmacol. 1981;19:387–92.

27. Server PS, Messerli FH. Hypertension management 2011: optimal combination therapy. Eur Heart J. 2011;32:2499–506. European Society of Cardiology

28. Xavier D, Noby M, Pradeep J, Prem P. Letter to the editor. Pattern of drug use in hypertension in a tertiary hospital; a cross sectional study in the inpatients ward. Indian J Pharm. 2001;33:456–7.

29. Al-Drabah E, Irshaid Y, Yasein N, Zmeili S. Prescription pattern of antihypertensive drugs in family practice clinics at Jordan University Hospital. Med Sci. 2013;2(1):469–88.

30. Ahmad N, Hassan Y, Tangiisuran B, Meng OL, Abd Aziz N, Khan AH. Guidelines adherence and hypertension control in an outpatient cardiology clinic in Malaysia. Trop J Pharm Res. 2012;11(4):665–72.

31. Abdulameer SA, Sahib MN, Aziz NA, Hassan Y, Abdul HA, Razzaq A, et al. Physician adherence to hypertension treatment guidelines and drug acquisition costs of antihypertensive drugs at the cardiac clinic: a pilot study. Patient Prefer Adherence. 2012;6:101–8.

32. Shobana J, Semere M, Sied M, Eyob T, Russom M. Prescribing pattern of anti hypertensive drugs among hypertension patients with cardiac complications in Eritrea. Lat Am J Pharm. 2012;6:101–8.

33. Jackson JH, Sobolski J, Krienke R, Wong KS, French-Tamas F, Nightengale B. Blood pressure control and pharmacotherapy patterns in the United States before and after release of the Joint National Committee on prevention, detection, evaluation and treatment of high blood pressure (JNC 7) guidelines. J Am Board Fam Med. 2008;21:512–21.

34. Ohta Y, Tsuchihashi T, Fujii K, Matsumura K, Ohya Y, Uezono K, et al. Improvement of blood pressure control in a hypertension clinic: a 10 year

follow up study. J Hum Hypertens. 2004;18:278.

35. Jeschke E, Thomas O, Horst CV, Matthias K, Angelina B, Claudia MW, et al. Evaluation of prescribing patterns in a German network of CAM physicians for the treatment of patients with hypertension: a prospective observational study. BMC Fam Pract. 2009;10:78.

36. Bog-Hansen E, Lindblad U, Ranstam J, Melander A, Rastam L. Antihypertensive drug treatment in a Swedish community: Skaraborg hypertension and diabetes project. Pharmacoepidemiol Drug Saf. 2002;11: 45–54.

37. Ma J, Lee KV, Stafford RS. Changes in antihypertensive prescribing during US outpatient visits for uncomplicated hypertension between 1993 and 2004. Hypertension. 2006;48:846–52.

38. Campbell NR, Tu K, Brant R, Duong-Hua M, McAlister FA. The impact of the Canadian hypertension education program on antihypertensive prescribing trends. Hypertension. 2006;47:22–8.

39. Guo JD, Liu GG, Christensen DB, Fu AZ. How well have practices followed guidelines in prescribing antihypertensive drugs: the role of health insurance. Value Health. 2003;6:18–28.

40. Adam AS, Soumerai SB, Ross-Degnan D. Use of antihypertensive drugs by medicare enrollees: does type of drug coverage matter? Health Aff. 2001;20: 276–86.

41. Ahluwalia JS, McNagny SE, Rask KJ. Correlates of controlled hypertension in indigent, inner-city hypertensive patients. J Gen Intern Med. 1997;12:7–14.

42. Blustein J. Drug coverage and drug purchases by medicare beneficiaries with hypertension. Health Aff. 2000;19:219–30.

43. Jackson MG, Drechsler-Martell CR, Jackson EA. Family practice resident's prescribing patterns. Drug Intell Clin Pharm. 1985;19:205–9.

44. Mohlala G, Peltzer K, Phaswana-Mafuya N, Ramlagan S. Drug prescription habits in public and private health facilities in 2 provinces in South Africa. East Mediterr Health J. 2010;16(3):324–8.

45. Holloway KA, Ivanovska V, Wagner AK, Vialle-Valentin C, Ross-Degnan. Have we improved use of medicines in developing and transitional countries and do we know how to? Two decades of evidence. Trop Med Int Health. 18(6): 656–64.

19

Pharmaceutical company spending on research and development and promotion in Canada, 2013-2016

Joel Lexchin[1,2] (iD)

Abstract

Background: Competing claims are made about the amount of money that pharmaceutical companies spend on research and development (R&D) versus promotion. This study investigates this question in the Canadian context.

Methods: Two methods for determining industry-wide figures for spending on promotion were employed. First, total industry spending on detailing and journal advertising for 2013-2016 was abstracted from reports from QuintilesIMS. Second, the mean total promotion spending for the years 2002-2005 was used to estimate total spending for 2013-2016. Total industry spending on R&D came from the Patented Medicine Prices Review Board (PMPRB). R&D to promotion spending using each method of determining the amount spent on promotion was compared for 2013-2016 inclusive. Data on the 50 top promoted drugs, the amounts spent, the companies marketing these products and their overall sales were abstracted from the QuintilesIMS reports. Spending on R&D and promotion as a percent of sales was compared for these companies.

Results: Industry wide, the ratio of R&D to promotion spending went from 1.43 to 2.18 when promotion was defined as the amount spent on detailing and journal advertising for the 50 most promoted drugs. Calculating total promotion spending from the mean of the 2002-2005 figures the ratio was 0.88 to 1.32 for the 50 most promoted drugs. For individual companies marketing one or more of the 50 most promoted drugs, mean R&D spending ranged from 3.7% of sales to 4.1% compared to mean promotion spending that went from 1.7 to 1.9%. The ratio of spending on R&D to promotion varied from 2.11 to 2.32. Eight to 10 companies per year spent more on promotion than on R&D.

Conclusions: Depending on the method used to determine promotion spending, industry-wide the ratio of R&D spending to promotion ranges from 1.45 to 2.18 (sales representatives and journal advertising only) or from 0.88 to 1. 32 (total promotion spending estimated based 2003-2005 data.) For the individual companies promoting one or more of the 50 most promoted drugs, 2.11 to 2.32 times more is spent on R&D compared to promotion. However these results should be interpreted cautiously because of data limitations.

Keywords: Canada, Expenditure, Pharmaceutical industry, Promotion, Research and development

Background

Pharmaceutical companies typically claim that one of the reasons for high drugs prices is because of the amount that they spend on research and development (R&D). According to the industry, it costs USD $2.6 billion to bring a drug to market [1]. Critics of the industry counter that companies are more focused on and spend more on promotion than on R&D. Gagnon and Lexchin produced figures that showed that in the United States (US) in 2004 the industry spent USD $57.5 billion on promotion versus USD $31.5 billion on R&D [2]. A report from the California-based Institute for Health and Socio-Economic Policy stated that in 2015 out of the top 100 pharmaceutical companies by sales, 64 spent twice as much on marketing and sales than on R&D, 58 spent three times, 43 spent five times as much and 27 spent 10 times the amount [3]. To date, arguments about promotion versus R&D spending have been based on American data. This study had two aims: first to estimate

Correspondence: jlexchin@yorku.ca
[1]School of Health Policy and Management, York University, 4700 Keele St., Toronto, ON M3J 1P3, Canada
[2]University Health Network, 200 Elizabeth St., Toronto, ON M5G 2C4, Canada

total industry-wide promotion and compare that to total industry-wide R&D spending and second, to look at the ratio of R&D versus promotional spending for individual companies marketing the most heavily promoted drugs in Canada.

Methods

Industry-wide

Two methods were used to determine industry-wide promotion spending. First, total spending on sales representatives and journal advertising, i.e., excluding all other types of promotion, for the top 50 most heavily promoted products from companies was available for the years 2013-2016 from the annual reports published by QuintilesIMS (formerly imshealth|brogan) [4–7].

Second, amounts for all types of promotion in Canada were available for the period 2002-2005 from Cammcorp International (Marc-Andre Gagnon, personal communication, January 15, 2011). The mean ratio of spending on detailing plus journal advertising to total promotion spending was calculated for that period and that ratio was then used to convert annual spending on detailing and journal advertising to total promotion spending for the years 2013-2016, assuming that the relative proportions spent on detailing plus advertising were the same in 2013-2016 as they were in 2002-2005. These calculated amounts constitute a floor for total promotional spending since the figures for 2013-2016 only cover the top 50 most promoted products. As an illustrative example, between 2002 and 2005 detailing plus advertising was a mean of 60.4% of total industry-wide promotional spending of $1.066 billion. In 2013, spending on detailing plus advertising for the 50 most heavily promoted drugs was $0.575 billion and therefore the calculated lower total amount was 0.575/ 60.4 × 100 = $0.952 billion. The calculation was repeated for the years 2014-2016.

Total R&D spending by all companies with a patented drug on the Canadian market for the same 4-year period was available from the annual reports from the Patented Medicine Prices Review Board (PMPRB), the federal body that sets a maximum introductory price for new patented medicines [8–11]. Ratios of spending on R&D to promotion

were calculated for each year using the two different methods of determining annual promotion spending.

Companies with the most heavily promoted drugs

The names of the 50 medications with the highest spending on promotion, the companies marketing these medications and the amount spent were abstracted for the years 2013 to 2016 inclusive from QuintilesIMS annual reports. These reports also contain total sales revenue for the top 50 companies in Canada and these figures along with figures on promotion spending was entered into an Excel spreadsheet. The amount spent on promotion by the top companies was summed and the mean percent of sales spent on promotion was also calculated for all of the top companies for each of the 4 years.

The percent of sales spent by companies on R&D was abstracted from the annual PMPRB reports for each of the companies with the most heavily promoted drugs and the amount spent on R&D for each company was calculated by multiplying this figure by the total sales of each company found in the QuintilesIMS reports. The combined amount and the mean percent of sales spent on R&D by the companies was calculated for each year.

Combined R&D spending and the mean percent of sales spent on R&D was compared to similar figures for promotion for the companies with the most heavily promoted drugs.

All of the data was publicly available and no patients were involved. Therefore, ethics approval was not necessary.

Results

Industry-wide

Total industry R&D spending, where industry is defined as all companies with a patented drug on the Canadian market, ranged from a low of $792,200,000 to a high of $918,200,000. Spending on sales representatives and journal advertising for the 50 most heavily promoted drugs went from a low of $421,434,000 to $562,926,000 and the ratio of R&D to promotion spending was 1.43 to 2.18. Total promotion spending on the 50 most heavily promoted drugs, calculated from the mean of the 2002-2005 figures, ranged from $697,000,000 to $932,000,000 and the ratio was 0.88 to 1.32 (Table 1).

Table 1 Spending on R&D[a] and promotion as a percent of sales industry-wide

Year	Total R&D spending ($000)	Promotion spending ($000)		Ratio R&D to promotion spending	
		Detailing and journal advertising top 50 drugs	Estimated total promotion based on data from 2002-2005	Promotion for top 50 drugs	Estimated total promotion
2013	798,300	550,871	912,000	1.45	0.88
2014	792,200	552,797	916,000	1.43	0.86
2015	869,100	562,926	932,000	1.54	0.93
2016	918,200	421,434	697,000	2.18	1.32

[a]Research and development

Table 2 Number of 50 most promoted drugs per company per year

Year	Number of drugs promoted						
	1	2	3	4	5	6	7
2013	10	5	3	3	1		
2014	10	6	3	2	1		
2015	10	7	1	2	2		
2016	10	6	2	2		1	1

Companies with the most heavily promoted drugs

In each of the 4 years, data was not available for a small number of the 50 most promoted drugs: 2013 – 4 drugs (no total sales figures), 2014 and 2015 – 4 drugs (no total sales figures) and 1 drug (no R&D as a percent of sales), 2016 – 1 drug (no total sales figure). (Complete data on individual companies for each year is available in Additional file 1: Table S1, Additional file 2: Table S2, Additional file 3: Table S3, Additional file 4: Table S4.)

R&D and promotion spending was available for 22 companies in each of the 4 years. (The individual companies selling the top 50 drugs varied from year to year and overall 26 unique companies had data for 1 to 4 years.) In 2016, the amount spent on promotion for one company included company promotion rather than promotion for an individual product. For the majority of companies (15-17 out of 22 in any given year) the amount spent on promotion was only available for 1 or 2 drugs (Table 2). Mean R&D spending ranged from 3.7% of sales to 4.1% compared to mean promotion spending that went from 1.7 to 1.9%. The ratio of spending on R&D to promotion varied from 2.11 to 2.32 (Table 3). Depending on the year, between 8 to 10 of the 22 companies spent more on promotion than on R&D (Table 3).

Figure 1 shows the distribution of spending on R&D versus promotion as a percent of sales by number of companies. Companies tended to cluster at the lower end for spending on promotion whereas they were at the higher end for spending on R&D. The largest amount spent by an individual company on R&D was 13.6% in 2016 and on promotion it was 7.8% in 2015.

Table 4 shows that for most companies there was significant variation in spending on both promotion and R&D on a year-to-year basis.

Discussion

Depending on the method used to determine promotion spending, industry-wide the ratio of R&D spending to promotion ranges from 1.45 to 2.18 (sales representatives and journal advertising only) or from 0.88 to 1.32 (total promotional spending) for the years 2013 to 2016. The amount spent on promotion used in calculating the former set of ratios is more accurate but is limited to just two types of promotion. The amount spent on promotion used in calculating the latter set of ratios is an estimate for all types of promotion but is less accurate. Both sets of ratios also only apply to the amount spent on the 50 most heavily promoted drugs. For the individual companies promoting one or more of the 50 most promoted drugs, 2.11 to 2.32 times more is spent on R&D compared to promotion. Even using the limited data on individual company promotion, 8-10 companies per year still spent less on R&D than they did on promotion.

However, all of these results should be interpreted cautiously for a number of reasons. First, the QuintilesIMS reports only provide figures for spending on sales representatives and journal advertising whereas companies engage in a number of other methods of promotion, among them, distributing free samples, hiring key opinion leaders to give talks, sponsoring meals and meetings and using social media. Second, the estimate for total promotional spending based on the mean of the 2002-2005 figures assumes that the proportion of the total used on journal advertising and detailing remained stable. Finally, for many companies promotion spending was based on the amount spent on just 1 or 2 drugs.

The reason for the abrupt decline in spending on detailing and journal advertising in 2016 compared to 2013-2015 requires further investigation. The variation in the year-to-year amount spent on both R&D and promotion by individual companies most likely reflects research priorities and how many drugs companies are aggressively marketing.

Table 3 Spending on R&D[a] and promotion as a percent of sales for companies with the most heavily promoted drugs

Year	Number of companies[b]	Number of drugs	Total sales ($000)	R&D spending ($000) (% sales)	Promotion spending ($000) (% sales)	Ratio of R&D to promotion spending	Number of companies spending more on promotion than on R&D
2013	22	46	12,761,798	565,670 (4.4)	243,420 (1.9)	2.32	9
2014	22	46	13,327,819	509,531 (3.8)	242,401 (1.8)	2.11	8
2015	22	45	13,215,385	487,223 (3.7)	230,157 (1.7)	2.18	9
2016	22	49	13,610,805	553,057 (4.1)	258,363 (1.9)	2.16	10

[a]Research and development
[b]Individual companies vary by year

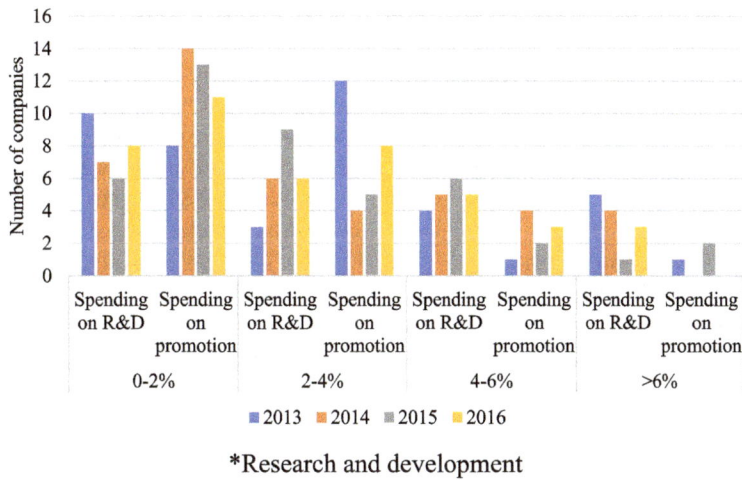

Fig. 1 Percent of sales spend on R&D* and promotion by number of companies. *Research and development

Table 4 Variation in promotion and research and development spending by individual company by year

Company	Promotion spending on drugs in 50 most promoted ($000)				Research and development spending ($000)			
	2013	2014	2015	2016	2013	2014	2015	2015
Abbott EPD	15,779	16,009	8104	–	0	0	0	–
Actavis	–	3034	2753	–	–	20	0	–
Allergan	–	–	–	2328	–	–	–	1751
Amgen	5816	5836	6515	6359	50,370	45,622	42,153	38,600
Astellas	3006	3097	8094	5612	4735	3447	6952	3851
AstraZeneca	20,066	35,416	33,655	41,304	13,781	24,273	41,143	61,468
Bayer	10,857	11,995	11,486	11,898	23,476	31,373	39,719	45,025
BGP Pharma	–	–	–	4809	–	–	–	0
BMS Pharma	20,081	13,132	7588	14,741	53,270	45,001	59,456	81,335
Boehringer Ingelheim	11,570	17,304	14,147	24,961	23,476	18,430	22,742	21,409
GlaxoSmithKline	19,384	30,547	13,328	27,567	88,350	77,648	53,413	43,326
Janssen	5636	12,666	16,839	6356	49,983	61,733	70,646	86,380
Leo	3847	–	–	–	939	–	–	–
Lilly	12,358	8261	7592	6150	53,672	26,620	22,277	36,710
Lundbeck	9956	3322	12,146	8900	888	2596	3126	0
Merck	27,682	13,065	18,441	36,963	19,962	26,505	21,667	32,582
Novartis	3460	7838	5376	12,002	106,013	78,553	51,916	44,701
Novo Nordisk	6536	4159	3517	3580	4563	10,857	7886	4548
Paladin	–	–	3113	–	–	–	265	–
Pfizer	24,429	12,009	12,178	14,162	24,643	14,174	8953	9738
Purdue	9996	3790	6099	2666	13,581	14,683	12,609	16,321
Sanofi-Aventis	3222	2870	–	3578	19,940	13,847	–	8450
Servier	7862	14,134	8893	7252	11.745	13,612	8067	7150
Shire	4145	6967	3287	3464	281	350	0	0
Takeda	14,099	13,415	19,582	5460	0	0	0	0
Valeant	3633	3535	7414	8251	0	0	14,231	9712

Beyond examining the amount of money spent on R&D and promotion, looking at the focus of that spending and the outcomes is another way of assessing the priorities that companies attach to each of these activities. Innovative Medicines Canada (IMC), the organization representing the research-based industry, signals the importance that it attaches to R&D on its website: "At present, there are more than 500 new products in development in Canada, including therapies focused on cancer treatments, infectious diseases and vaccines. These products have the potential to help Canadians and people all over the world live longer and healthier lives" [12]. However, industry spending on R&D in Canada has been declining ever since 1997/1998 when it peaked at 11.5% of sales and it now stands at 4.4% [11]. Out of 564 new patented medicines introduced into Canada from 2010 to 2016 inclusive, only 37 (6.6%) were rated by the PMPRB as breakthroughs or substantial therapeutic improvements [11]. Although most products that fail in the clinical development stage do so because of a lack of efficacy or for safety reasons, 57% and 17% respectively, 22% are stopped for commercial reasons [13] indicating that products that might be both safe and efficacious are not brought to market.

Industry is also positive about the role of promotion, especially the activities of sales representatives. This orientation is reflected in a statement about the role of pharmaceutical sales representatives issued by Rx&D, the predecessor to IMC: "Provider-supported detailing generates awareness about new treatments and provides science-based and Health Canada approved advice on how to administer these medications" [14]. Previous research that examined the most heavily promoted products in Canada, showed that the vast majority of spending went to medications that offered little to no additional therapeutic value over existing therapies [15]. The comprehensiveness of the safety information provided by sales representatives when they visit doctors was investigated in a study involving primary care practitioners in Vancouver and Montreal. "Minimally adequate safety information" defined a priori as the mention of one or more of the following: approved indications, serious adverse events, common non-serious adverse events and contraindications *and* no unapproved indications or unqualified safety claims (e.g., "this drug is safe") was provided in 5/412 (1.2%) of promotions in Vancouver and 7/423 (1.7%) in Montreal. Representatives did not provide any information about harms (a serious adverse event, a common adverse event or a contraindication) in two-thirds of interactions [16].

It would appear that regardless of the amount of money spent on these two activities – R&D or promotion – that commercial objectives are one of the main considerations behind how pharmaceutical companies direct their expenditures.

Limitations

These results only apply to companies that market the top 50 most promoted drugs in Canada in any given year. Results for other companies may vary. The pharmaceutical industry also disputes the R&D figures in the annual PMPRB reports because these figures are based on the definition of R&D used by Revenue Canada, whereas according to the industry other types of investment should also be included, increasing the amount of R&D spending [17].

Conclusion

Based on the available data, individual pharmaceutical companies in Canada, on average, are spending more on R&D than on promotion; however, the reverse is true for a minority of companies. For the industry as a whole, more may be spent on promotion versus R&D although a definite conclusion would require access to more complete data.

Abbreviations
IMC: Innovative Medicines Canada; PMPRB: Patented Medicine Prices Review Board; R&D: Research and development

Acknowledgements
None.

Funding
There was no funding for this study.

Authors' contributions
JL conceived of the idea for this study, gathered the data, wrote and revised the manuscript and read and approved the final manuscript.

Competing interests
In 2015-2017, Joel Lexchin was a paid consultant on two projects: one looking at indication-based prescribing (United States Agency for Healthcare Research and Quality) and a second deciding what drugs should be provided free of charge by general practitioners (Government of Canada, Ontario Supporting Patient Oriented Research Support Unit and the St Michael's Hospital Foundation). He also received payment for being on a panel that discussed a pharmacare plan for Canada (Canadian Institute, a for-profit organization). He is member of the Foundation Board of Health Action International.

References
1. DiMasi J, Grabowski H, Hansen R. Innovation in the pharmaceutical industry: new estimates of R&D costs. J Health Econ. 2016;47:20–33.
2. Gagnon M-A, Lexchin J. The cost of pushing pills: a new estimate of pharmaceutical promotion expenditures in the United States. PLoS Med. 2008;5(1):e1.
3. Institute for Health & Socio-Economic Policy. The R&D smokescreen: the prioritization of marketing & sales in the pharmaceutical industry: IHSP; 2016. http://nurses.3cdn.net/e74ab9a3e937fe5646_afm6bh0u9.pdf. Accessed 12 Nov 2017

4. Canadian pharmaceutical industry review 2013. IMS Brogan, Montreal. 2014. http://imsbrogancapabilities.com/YIR_2013_FINAL. Accessed 12 Nov 2017.
5. Canadian pharmaceutical industry review 2014. IMS Brogan, Montreal. 2015. http://imsbrogancapabilities.com/YIR_2014_FINAL. Accessed 12 Nov 2017.
6. Canadian pharmaceutical industry review 2015. IMS Brogan, Montreal. 2016. http://imsbrogancapabilities.com/YIR_2015_FINAL. Accessed 12 Nov 2017.
7. Canadian pharmaceutical industry review 2016. QuintilesIMS, Montreal. 2017 http://imsbrogancapabilities.com/YIR_2016_FINAL. Accessed 12 Nov 2017.
8. Patented Medicine Prices Review Board: Annual report 2013. PMPRB, Ottawa. 2014.
9. Patented Medicine Prices Review Board: Annual report 2014. PMPRB, Ottawa. 2015.
10. Patented Medicine Prices Review Board: Annual report 2015. PMPRB, Ottawa. 2016.
11. Patented Medicine Prices Review Board: Annual report 2016. PMPRB, Ottawa. 2017.
12. IMC. Research and development. Innovative medicines Canada, Ottawa. 2017. http://innovativemedicines.ca/innovation/research-and-development/. Accessed 12 Nov 2017.
13. Hwang T, Carpenter D, Lauffenburger J, Wang B, Franklin J, Kesselheim A. Failure of investigational drugs in late-stage clinical development and publication of trial results. JAMA Intern Med. 2016;176:1826–33.
14. Rx&D. Where we stand: detailing. Ottawa, Canada's research-based pharmaceutical companies. 2010.
15. Lexchin J. The relationship between promotional spending on drugs and their therapeutic gain: a cohort analysis. CMAJ Open. 2017;5:E724–8.
16. Mintzes B, Lexchin J, Sutherland J, Beaulieu M-D, Wilkes M, Durrieu G, Reynolds E. Pharmaceutical sales representatives and patient safety: a comparative prospective study of information quality in Canada, France and the United States. J Gen Intern Med. 2013;28:1368–75.
17. Ernst & Young LLP. Innovative medicines Canada data analytics and members' economic footprint and impact in Canada. Vancouver: EY; 2017.

20

A bibliometric analysis of the global research on biosimilars

Akram Hernández-Vásquez[1]*(iD), Christoper A. Alarcon-Ruiz[2], Guido Bendezu-Quispe[3], Daniel Comandé[4] and Diego Rosselli[5]

Abstract

Background: Biosimilars could be a promising option to help decrease healthcare costs and expand access to treatment. There is no previous evidence of a global bibliometric analysis on biosimilars. Therefore, we aimed to assess the quantity and quality of worldwide biosimilars research.

Methods: We performed a bibliometric analysis using documents about biosimilars published until December 2016 in journals indexed in Scopus. We extracted the annual research, languages, countries, journals, authors, institutions, citation frequency, and the metrics of journals. The data were quantitatively and qualitatively analyzed using Microsoft Excel 2013. Additional information about authors' participation was obtained using the R-package Bibliometrix. Publication activity was adjusted for the countries by population size. Also, author co-citation analysis and a term co-occurrence analysis with the terms included in the title and abstract of publications was presented as network visualization maps using VOSviewer.

Results: A total of 2330 biosimilar-related documents identified in the Scopus database, most of them were articles (1452; 62.32%). The number of documents published had an exponential increased between 2004 and 2016 ($p < 0.001$). The United States was the country with the highest production with 685 (29.40%) documents followed by Germany and UK with 293 (12.58%) and 248 (10.64%), respectively. Switzerland (11.05), Netherlands (5.85) and UK (3.83) showed the highest per capita ratio. The highest citation/article ratio were for the Netherlands (28.06), Spain (24.23), and France (20.11). *Gabi Journal* published 73 (3.13%) documents; both *Biopharm International* and *Pharmaceutical Technology* and *Mabs*, 41 (1.76%). Three out of top ten journals were Trade publications. Amgen Incorporated from the USA was the most prolific institution with 51 documents followed by Pfizer Inc. with 48. Terms about specific diseases and drugs were found in recent years, compared with terms such as legislation, structure, protein, dose and generic in the early years.

Conclusions: Research production and publication of documents on biosimilars are increasing. The majority of publications came from high-income countries. The trends in terminology use are according to state of the art in the topic, and reflects the interest in the utilization of biosimilars in diseases who are expected to obtain benefits of its use.

Keywords: Biosimilar pharmaceuticals, Bibliometrics, Biomedical research (source: MeSH NLM)

Background

A biosimilar, or "similar biological product", is a highly similar product to an already approved biological product regarding structure, function, potency, quality, clinical efficacy and safety [1]. Currently, there are already 5 and 39 biosimilars products approved in the United States [2] and Europe [3], respectively. The number of approved biosimilars might increase in the next year due to manifest interest from different healthcare systems and international organizations [4].

The development of biological products represented a significant advance in the therapy of many diseases that did not have effective treatments. Nonetheless, these products require a vast expenditure of money and resources to develop, leading to an increase in the cost of these therapies for both patients and the health sector [5, 6]. The field of biosimilars could be a promising option to help decrease healthcare costs and expand access to treatment [7] particularly when many patents have already expired or will do so soon [8].

* Correspondence: akram.hernandez.v@upch.pe
[1]Universidad Privada del Norte, Lima, Peru
Full list of author information is available at the end of the article

Few studies had evaluated the clinical evidence in support of different biosimilars: there are only three cancer related-biosimilars products whose safety/efficacy have been published [9], while five biosimilars for chronic inflammatory diseases have six clinical trials comparing them with their reference drug [10]. This situation of scarce evidence may lead physicians [11], pharmacists [12] and patients to have low confidence their safety and efficacy [13].

Bibliometric analysis is a useful method to objectively measure current research of a certain subject and its international scientific influence as an aspect of scientific quality [14]. However, to our knowledge, there is no previous evidence of a global bibliometric analysis on biosimilars. Our study aimed to assess the quantity and quality of worldwide biosimilars research.

Methods
Study design
We performed a bibliometric analysis using documents published until December 2016 in journals indexed in Scopus (https://www.scopus.com/). While there are a variety of document types, only articles, reviews, editorials and letters were included.

Source of information
Scopus (Elsevier BV Company, USA) is the largest abstract and citation database of scientific peer-review literature including more than 22,000 titles from international publishers. We decided to use this database because it includes all MEDLINE documents and includes further characteristics such as country of all the authors and citations per document, information that is relevant for this study [15–17].

Search strategy
A literature search was conducted by a research librarian in Scopus for publications on a single day, October 18, 2017, and used the following MeSH and free terms in the title and abstract field: biosimilar pharmaceutical OR biosimilar*. The validity of the search strategy was tested by manually reviewing retrieved articles.

Data analysis
All data were collected by two authors and downloaded in csv format (Additional file 1: Dataset). The data were imported to Microsoft Excel 2013 and quantitatively and qualitatively analyzed. The Scopus database presents some disadvantages for bibliometric applications [17]. For this reason, it was necessary to standardize the data. We detected documents mistakenly attributed to the domain of author name and affiliation. Therefore, a standardization was carried out manually by the authors.

Bibliometric indicators were extracted from the data and with the option "Analyze Results" in Scopus, including annual research, languages, countries, journals, authors, institutions, and citation frequency. Scopus Journal Metrics was used to extract the metrics of journals. The contributions of countries were evaluated based on paper and citation numbers, and the research output of each country was adjusted according to population size (https://www.cia.gov/library/publications/the-world-factbook/geos/ag.html). To describe more information about author participation in research production about biosimilars, we use the open-source Bibliometrix R-package (http://www.bibliometrix.org/) to obtain the mean of articles per author, the mean of authors per article, the mean of articles' citation and the number of articles with only one or more than one author.

Author co-citation analysis (ACA) to analyze the relations among highly cited references and productive authors, and a term co-occurrence analysis with the terms included in the title and abstract of publications was presented as network visualization maps using VOSviewer version 1.6.6 (Leiden University, Leiden, Netherlands) techniques [18].

Research ethics
The data were downloaded from Scopus and as secondary data, did not involve any interactions with human subjects. There were no ethical questions about the data. Approval of an ethics committee was not necessary.

Results
A total number of 2330 documents indexed on Scopus were retrieved from 2004 to 2016. The majority of papers were articles (1452; 62.32%) followed by reviews (642; 27.55%), editorials (138; 5.92%), and letters (98; 4.21%). In 2004, three publications were identified compared to 521 in 2016 (Fig. 1); this increase in the amount of papers was statistically significant ($p < 0.001$). In general, 83 countries contributed to research articles about biosimilars. Table 1 listed the top ten countries, which represented 84.12% of the total. Seven of the top ten publishing countries are European. United States was the country with the highest production with 685 (29.40%) documents followed by Germany and UK with 293 (12.58%) and 248 (10.64%), respectively. European countries such as Switzerland (11.05), Netherlands (5.85) and UK (3.83) showed the highest per capita ratio. The highest citation/article ratio were for the Netherlands (28.06), Spain (24.23), and France (20.11).

The analysis of the subject area, Table 2 shows that most documents were included in the broad category "Medicine" with 1453, followed by "Pharmacology, toxicology and pharmaceutics" with 946 and "Biochemistry, Genetics and Molecular biology" with 607.

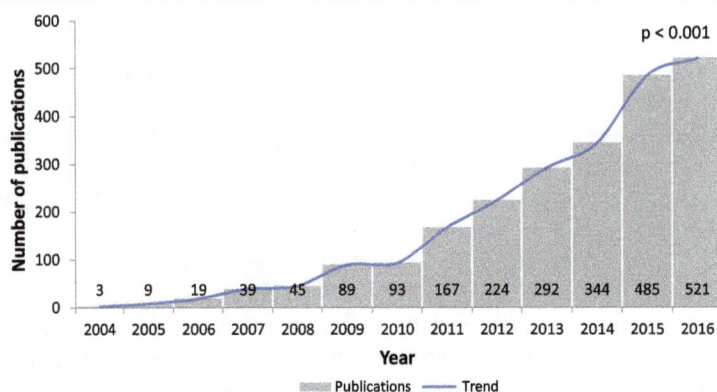

Fig. 1 Annual scientific documents of biosimilar research, Scopus 2004–2016

The total of documents retrieved were published in 803 journals, but top ten journals account for 18.82% of the total (Table 3). The top journals included in first place *Gabi Journal* with 73 (3.13%) documents, followed by *Biopharm International* and *Pharmaceutical Technology* and *Mabs* both with 41 (1.76%). Three out of ten titles were Trade publications. *Mabs* journal had the greatest SJR 2016 (1.62).

Table 4 presents a ranking of the Top ten institutions that published in biosimilars. Amgen Incorporated from the USA was the most prolific institution with 51 documents followed by Pfizer Inc. with 48. Seven of this top 10 list are European institutions, the others from USA. Four institutions were pharmaceutical companies. Based on the citations, academic institutions obtained higher positions compared to pharmaceutical companies being Medizinische Universitat Wien the institution with the highest number of citations and citations per articles ratio.

There were 6344 authors in the documents on biosimilars. The mean of articles per author was 0.4 and there were 420 documents with only one author. A co-authorship analysis that included authors with at least five publications is shown in Fig. 2. There were 143 authors; each circle represents one author, the closer the circles the closer the collaboration.

We show the top 10 cited articles in biosimilars in Table 5. The article "EULAR recommendations for the management of rheumatoid arthritis with synthetic and biological disease-modifying antirheumatic drugs: 2013 update" published in 2014 received the highest citation (962) within the retrieved documents. The top 10 include five articles and five reviews. All of the top ten cited articles were published in scientific journals. In general, the mean of citations per article was 9.6.

In the analysis of terms co-occurrence (Fig. 3), we used words in the titles and abstracts related to specific diseases and drugs. Rheumatoid arthritis, ulcerative colitis, rheumatism, infliximab, etanercept, and tofacitinib were found in recent years, compared with terms such as legislation, structure, protein, dose and generic in the early years.

Discussion

Biosimilars' cost-saving potential is their best attribute, making them an attractive option in the close future [19]. Also, the mandatory research that they have to do prior of their approval, and their large utility in diverse diseases, such as cancer, hemophilia, autoimmune diseases, and rare genetic conditions, make biosimilars an

Table 1 Top ten countries with more publications on biosimilars, and there average citation rate. Scopus 2004–2016

Rank	Country	Number of documents	% of articles	Number of articles per million inhabitants	Citations (up 2016)	Citations/Article
1	United States	685	29.40	2.10	6768	9.88
2	Germany	293	12.58	3.64	4373	14.92
3	United Kingdom	248	10.64	3.83	3824	15.42
4	Italy	149	6.39	2.40	2097	14.07
5	France	132	5.67	2.10	2654	20.11
6	Netherlands	100	4.29	5.85	2806	28.06
7	Spain	91	3.91	1.86	2205	24.23
8	Switzerland	91	3.91	11.05	1783	19.59
9	India	86	3.69	0.07	338	3.93
10	Canada	85	3.65	2.39	794	9.34

Table 2 Subject areas for documents published on biosimilars, Scopus, 2004–2016

Rank	Subject area	Documents published	% of documents
1	Medicine	1453	37.92
2	Pharmacology, Toxicology and Pharmaceutics	946	24.69
3	Biochemistry, Genetics and Molecular Biology	607	15.84
4	Immunology and Microbiology	219	5.72
5	Health Professions	165	4.31
6	Chemistry	137	3.58
7	Chemical Engineering	136	3.55
8	Business, Management and Accounting	68	1.77
9	Engineering	62	1.62
10	Mathematics	39	1.02

interesting field to make research. This explains the growing interest by many groups, including patients, health insurers, and providers, as well as the pharmaceutical industry. This interest is evidenced in the exponential increased of documents published on biosimilars between 2004 and 2016. High-income countries seem to dominate research in the field of biosimilars where the United States and Western European countries contributed to most of the world's research on biosimilars, and receive the most of the citations.

Authors from the United States published the highest number of scientific publications and received more citation compared to other countries. This result is not surprising, since the US leads the rankings in worldwide research, including medicine [20–22]. Majority of top-ranking countries were European. Although Switzerland, Netherlands, and United Kingdom do not have as many papers but go to the top of the list when we adjust by population. On the other hand, Netherlands, Spain, and France have the greatest citation per article. Those

situations are similar in other biomedical fields: Rheumatology [20], arthroscopy [23], foot and ankle [24], and probiotics in pediatrics [25], but it differs from endocrinology and metabolism field [26] and research on tramadol [27]. It would perhaps be better to adjust by the number of researchers, instead of inhabitants, but this information is not easily accessible [26].

"Gabi Journal" and "Mabs" were the most productive peer-review journals in the topic of biosimilars. Besides, "Biopharm International", a trade publication journal, occupied the second most productive journal on biosimilars. It is remarkable that three trade publication journals, perhaps showing the industry's interest in promoting their products, were in the top 10 most productive journals, but they do not receive that many citations. This may reflect the fact that they might be considered less trustful, or that they are not necessarily targeted at researchers [28]. Both "Mabs" and "Expert Opinion on Biological Therapy" are rated much higher in CiteScore 2017, SJR 2016, and SNIP 2016, despite having less publications. These suggest that at least in the field of biosimilars quantity is not necessarily correlated with quality. This situation differs from other biomedical fields like spine surgery [29].

Only three of the top 10 institutions were from America, the other seven were from Europe. This reflects the fact that biosimilars are a subject of interest in many different countries. Additionally, institutions with most citations and mean citation rate were from universities, which might indicate its better quality. Also, there is less risk that universities have conflicts of interest in developing research papers in biosimilars, so their results might be more trustful.

The top five most cited papers were original articles. The top two were guidelines for management of clinical conditions (rheumatoid arthritis and febrile neutropenia). This could be explained because three biosimilars are available to treat rheumatoid arthritis and others are in the way to approval [30], and the recent

Table 3 Top ten journals publishing on biosimilars (*N* = 2330). Scopus 2004–2016

Rank	Source title	Publication type	Documents published	% of articles	CiteScore 2016	SJR 2016	SNIP 2016
1	Gabi Journal	Journal	73	3.13	0.28	0.23	0.08
2	Biopharm International	Trade Publication	41	1.76	0.17	0.16	0.08
3	Mabs	Journal	41	1.76	4.66	1.62	1.25
4	Biodrugs	Journal	40	1.72	2.98	1.01	1.13
5	Bioprocess International	Trade Publication	39	1.67	0.26	0.23	0.25
6	Pharmaceutical Technology	Journal	39	1.67	0.09	0.14	0.16
7	Biologicals	Journal	34	1.46	1.65	0.62	0.74
8	Contract Pharma	Trade Publication	30	1.29	0.02	0.12	0
9	Journal of Generic Medicines	Journal	28	1.20	0.12	0.14	0.39
10	Expert Opinion on Biological Therapy	Journal	27	1.16	3.14	1.14	0.75

Table 4 Top ten institutions publishing on biosimilars, and their citations. Scopus 2004–2016

Rank	Institution Name	Country	Number of papers	Citations	Citations/Article
1	Amgen Incorporated	United States	51	394	7.73
2	Pfizer Inc.	United States	48	201	4.19
3	Utrecht University	Netherlands	44	898	20.41
4	Duke University	United States	37	763	20.62
5	Sandoz International GmbH	Germany	33	460	13.94
6	Medizinische Universitat Wien	Austria	23	1538	66.87
7	KU Leuven	Belgium	22	227	10.32
8	Erasmus University Medical Center	Netherlands	20	929	46.45
9	Universita degli Studi di Milano	Italy	20	152	7.6
10	Novartis International AG	Switzerland	19	174	9.

approval process of granulocyte-colony stimulating factor biosimilars, a useful drug to treat febrile neutropenia [31]. Moreover, clinical practice guidelines from any field generally have a lot of cites. The fourth and fifth most cited articles were randomized controlled clinical trials of the infliximab biosimilar CT-P13. This is the first biosimilar monoclonal antibody approved by the European Medicines Agency [32]. Overall, those two clinical trials help to understand and accept their interchangeability with infliximab as a feasible and safe strategy to be applied in real-life clinical practice [33]. On the other side, there were five reviews in the top 10.

Mostly, they try to better explain biosimilars to health professionals, especially clinician [34], that could have some reluctance about the use of biosimilars [35]. These reviews focus on improving the uptake of biosimilars, educating the physicians, and motivating to adopt them in routine clinical practice [36].

Words included in the title and abstracts of biosimilars research papers and their main year when they were published were: Legislation (2011), enzyme (2012), structure, protein, dose, antibody, interchangeability (2013), glycosylation, receptor, phase, adverse event (2014), and rheumatoid arthritis, ulcerative colitis,

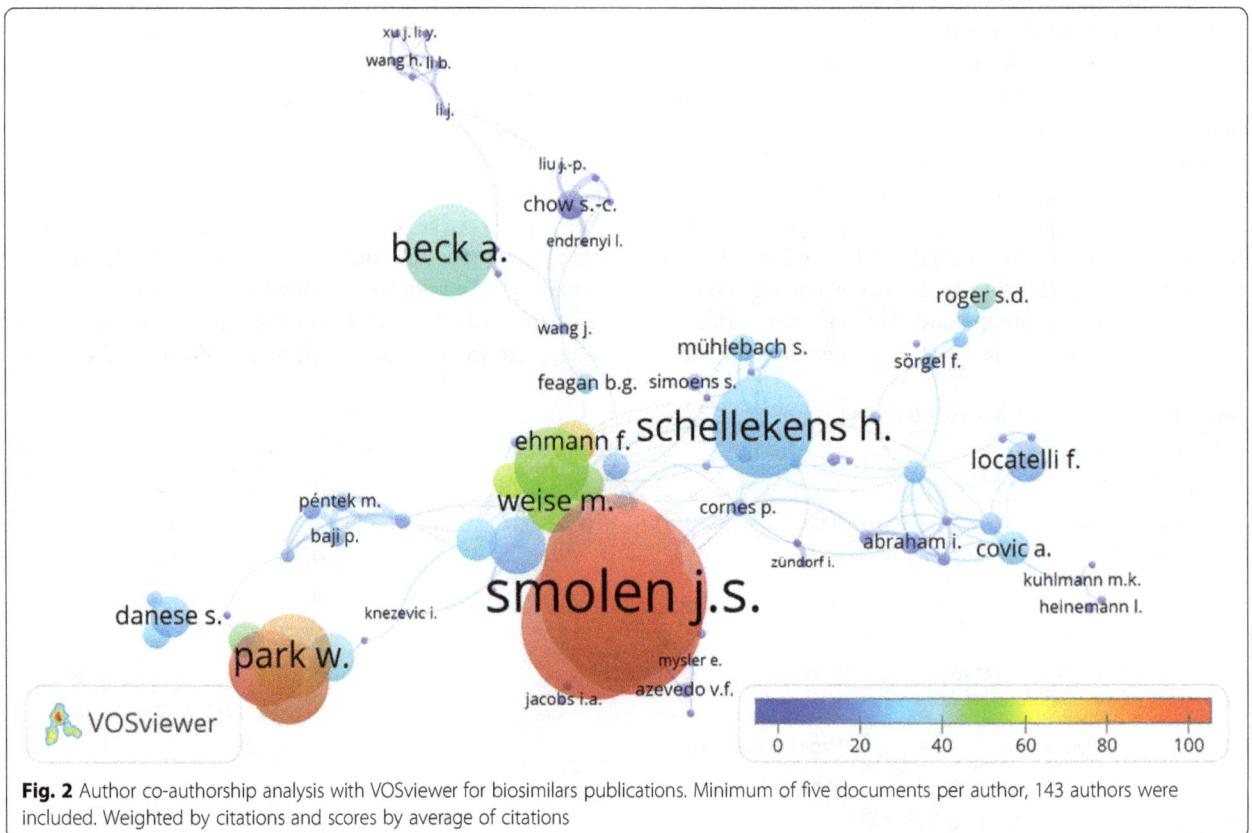

Fig. 2 Author co-authorship analysis with VOSviewer for biosimilars publications. Minimum of five documents per author, 143 authors were included. Weighted by citations and scores by average of citations

Table 5 Top 10 cited documents of biosimilars research. Scopus 2004–2016

Rank	Title	Year	Journal name	Cited by	Type of document
1	EULAR recommendations for the management of rheumatoid arthritis with synthetic and biological disease-modifying antirheumatic drugs: 2013 update	2014	Annals of the Rheumatic Diseases	962	Article
2	2010 update of EORTC guidelines for the use of granulocyte-colony stimulating factor to reduce the incidence of chemotherapy-induced febrile neutropenia in adult patients with lymphoproliferative disorders and solid tumours	2011	European Journal of Cancer	498	Article
3	Biopharmaceutical benchmarks 2014	2014	Nature Biotechnology	275	Article
4	A randomised, double-blind, parallel-group study to demonstrate equivalence in efficacy and safety of CT-P13 compared with innovator infliximab when coadministered with methotrexate in patients with active rheumatoid arthritis: The PLANETRA study	2013	Annals of the Rheumatic Diseases	269	Article
5	A randomised, double-blind, multicentre, parallel-group, prospective study comparing the pharmacokinetics, safety, and efficacy of CT-P13 and innovator infliximab in patients with ankylosing spondylitis: The PLANETAS study	2013	Annals of the Rheumatic Diseases	250	Article
6	Analytical tools for characterizing biopharmaceuticals and the implications for biosimilars	2012	Nature Reviews Drug Discovery	215	Review
7	PEG-modified biopharmaceuticals	2009	Expert Opinion on Drug Delivery	201	Review
8	The challenge of biosimilars	2008	Annals of Oncology	178	Review
9	Sublingual immunotherapy: World Allergy Organization position paper 2013 update	2014	World Allergy Organization Journal	172	Review
10	Biosimilars: What clinicians should know	2012	Blood	158	Review

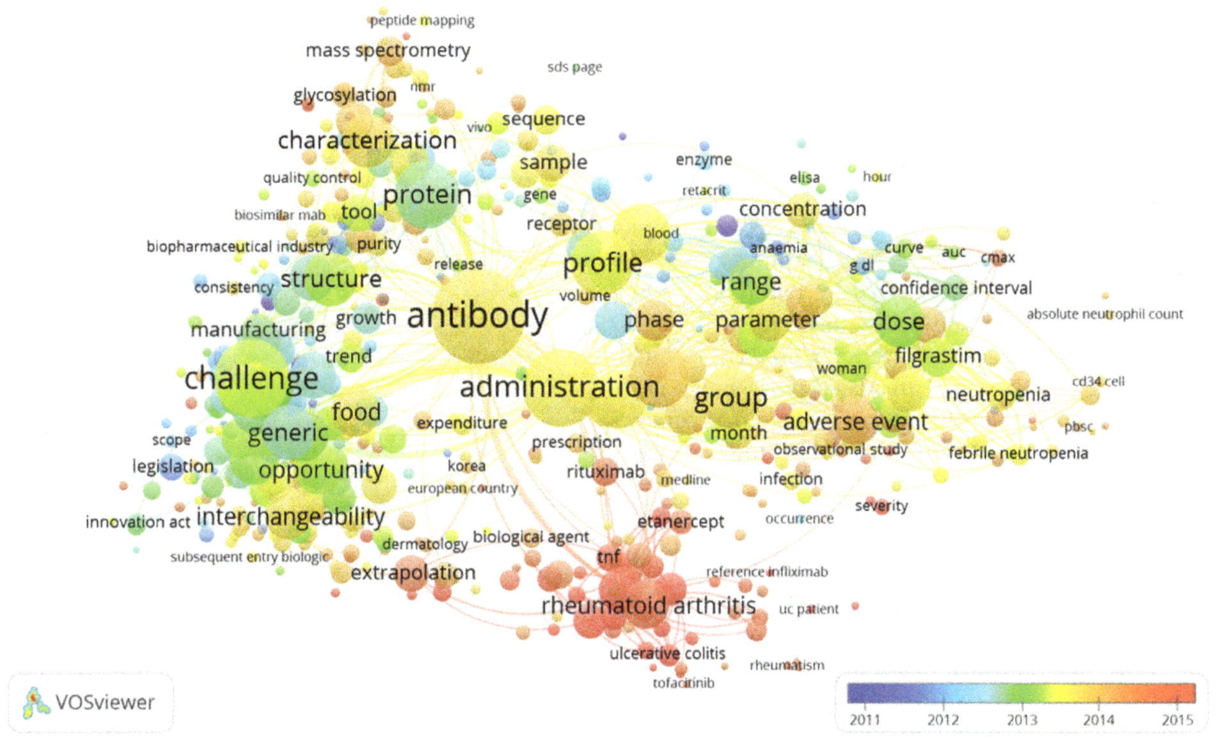

Fig. 3 Terms co-occurrence analysis of tittles and abstracts (overlay visualization) and their temporal evolution with VOSviewer for biosimilars publications. Binary counting method, choose threshold (10 terms). Term "conclusion" was excluded

extrapolation, rituximab, etanercept (2015). This suggests that the emphasis of biosimilars research responds to a subject that is very new to researchers and should follow the law of the development of a new discipline. This find is similar to a report in a previous bibliometric analysis on exomes [37]. In the field of biosimilars, there are requirements for their approval, including to demonstrate similarity, safety, and effectiveness [38]. These terms were more frequently found in the early.

The present research shows an overall view about biosimilars research and their distribution mostly in high-income countries where they have policies to their approval. Although markets like BRICS (Brazil, Russia, India, China, and South Africa), MIST (Mexico, Indonesia, South Korea, and Turkey) [39], and Latin America [40] provides an emerging future to biosimilars, they do not represent an important influence in biosimilars research. Also, the present study like previous bibliometric analyses has some limitations. First, our study did not include articles published in non-Scopus databases. However, Scopus is a reliable and significant source for bibliometric studies in general. Second, it is difficult to distinguish articles that focus on biosimilars from those that only mention the term or tangentially address it. However, using correct keywords and given its original subject, this study still provides a comprehensive picture of biosimilar research productivity, which could be used to track overall trends and identify topics of interest.

Conclusions

In summary, the results of the present study showed that documents published in journals about biosimilars are increasing. The majority of publications came from high-income countries, being the US the most productive country in biosimilars followed by European countries. To the best of our knowledge, this is the first study conducted in the analysis of research production and citations in biosimilars. The trends in terminology use are according to state of the art in the topic that comes from issues of safety and efficacy to the study of new biosimilar products in specific diseases.

Abbreviations
MeSH: Medical subject heading; SNIP: SCImago journal rank; SRJ: Source normalised impact per paper; UK: United Kingdom; USA: United States of America

Funding
This research received no specific grant from any funding agency.

Authors' contributions
AHV conceived the idea for the study; AHV and DC collected the data; AHV and GBQ did the statistical analysis; AHV, GBQ, CAAR and DR drafted the manuscript; all authors contributed in the writing and preparation of the manuscript. All authors read and approved the final manuscript.

Competing interests
The authors declare that they have no competing interests.

Author details
[1]Universidad Privada del Norte, Lima, Peru. [2]Facultad de Medicina, Universidad Ricardo Palma, Lima, Peru. [3]Universidad Peruana Cayetano Heredia, Lima, Peru. [4]Institute for Clinical Effectiveness and Health Policy (IECS), Buenos Aires, Argentina. [5]Departamento de Epidemiología Clínica y Bioestadística, Facultad de Medicina, Pontificia Universidad Javeriana, Bogotá, Colombia.

References
1. Declerck P, Danesi R, Petersel D, Jacobs I. The language of Biosimilars: clarification, definitions, and regulatory aspects. Drugs. 2017;77(6):671–7.
2. US Food and Drug Administration. Purple Book: Lists of Licensed Biological. US Department of Health and Human Services, Food and Drug Administration, Center for Biologics Evaluation and Research (CBER). 2017 [cited 2017 August 13]. Available from: https://www.fda.gov/downloads/Drugs/DevelopmentApprovalProcess/HowDrugsareDevelopedandApproved/ApprovalApplications/TherapeuticBiologicApplications/Biosimilars/UCM560162.pdf.
3. Biosimilars approved in Europe. Generics and Biosimilars Initiative July 7, 2017 [cited 2017 August 13]. Available from: http://www.gabionline.net/Biosimilars/General/Biosimilars-approved-in-Europe.
4. Bennett S. WHO to begin pilot prequalification of biosimilars for cancer treatment. 2017 [cited 2017 November 05]. Gineva: World Health Organization; [Nov 05, 2017]. Available from: http://www.who.int/mediacentre/news/releases/2017/pilot-prequalification-biosimilars/en/.
5. Blackstone E, Fuhr J. Innovation and competition: will biosimilars succeed? Biotechnol Healthcare. 2012;9(1):24–7.
6. Prince FH, van Suijlekom-Smit LW. Cost of biologics in the treatment of juvenile idiopathic arthritis: a factor not to be overlooked. Paediatr Drugs. 2013;15(4):271–80.
7. Boccia R, Jacobs I, Popovian R, de Lima LG, Jr. Can biosimilars help achieve the goals of US health care reform? Cancer Manag Res. 2017;9:197–205.
8. Ventola CL. Biosimilars. Part 1: proposed regulatory criteria for FDA approval. P T. 2013;38(5):270–4. 277, 287
9. Jacobs I, Ewesuedo R, Lula S, Zacharchuk C. Biosimilars for the treatment of Cancer: a systematic review of published evidence. BioDrugs. 2017;31(1):1–36.
10. Olteanu R, Zota A, Constantin M. Biosimilars: an update on clinical trials (review of published and ongoing studies). Acta Dermatovenerol Croat. 2017;25(1):57–66.
11. Cohen H, Beydoun D, Chien D, Lessor T, McCabe D, Muenzberg M, et al. Awareness, knowledge, and perceptions of Biosimilars among specialty physicians. Adv Ther. 2017;33(12):2160–72.
12. Beck M, Michel B, Rybarczyk-Vigouret MC, Leveque D, Sordet C, Sibilia J, et al. Knowledge, behaviors and practices of community and hospital pharmacists towards biosimilar medicines: results of a French web-based survey. MAbs. 2017;9(2):383–90.
13. Jacobs I, Singh E, Sewell KL, Al-Sabbagh A, Shane LG. Patient attitudes and understanding about biosimilars: an international cross-sectional survey. Patient Preference Adherence. 2016;10:937–48.
14. Van Raan T. The use of bibliometric analysis in research performance assessment and monitoring of interdisciplinary scientific developments. Technikfolgenabschautzung - Theorie und Praxis. 2003;1:20–9.
15. Falagas ME, Pitsouni EI, Malietzis GA, Pappas G. Comparison of PubMed, Scopus, web of science, and Google scholar: strengths and weaknesses. FASEB J. 2008;22(2):338–42.

16. Kulkarni AV, Aziz B, Shams I, Busse JW. Comparisons of citations in web of science, Scopus, and Google scholar for articles published in general medical journals. JAMA. 2009;302(10):1092–6.

17. Agarwal A, Durairajanayagam D, Tatagari S, Esteves SC, Harlev A, Henkel R, et al. Bibliometrics: tracking research impact by selecting the appropriate metrics. Asian J Androl. 2016;18(2):296–309.

18. van Eck NJ, Waltman L. Software survey: VOSviewer, a computer program for bibliometric mapping. Scientometrics. 2010;84(2):523–38.

19. Nabhan C, Parsad S, Mato AR, Feinberg BA. Biosimilars in oncology in the United States: a review. JAMA Oncol. 2017;4(2):241–7.

20. Cheng T, Zhang G. Worldwide research productivity in the field of rheumatology from 1996 to 2010: a bibliometric analysis. Rheumatology. 2013;52(9):1630–4.

21. Li Q, Jiang Y, Zhang M. National representation in the emergency medicine literature: a bibliometric analysis of highly cited journals. Am J Emerg Med. 2012;30(8):1530–4.

22. Zhang WJ, Ding W, Jiang H, Zhang YF, Zhang JL. National representation in the plastic and reconstructive surgery literature: a bibliometric analysis of highly cited journals. Ann Plast Surg. 2013;70(2):231–4.

23. Liang Z, Luo X, Gong F, Bao H, Qian H, Jia Z, et al. Worldwide research productivity in the field of arthroscopy: a bibliometric analysis. Arthroscopy. 2015;31(8):1452–7.

24. Luo X, Liang Z, Gong F, Bao H, Huang L, Jia Z. Worldwide productivity in the field of foot and ankle research from 2009-2013: a bibliometric analysis of highly cited journals. J Foot Ankle Res. 2015;8:12.

25. Sweileh WM, Shraim NY, Al-Jabi SW, Sawalha AF, Rahhal B, Khayyat RA, et al. Assessing worldwide research activity on probiotics in pediatrics using Scopus database: 1994-2014. World Allergy Organ J. 2016;9:25.

26. Zhao X, Ye R, Zhao L, Lin Y, Huang W, He X, et al. Worldwide research productivity in the field of endocrinology and metabolism–a bibliometric analysis. Endokrynologia Polska. 2015;66(5):434–42.

27. Sweileh WM, Shraim NY, Zyoud SH, Al-Jabi SW. Worldwide research productivity on tramadol: a bibliometric analysis. SpringerPlus. 2016;5(1):1108.

28. Oklahoma State University. Article Types and indentification: Trade Publications [Internet]. Oklahoma: Oklahoma State University, Library; 2016 [cited 2017 Sep 23]. [Available from: info.library.okstate.edu/c.php?g=151701&p=998800.

29. Wei M, Wang W, Zhuang Y. Worldwide research productivity in the field of spine surgery: a 10-year bibliometric analysis. Eur Spine J. 2016;25(4):976–82.

30. Rein P, Mueller RB. Treatment with biologicals in rheumatoid arthritis: an overview. Rheumatol Ther. 2017;4(2):247–61.

31. Schulz M, Bonig H. Update on biosimilars of granulocyte colony-stimulating factor - when no news is good news. Curr Opin Hematol. 2016;23(1):61–6.

32. McKeage K. A review of CT-P13: an infliximab biosimilar. BioDrugs. 2014;28(3):313–21.

33. Becciolini A, Raimondo MG, Crotti C, Agape E, Biggioggero M, Favalli EG. A review of the literature analyzing benefits and concerns of infliximab biosimilar CT-P13 for the treatment of rheumatologic diseases: focus on interchangeability. Drug Des, Dev Ther. 2017;11:1969–78.

34. Eleryan MG, Akhiyat S, Rengifo-Pardo M, Ehrlich A. Biosimilars: potential implications for clinicians. Clin Cosmet Investig Dermatol. 2016;9:135–42.

35. van Overbeeke E, De Beleyr B, de Hoon J, Westhovens R, Huys I. Perception of originator biologics and Biosimilars: a survey among Belgian rheumatoid arthritis patients and rheumatologists. BioDrugs. 2017;31(5):447–59.

36. Gyawali B. Biosimilars in oncology: everybody agrees but nobody uses? Recenti Prog Med. 2017;108(4):172–4.

37. Wang Y, Wang Q, Wei X, Shao J, Zhao J, Zhang Z, et al. Global scientific trends on exosome research during 2007-2016: a bibliometric analysis. Oncotarget. 2017;8(29):48460–70.

38. Sullivan PM, DiGrazia LM. Analytic characterization of biosimilars. Am J Health Syst. 2017;74(8):568–79.

39. Farhat F, Torres A, Park W, de Lima LG, Mudad R, Ikpeazu C, et al. The concept of Biosimilars: from characterization to evolution-a narrative review. Oncologist. 2017;22:1–7.

40. Garcia R, Araujo DV. The regulation of Biosimilars in Latin America. Curr Rheumatol Rep. 2016;18(3):16.

21

Insights into early stage of antibiotic development in small- and medium-sized enterprises: a survey of targets, costs, and durations

Christine Årdal[1][*] ⓘ, Enrico Baraldi[2], Ursula Theuretzbacher[3], Kevin Outterson[4], Jens Plahte[5], Francesco Ciabuschi[6] and John-Arne Røttingen[7]

Abstract

Background: Antibiotic innovation has dwindled to dangerously low levels in the past 30 years. Since resistance continues to evolve, this innovation deficit can have perilous consequences on patients. A number of new incentives have been suggested to stimulate greater antibacterial drug innovation. To design effective solutions, a greater understanding is needed of actual antibiotic discovery and development costs and timelines. Small and medium-sized enterprises (SMEs) undertake most discovery and early phase development for antibiotics and other drugs. This paper attempts to gather a better understanding of SMEs' targets, costs, and durations related to discovery and early phase development of antibacterial therapies.

Methods: DRIVE-AB, a project focused on developing new economic incentives to stimulate antibacterial innovation, held a European stakeholder meeting in February 2015. All SMEs invited to this meeting ($n = 44$) were subsequently sent a survey to gather more data regarding their areas of activity, completed and expected development costs and timelines, and business models.

Results: Twenty-five companies responded to the survey. Respondents were primarily small companies each focusing on developing 1 to 3 new antibiotics, focused on pathogens of public health importance. Most have not yet completed any clinical trials. They have reported ranges of discovery and development out-of-pocket costs that appear to be less expensive than other studies of general pharmaceutical research and development (R&D) costs. The duration ranges reported for completing each phase of R&D are highly variable when compared to previously published general pharmaceutical innovation average durations. However, our sample population is small and may not be fully representative of all relevant antibiotic SMEs.

Conclusions: The data collected by this study provide important insights and estimates about R&D in European SMEs focusing on antibiotics, which can be combined with other data to design incentives to stimulate antibacterial innovation. The variation implies that costs and durations are difficult to generalize due to the unique characteristics of each antibiotic project and depend on individual business strategies and circumstances.

Keywords: Antimicrobial innovation, Antibacterial innovation, DRIVE-AB, Pharmaceutical research and development

---

* Correspondence: christine.ardal@fhi.no
[1]Norwegian Institute of Public Health, Postboks 4404 Nydalen, 0403 Oslo, Norway
Full list of author information is available at the end of the article

Background

The world is facing an emerging threat of greater antibiotic resistance [1]. New antibacterial technologies are needed to treat pathogens as they become increasingly resistant to existing antibiotics [1, 2]. Yet, the last new classes of antibiotics to meet unmet needs were discovered in the 1980s [3, 4]. Only about five large pharmaceutical companies invest in antibacterial research & development (R&D) today [5]. However, many more small to medium-sized enterprises (SMEs) have been contributing to the R&D pipeline in this field and are currently the most significant participants in discovery and pre-clinical development activities [6, 7]. Seven out of the eight most recently approved antibiotics were based on key research and early development performed at SMEs [8]. Thus SMEs are key actors in any scheme to reinvigorate antibacterial drug innovation.

Antibacterial innovation is receiving significant political attention of late, including in the G7 and G20 groups of countries [9], the World Health Organization [10] and the United Nations General Assembly [11]. The United Kingdom has provided political momentum to increase antibacterial innovation by commissioning the AMR Review, led by the economist, Lord Jim O'Neill, to propose potential solutions, which were completed in May 2016 [12]. Europe's Innovative Medicines Initiative (IMI) has financed a project, DRIVE-AB (i.e., Driving reinvestment in research and development for antibiotics and advocating their responsible use, www.drive-ab.eu), a consortium of 16 public sector partners and seven pharmaceutical companies, which aimed to transform the way policymakers stimulate innovation, sustainable use and equitable access of novel antibacterial products to meet public health needs. This article is a part of DRIVE-AB's research efforts.

A variety of economic incentives have been proposed to stimulate antibacterial drug innovation [12–15]. Since many large pharmaceutical companies have exited the antibiotic field citing unsatisfactory commercial returns [16], the incentives are aimed at stimulating greater private sector involvement by increasing publicly sponsored rewards at the time of regulatory approval so that antibacterial innovation becomes an attractive business case. Determining the appropriate reward amount is a challenging task since it needs to sway innovators and investors to increase their private investments in antibacterial R&D while at the same time ensuring that the public sector is receiving value for money and meeting the important public health goals of sustainable use and equitable access. Knowledge on R&D costs, timelines, and profit expectations of pharmaceutical and venture capital companies is important in order to design and scale up effective solutions. Such knowledge about SMEs is of particular importance, given their position as the primary early-stage antibiotic innovators.

Actual pharmaceutical R&D costs are deemed highly confidential and controversial. Few researchers have been allowed access to this type of data, with the one main exception of DiMasi and colleagues at Tufts University, whose results are based upon data from ten, large pharmaceutical companies focusing on a range of therapeutic areas [17]. The study has been subject to much debate due to a lack of transparency and the resulting implications for pricing of pharmaceuticals [18].

This article is meant to shed some light on the targets, costs and durations of early phase development (up to Phase II clinical trials) for antibiotic innovation (see Table 1) in European SMEs.

Methods

Forty-four (44) European-based SMEs were invited to attend a stakeholder meeting in London in February 2015, with a purpose to understand the environment in which SMEs operate, their motivations, and the challenges they face in undertaking antibiotic R&D. The list of companies and contacts was gathered through expert advice and personal contacts of all known European SMEs with at least one antibacterial project in their pipelines. Out of the 44 SMEs invited, representatives of twenty-six (26) companies attended the meeting. The companies varied in size, from virtual companies with no full-time employees to those with dozens of employees. The attendees were divided into four groups with rapporteurs assigned to each group. Each group followed a discussion guide which included challenges faced by antibacterial drug-focused SMEs, financial barriers to investment, the role of SMEs in relation to other R&D organizations, and brainstorming on potential incentives to address SME challenges. Findings from the group work were then discussed in plenary. A final meeting report has been produced which includes the discussion questions, as well as the list of the attending SMEs [19].

A survey (see Additional file 1) was sent on March 5, 2015 to these 44 antibacterial-focused SMEs to gather more specific data regarding their areas of activity, development costs and timelines by R&D phase, and business models. Technology Readiness Levels (TRL) [20] are also given in Table 1 in order to ease comparison of this article's results with other articles. Reminder e-mails were sent on April 8, 2015 and May 5, 2015. Since the survey asks respondents to share confidential information, such as development costs, it was decided that the answers would be best formatted as multiple choice ranges. The intention was to both receive an acceptable response rate as well as to allow participants to complete the survey in about 30 min or less. The ranges for development costs and timelines were based on existing studies from pharmaceutical R&D [17, 21]. Survey participants were asked to select the range that

Table 1 Phases of R&D and Technology Readiness Levels (TRLs) in drug development

R&D Phase	Description	TRL
Research - Discovery activities, hit generation and testing	Generation of chemical starting points (hits) from screens or other drug discovery strategies	2
Research - Lead compound identification	Hits are evaluated and undergo limited optimization to identify promising lead compounds with meaningful activity against the target pathogens and possess the properties needed to make an effective and safe drug	3
Research - Lead compound optimization	Modifying and testing lead compound series to improve compound properties; selecting a candidate drug for further preclinical studies	4
Development - Preclinical testing	Conducting required toxicity and efficacy in vitro and vivo studies under good laboratory practice (GLP) protocols, and chemistry, manufacturing and control (CMC) studies	5
Development - Phase I clinical trials	Testing the candidate drug in healthy volunteers to determine pharmacokinetics, safe dose ranges and identify common toxicity; pharmacokinetic data feed into pharmacokinetic/ pharmacodynamic (PK/PD) models to determine the most appropriate doses for the next phase	6
Development - Phase II clinical trials	Testing the candidate drug in a small number of patients to obtain preliminary efficacy data and more short term safety information; refining PK/PD models	7
Development - Phase III clinical trials	Testing on a larger number of patients to document efficacy, determine non-inferiority activity (or rarely superiority) and safety compared to other indicated drugs	8

represented the value that it took for the company to complete the identified R&D phase. Therefore, the results for the clinical trials should not be viewed as a value for completing one clinical trial but rather for finishing all of the clinical trials that the company expects to perform for the identified phase for their main antibacterial project. An "antibacterial project" is the R&D surrounding one specific antibiotic candidate or antibacterial technology.

Results

Twenty-five (25) SMEs responded to our survey (a response rate of 57%). These can be classified mostly as small companies since only one company has more than 100 employees. 54% of the respondents ($n = 13$) had no revenues in 2014. 68% of the respondents ($n = 17$) focused on 1 to 3 internal antibacterial projects. In addition, 40% of the respondents ($n = 10$) outsourced more than half of their R&D budget to external organizations.

The stakeholder meeting identified three main sources of discovery of companies' antibacterial projects, either they were discovered: (1) in an academic setting which led to the establishment of a spin-off company, (2) independently by an expert in this field who subsequently formed a new company, or (3) in a large pharmaceutical company and subsequently spun-off as an SME. 80% of the survey respondents ($n = 20$) identified their own research as the source of their lead antibacterial project. In a separate question, 20% ($n = 4$) reported that they are spin-offs from universities or research institutes and another 20% (n = 4) spin-offs from a large, multinational pharmaceutical companies.

Type of products and clinical targets pursued

Companies at the stakeholder meeting expressed that they entered the antibacterial market because there are significant public health opportunities in new antibacterial

products with little competition. Several of these stakeholders also claimed that these opportunities are linked to significant unmet public health needs. The research focus of the survey respondents is largely small molecule development, i.e., traditional antibiotics. 76% ($n = 19$) perform R&D for small molecules, and 44% ($n = 11$) focus on antibodies, adjunctive antibacterial technologies including phage-based therapies and preventive vaccines. (Five companies have both small molecules and adjunctive programs.) Most companies focus solely on human health, but 28% ($n = 5$) also target animal health and/or environmental issues. The overwhelming majority of survey respondents claimed that they are involved in research and development of novel products, with 56% ($n = 14$) pursuing a novel class and 20% (n = 5) a novel mode of action.

Participants at the stakeholder meeting agreed that the increasing resistance problem is the primary market opportunity for antibacterial R&D, and SMEs aim, therefore, to meet therapeutic needs caused by emerging resistance against existing antibiotics. 44% ($n = 11$) of respondents stated that the focus of their main antibacterial project is a narrow-spectrum target and 36% ($n = 9$) a pathogen-specific approach. 80% ($n = 20$) of respondents reported their main antibacterial project targets, including *Acinetobacter baumannii*, *Pseudomonas aeruginosa*, *Escherichia coli*, *Klebsiella pneumoniae*, *Neisseria gonorrhoeae*, *Clostridium difficile*, and/or *Staphylococcus aureus*.

SMEs focused on pharmaceutical innovation typically perform discovery and early phase development work (up to Phase II clinical trials). SMEs at the stakeholder meeting stated that they struggled to find an exit strategy or pathways to commercialize their products due to the paucity of large, pharmaceutical companies actively pursuing R&D on antibacterial products. Many did not see a realistic way to commercialize products by themselves, but were considering taking on this role due to the few commercialization options. When asked to select among multiple exit strategies, 71% ($n = 17$) of respondents expressed hope to be acquired, 63% ($n = 15$) expressed hope to out-license their products, and only 17% ($n = 4$) would consider commercializing their products on their own. This in turn translates into their expectations on the extent of their development work. 36% ($n = 9$) of respondents aimed to complete Phase II clinical trials before out-licensing or selling their main antibacterial projects, whereas 24% ($n = 6$) aimed to complete Phase I clinical trials. And 24% ($n = 6$) aimed to out-license or sell prior to clinical trials.

Discovery and development costs and timelines

Respondents to the survey were asked to report discovery and development costs concerning three stages of their main antibacterial project – for each completed phase, the current phase, and the next phase. They were requested not to include opportunity cost or the costs of other candidate products. Therefore, the development cost should represent the out-of-pocket cost in order to complete the particular R&D phase for one antibacterial project. They were also asked about the duration for each phase, both completed and current. We were not able to measure the important component of the quality and scope of the work, for example whether the preclinical testing met bare minimum standards or was more extensive in order to better characterize the project.

The following development costs and timelines relate only to those who reported performing R&D on small molecules ($n = 19$) in order to report similar activities. Figure 1 shows the current phase of R&D for the main antibacterial project by the SMEs focusing on small molecules.

Lead compound identification

Eight SMEs have reported that they have completed lead compound identification. This may seem contradictory since 18 companies have reported that they are currently beyond lead compound identification. We can only presume that these ten companies either chose not to report the data or that they acquired the main antibacterial project after lead compound identification had

already been performed. One company, at the time of the survey, was currently performing lead compound identification.

All eight companies reported that it took four years or less, including three that reported it took a year or less. Development costs ranged widely from € 100,001–250,000 ($n = 3$) to more than € 1 million (n = 3) (see Fig. 2) with the remaining two companies falling in between these two ranges. The company currently performing lead compound identification at the time of the survey expected it to take in total 6 months to one year and cost less than € 1 million. Three out of the eight claimed that the main antibacterial project represented a novel class and three claimed a novel mode of action. However, neither duration nor the cost of research seemed to have been influenced by novelty, meaning that the novel products were spread across all cost and duration ranges. Therefore, we can estimate that SMEs may spend from € 100,001 to more than € 1,000,000 on lead compound identification which can take as short as 6 months or as long as 4 years.

Lead compound optimization

Four companies reported that they have completed lead compound optimization. Seven companies reported, at the time of the survey, that they were currently performing lead compound optimization. One company, at the time of the survey, was performing the previous R&D phase (lead compound identification) and estimated costs for lead compound optimization.

Among the four companies that have completed this phase, one took less than a year, another took one to two years, and the remaining two took two to four years. Amongst the seven companies, at the time of the survey, currently performing this phase, one company expects it to take less than six months, another predicts it will take six months to one year, four expect it to take one to two years, and the remaining company expects two to four years.

Three out of the four companies that have completed the phase reported the costs incurred. One reported costs less than € 1 million and the other two companies between € 1–5 million. Among the eight companies with expected costs, six expected that the phase will cost

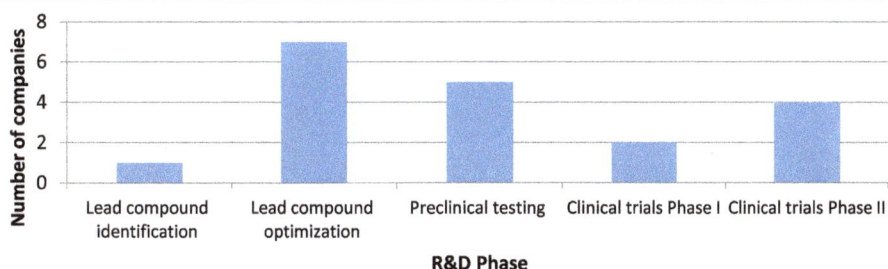

Fig. 1 Current phase of R&D for the main antibacterial project

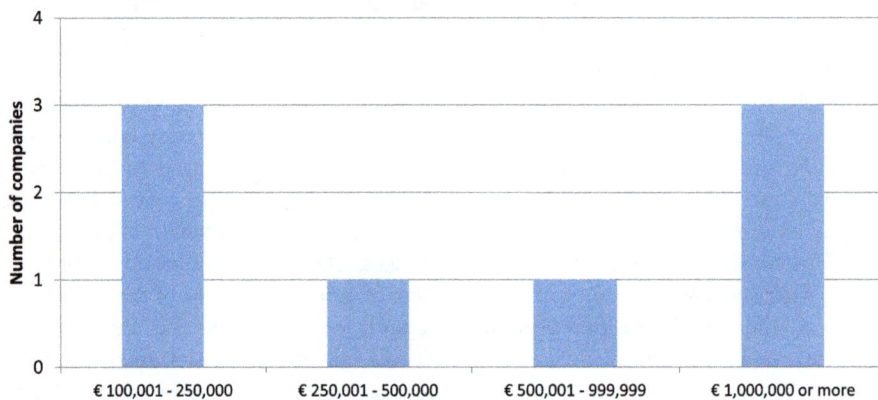

Fig. 2 Out-of-pocket cost of lead compound identification per main antibiotic project

between € 1–5 million, whereas two others estimated less than € 1 million. See Fig. 3 for the completed and expected costs by number of SMEs.

Out of the twelve companies in total reporting for lead compound optimization, seven claimed that the main antibacterial project represented a novel class and four claimed a novel mode of action. (The remaining company was performing R&D on a known class.) However, neither duration nor cost seemed to be influenced by novelty, meaning that the products described as novel were spread across all cost and duration ranges. The majority of SMEs have spent (or plan to spend) from € 1 to 5 million on lead compound optimization which can take as short as 6 months or as long as 4 years.

Preclinical testing

Four companies reported that they have completed preclinical testing. Five companies reported, at the time of the survey, that they were currently performing preclinical testing. Seven companies, at the time of the survey, were at the phase of lead compound optimization (before preclinical testing) and therefore estimated the costs for preclinical testing.

Among the four companies that have completed the phase, only three reported time durations. All took from one to two years. Amongst the five companies, at the time of the survey, currently performing the phase, one

expects it to take six months to one year, and the remaining four expect it to take one to two years.

Amongst the four companies that have completed the phase, one reported costs less than € 1 million and the remaining three between € 1–5 million. Among the twelve companies with expected costs (i.e., those currently performing preclinical testing or the previous phase, lead optimization), two expect that the phase will cost less than € 1 million, eight between € 1–5 million, and two between € 5–10 million. See Fig. 4 for the completed and expected costs by number of SMEs.

Out of the 16 companies in total reporting for preclinical testing, nine claimed that the main antibacterial project represented a novel class and three claimed a novel mode of action. (The remaining four companies are performing R&D on known classes.) However, neither duration nor cost seemed to have been influenced by novelty, meaning that the novel products were generally spread across all cost and duration ranges. Both two out of three of the least expensive projects (less than € 1 million) and the two most expensive projects (estimated to cost € 5–10 million) represent novel classes. The shortest duration (6 months to one year) was to complete preclinical testing for a project related to a known class. The majority of SMEs have spent (or plan to spend) from between € 1 and 5 million on preclinical testing which can take approximately one to two years.

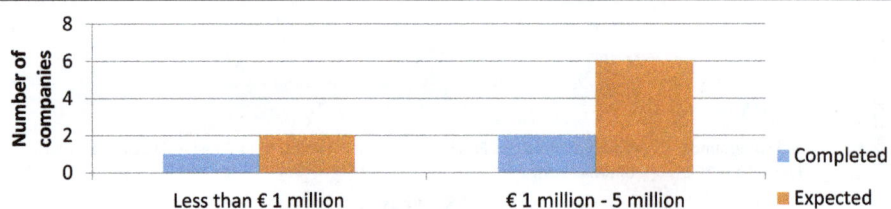

Fig. 3 Out-of-pocket costs of lead compound optimization – completed and expected – per main antibiotic project

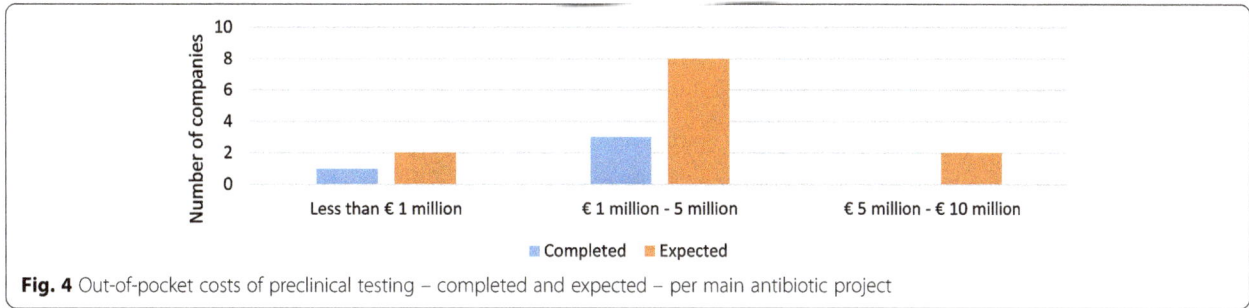

Fig. 4 Out-of-pocket costs of preclinical testing – completed and expected – per main antibiotic project

Phase I clinical trials

Six companies reported that they have completed Phase I clinical trials. Two companies reported, at the time of the survey, that they were currently performing Phase I clinical trials. Five companies, at the time of the survey, were performing the previous R&D phase (preclinical trials) and estimated costs for Phase I clinical trials.

Among the six companies that have completed the phase, three reported that it took six months to a year to complete Phase I clinical trials, two reported between one to two years, with the remaining reporting five or more years. Amongst the two companies, at the time of the survey, currently performing the phase, one expects it to take less than six months and the other six months to a year.

Among the six companies that have completed the phase, two reported costs less than € 1 million, three between € 1–5 million, and the remaining between € 10–15 million. Among the seven companies with expected costs, one expects that the phase will cost less than € 1 million, four between € 1–5 million, and two between € 5–10 million. See Fig. 5 for the completed and expected costs by number of SMEs.

Out of the 13 companies in total reporting for Phase I clinical trials, seven claimed that the main antibacterial project represented a novel class and two claimed a novel mode of action. (The remaining four represented R&D on known classes.) However, neither duration nor cost seemed to have been influenced by novelty, meaning that the products described as novel were spread

across all cost and duration ranges. The one company that reported a duration of five years or more is developing a novel class. The majority of SMEs have spent (or plan to spend) from € 1 to 10 million on Phase I clinical trials which can take six months to two years.

Phase II clinical trials

Only one company has completed Phase II clinical trials. In order to safeguard the anonymity of results since few European antibacterial-related SMEs have completed Phase II clinical trials we have combined the completed and expected figures for Phase II. Three companies, at the time of the survey, were performing Phase II clinical trials, and two companies were performing Phase I clinical trials and reported the estimated costs for Phase II as well.

Four companies reported duration data, two reported that it took one to two years to complete Phase II clinical trials and the other two reported between two to four years. Among the six companies reported cost data, one reported costs less than € 1 million, one between € 1–5 million, two between € 10–20 million, and the remaining one more than €20 million (Fig. 6).

Out of the six companies in total reporting for Phase II clinical trials, four claimed that the main antibacterial project represented a novel class and one claimed a novel mode of action. (The remaining company is performing R&D on a known class.) However, neither duration nor cost seemed to have been influenced by novelty, meaning that the products described as novel

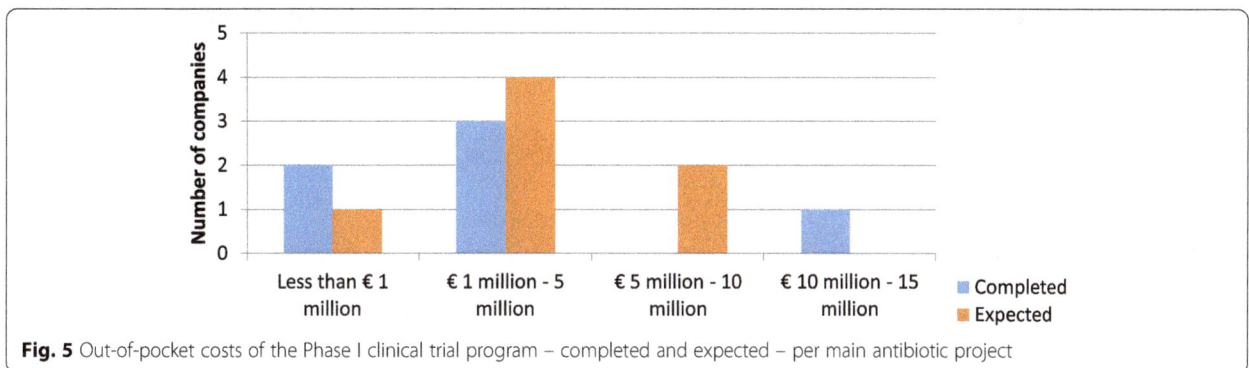

Fig. 5 Out-of-pocket costs of the Phase I clinical trial program – completed and expected – per main antibiotic project

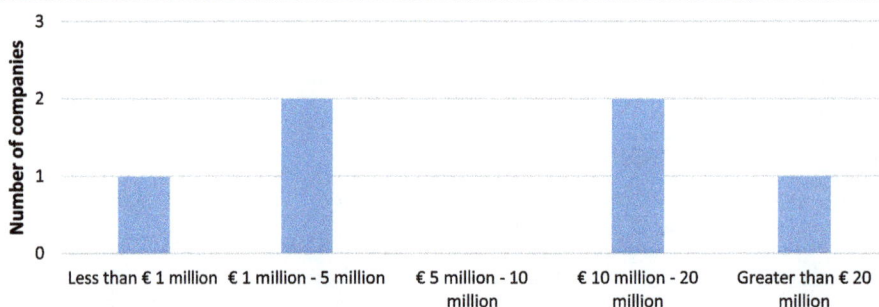

Fig. 6 Out-of-pocket costs of Phase II clinical trials – completed and expected – per main antibiotic project

were generally spread across all cost and duration ranges with the notable exception that the most expensive assertion (more than €20 million) was related to trials for a known class. The majority of SMEs have spent (or plan to spend) from € 1 to 20 million on Phase II clinical trials which can take one to four years.

Discussion

The results from our stakeholder meeting and survey provided data regarding development targets, development costs and timelines of European antibacterial-focused SMEs. These may not be a full representation of antibacterial SMEs in general since the sample population is small, and it becomes even smaller when the data are further sub-divided by R&D phase. Additionally, our findings report both actual and expected out-of-pocket costs within fairly broad ranges (as indicated in each of the previous figures). Expected costs may change over time. However, the results provided important insights into the therapeutic targets, R&D costs and R&D phase durations of European SMEs operating in antibiotic development.

DRIVE-AB and other initiatives need estimation of cost and duration to be made in order to effectively calculate adequate rewards. An "adequate" reward is one where the publicly-sponsored reward will generate a positive return on investment (or net present value) for the innovator without the public sector over-paying. Based on our results we propose the ranges in Table 2 to estimate development costs of antibiotics for SMEs.

(We state antibiotics here since these results focus solely on small molecule R&D.) To generate these ranges, for most values, we have selected the lowest and highest figures reported by the majority of SMEs who claim to be developing novel classes or modes of action. For lead compound identification, the higher boundary value is "more than € 1 million". This is unfortunate since it does not give us a definitive value as we expected the average value to be smaller when designing the survey. Therefore, our proposed maximum cost is taken from the general pharmaceutical R&D cost fig. [22] which is USD 2.5 million. (The Euro as per the current date of this article is slightly higher than the US dollar. We have given an equivalent in Euros since otherwise this figure appears to give an incorrect impression of precision).

In order to give a perspective regarding our proposed minimum and maximum costs per R&D phase we include two other studies [17, 22] which look across all therapeutic areas (which we call "general pharmaceutical R&D costs") and the antibacterial-specific costs reported by Sertkaya et al. (Table 2) [23]. Paul et al. utilized industry benchmarking data as well as internal data from the pharmaceutical company, Eli Lilly and Company, therefore, representing large pharmaceutical company costs only [22]. DiMasi et al. utilized data from ten multinational pharmaceutical companies. Sertkaya et al. interviewed about ten experts in antibacterial drug development and company representatives to gather their data regarding costs, in addition to reviewing the published literature [23]. For Phase II clinical trials

Table 2 Proposed minimum and maximum out-of-pocket cost per R&D phase for SME antibiotic innovation for DRIVE-AB models

R&D Phase	General Pharmaceutical R&D Costs	Sertkaya et al. [23]	Proposed Minimum Cost	Proposed Maximum Cost
Lead compound identification	USD 2.5 million [22]	(Used general pharmaceutical cost)	€ 100,000	€ 2.5 million
Lead compound optimization	USD 10 million [22]	(Used general pharmaceutical cost)	€ 1 million	€ 5 million
Preclinical testing	USD 5 million [22]	(Used general pharmaceutical cost)	€ 1 million	€ 5 million
Phase I clinical trials	USD 25 million [17]	USD 10 million	€ 1 million	€ 10 million
Phase II clinical trials	USD 35 million [17]	USD 9–16 million	€ 1 million	€ 20 million

Sertkaya et al. estimated the cost by indication, therefore, a range is given [23].

Our findings suggest that SMEs expect to perform antibacterial drug development less expensively than large pharmaceutical companies. One interpretation is that SMEs are leaner in structure and more cost-effective in their R&D activities. An alternative explanation may be that SMEs focus mainly on the essential studies that are minimally required by regulatory agencies for entry into limited Phase 2 studies and that they conduct additional studies at later time points. Total costs may be higher than those reported by SMEs here as the company that intends to commercialize the antibiotic may need to back-fill missing data to get licensure. Larger companies may include additional supporting studies or study variables to increase confidence in study results and reduce future risk of failure while a smaller company might be willing to take greater risk while anticipating an exit prior to regulatory approval. Recent changes in the regulatory landscape have significantly influenced costs and duration of later phases of clinical development with the option of abbreviated special pathways with smaller trial sizes. SMEs may also be anticipating these cost savings from regulatory changes; however, these should mostly be related to Phase III clinical trials which are not included in our study. Lastly, as stated clearly throughout the paper, a large percentage of the data is estimated amounts which may vary when faced with real-world obstacles. While the sample companies are inexperienced with performing more advanced development work, at least some SME executives have substantial drug development experience from previous employment.

Table 3 estimates the durations of R&D phases for antibiotic R&D. Again, to generate these ranges for most values we use the higher and lower boundaries of the values reported by the majority of the SMEs claiming to develop either novel classes or modes of action.

Our duration ranges demonstrate a great deal of variation. The range generally contains the estimates from both the general pharmaceutical innovation and Sertkaya et al., with the exception of Phase I clinical trials. Indeed,

in each R&D stage, the duration and costs reported by the surveyed companies vary by a factor of 10 or even more (see e.g., Fig. 5, with costs ranging between €1 million and 10–15 million; or Fig. 6 with a range between 1 and over 20 million). While this large variation implies that that our figures on costs and duration are difficult to generalize, it also suggests that the cost and duration of each antibiotic project depends on many specific factors, such as scientific and technical challenges, the presence or absence of prior data on the specific compound (or compound family), and a range of external factors, including an SME's availability of funds and experienced leading staff. This variation in durations has also been exemplified in Deak et al., which examined all eight antibiotics approved in the U.S. from 2010 to 2015 [8].

From the stakeholder meeting's roundtable discussion, several instances emerged of SMEs which were obliged to keep R&D on hold, generally during clinical trials but also in other phases. The barriers reported to cause delays in R&D activities include difficulty in securing funding and partners, preparing initial public offerings, manufacturing and quality control issues.

Regarding targets, both the stakeholder meeting and the survey confirmed that SMEs are focusing their R&D efforts on therapeutic needs caused by emerging resistance against existing antibiotics.

Conclusions

In conclusion, our results indicate that SMEs seek to deliver antibiotic discovery, preclinical and early clinical development at costs lower than large pharmaceutical companies have reported in the past. Costs for Phase III studies were not assessed. Duration appears to be highly variable but largely in line with other estimates.

DRIVE-AB delivered its final recommendations in January 2018. All recommendations were extensively discussed in consultations with a broad range of stakeholders including policymakers, healthcare insurers (both national and private), medicines regulatory authorities, SMEs, national research funding agencies, academic research institutions, and more. Although principally European in focus, DRIVE-AB actively engaged stakeholders globally

Table 3 Proposed minimum and maximum durations per R&D phase for SME antibiotic innovation for DRIVE-AB models

R&D Phase	General Pharmaceutical Innovation Durations	Sertkaya et al. [23]	Proposed Minimum Duration	Proposed Maximum Duration
Lead compound identification	1.5 years [22]	(Used general pharmaceutical duration)	6 months	4 years
Lead compound optimization	2 years [22]	(Used general pharmaceutical duration)	6 months	4 years
Preclinical testing	1 year [22]	(Used general pharmaceutical duration)	1 year	2 years
Phase I clinical trials	33 months [17]	0.9 years	6 months	2 years
Phase II clinical trials	39 months [17]	0.8–1.5 years	1 year	4 years

to ensure that its recommendations can be integrated in a broader context to ensure sustainable access to efficacious antibiotics and ultimately combatting resistance.

DRIVE-AB performed a computer simulation on different innovation incentives and combined several estimates of costs and durations such as those reviewed in this paper in order to calculate potential profits. It was valuable to have direct data from SMEs in order to develop realistic reward models. Despite the abovementioned limitations, the findings in this paper provide further insights that can help devising more precise policy tools for simulating pharmaceutical innovation taking into account their costs and durations. Similar research regarding SMEs outside of Europe would be beneficial.

Abbreviations

DRIVE-AB: A research project name - Driving reinvestment in research and development for antibiotics and advocating their responsible use; IMI: The European Union's Innovative Medicines Initiative; R&D: Research and development; SME: Small and medium-sized enterprises; TRL: Technology Readiness Levels

Acknowledgements

We would like to thank all SME participants who attended the stakeholder meeting and completed the survey.

Funding

All authors received funding from the DRIVE-AB project (www.drive-ab.eu). DRIVE-AB is supported by the Innovative Medicines Initiative (IMI) Joint Undertaking resources of which are composed of financial contribution from the European Union's Seventh Framework Programme (FP7/2007–2013) and EFPIA (European Federation of Pharmaceutical Industries and Associations) companies' in kind contribution. DRIVE-AB is part of IMI's New Drugs for Bad Bugs (ND4BB) programme. No authors receive any funding from the pharmaceutical industry. CÅ, JP, and J-AR are partially financed by the Norwegian Research Council (grant number 234608). KO is partially funded by the US Department of Health & Human Services (grant number IDSEP160030–01-00). The funders had no role in the design of the study, the collection, analysis, and interpretation of data, or in writing the manuscript.

Authors' contributions

The stakeholder meeting was organized by UT with inputs from the other authors. CÅ, EB, UT, and FC were present at the stakeholder meeting. UT, EB, and others wrote the final report from the meeting with input from all authors. The survey was designed by EB and CÅ with input from all authors. The survey data was assessed by CÅ and EB. All authors have participated in the drafting and revision of this article. All authors read and approved the final manuscript.

Competing interests

The authors declare that they have no competing interests.

Author details

[1]Norwegian Institute of Public Health, Postboks 4404 Nydalen, 0403 Oslo, Norway. [2]Uppsala University, Box 513, 751 20 Uppsala, Sweden. [3]Center for Anti-Infective Agents, Vienna, Austria. [4]Boston University, 765 Commonwealth Avenue, Boston, MA 02215, USA. [5]Norwegian Institute of Public Health, Postboks 4404 Nydalen, 0403 Oslo, Norway. [6]Uppsala University, Box 513, 751 20 Uppsala, Sweden. [7]Norwegian Institute of Public Health, University of Oslo, Postboks 4404 Nydalen, 0403, Boks 1072 Blindern, 0316 Oslo, Norway.

References

1. Laxminarayan R, Duse A, Wattal C, Zaidi AK, Wertheim HF, Sumpradit N, Vlieghe E, Hara GL, Gould IM, Goossens H, et al. Antibiotic resistance-the need for global solutions. Lancet Infect Dis. 2013;13(12):1057–98.
2. Laxminarayan R, Matsoso P, Pant S, Brower C, Røttingen J-A, Klugman K, Davies S. Access to effective antimicrobials: a worldwide challenge. Lancet. 2016;387(10014):168–75.
3. Silver LL. Challenges of antibacterial discovery. Clin Microbiol Rev. 2011; 24(1):71–109.
4. Laxminarayan R. Antibiotic effectiveness: Balancing conservation against innovation. Science. 2014;345(6202):1299–301.
5. Harbarth S, Theuretzbacher U, Hackett J, Adriaenssens N, Anderson J, Antonisse A, Årdal C, Baillon-Plot N, Baraldi E, Bhatti T. Antibiotic research and development: business as usual? J Antimicrob Chemother. 2015;70(6):1604–7.
6. Antibiotics Currently in Clinical Development [http://www.pewtrusts.org/en/multimedia/data-visualizations/2014/antibiotics-currently-in-clinical-development].
7. Theuretzbacher U. Market watch: Antibacterial innovation in European SMEs. Nat Rev Drug Discov. 2016;15:812–3.
8. Deak D, Outterson K, Powers JH, Kesselheim AS. Progress in the Fight Against Multidrug-Resistant Bacteria? A Review of US Food and Drug Administration–Approved Antibiotics, 2010–2015. Ann Intern Med. 2 016; 165:363–72.
9. G7 Health Ministers. Declaration of the G7 Health Ministers. Berlin: G7; 2015.
10. World Health Organization. WHO 67.25 Antimicrobial resistance. Geneva: World Health Organization; 2014.
11. United Nations. Political declaration of the high-level meeting of the General Assembly on antimicrobial resistance. New York: United Nations; 2016.
12. AMR Review. Tackling Drug-Resistant Infections Globally: Final Report and Recommendations. London: The Review on Antimicrobial Resistance; 2016.
13. Renwick MJ, Brogan DM, Mossialos E. A systematic review and critical assessment of incentive strategies for discovery and development of novel antibiotics. The Journal of antibiotics. 2016;69(2):73–88.
14. Rex JH, Outterson K. Antibiotic reimbursement in a model delinked from sales: a benchmark-based worldwide approach. Lancet Infect Dis. 2016;16(4):500–5.
15. Outterson KPJ, Daniels GW, McClellan MB. Repairing the broken market for antibiotic innovation. Health Aff. 2015;35(2):277–85.
16. Kinch MS, Patridge E, Plummer M, Hoyer D. An analysis of FDA-approved drugs for infectious disease: antibacterial agents. Drug Discov Today. 2014; 19(9):1283–7.
17. DiMasi JA, Grabowski HG, Hansen RW. Innovation in the pharmaceutical industry: new estimates of R&D costs. J Health Econ. 2016;47:20–33.
18. Light DW, Warburton R. Demythologizing the high costs of pharmaceutical research. BioSocieties. 2011;6(1):34–50.
19. DRIVE-AB: DRIVE-AB Stakeholder Meeting Report. In.; 2015.
20. Technology Readiness Levels (TRLs). https://www.medicalcountermeasures.gov/federal-initiatives/guidance/integrated-trls.aspx.
21. Maurer S: The right tool (s): designing cost-effective strategies for neglected disease research. Report to WHO Commission on Intellectual Property Rights, Innovation and Public Health. March 29, 2005. In.; 2005.
22. Paul SM, Mytelka DS, Dunwiddie CT, Persinger CC, Munos BH, Lindborg SR, Schacht AL. How to improve R&D productivity: the pharmaceutical industry's grand challenge. Nat Rev Drug Discov. 2010;9(3):203–14.
23. Sertkaya A, Eyraud JT, Birkenbach A, Franz C, Ackerley N, Overton V, Outterson K: Analytical framework for examining the value of antibacterial products. 2014.

22

Provider preferences for postoperative analgesia in obese and non-obese patients undergoing ambulatory surgery

Anthony H. Bui[1], David L. Feldman[1,2], Michael L. Brodman[1], Peter Shamamian[3], Ronald N. Kaleya[4], Meg A. Rosenblatt[1], Debra D'Angelo[2], Donna Somerville[2], Santosh Mudiraj[2], Patricia Kischak[2] and I. Michael Leitman[1,5]* ⓘⒹ

Abstract

Background: Few guidelines exist on safe prescription of postoperative analgesia to obese patients undergoing ambulatory surgery. This study examines the preferences of providers in the standard treatment of postoperative pain in the ambulatory setting.

Methods: Providers from five academic medical centers within a single US city were surveyed from May–September 2015. They were asked to provide their preferred postoperative analgesic routine based upon the predicted severity of pain for obese and non-obese patients. McNemar's tests for paired observations were performed to compare prescribing preferences for obese vs. non-obese patients. Fisher's exact tests were performed to compare preferences based on experience: > 15 years vs. ≤15 years in practice, and attending vs. resident physicians.

Results: A total of 452 providers responded out of a possible 695. For mild pain, 119 (26.4%) respondents prefer an opioid for obese patients vs. 140 (31.1%) for non-obese ($p = 0.002$); for moderate pain, 329 (72.7%) for obese patients vs. 348 (77.0%) for non-obese ($p = 0.011$); for severe pain, 398 (88.1%) for obese patients vs. 423 (93.6%) for non-obese ($p < 0.001$). Less experienced physicians are more likely to prefer an opioid for obese patients with moderate pain: 70 (62.0%) attending physicians with > 15 years in practice vs. 86 (74.5%) with ≤15 years ($p = 0.047$), and 177 (68.0%) attending physicians vs. 129 (83.0%) residents ($p = 0.002$).

Conclusions: While there is a trend to prescribe less opioid analgesics to obese patients undergoing ambulatory surgery, these medications may still be over-prescribed. Less experienced physicians reported prescribing opioids to obese patients more frequently than more experienced physicians.

Background

There is growing concern regarding overprescription of narcotic pain medication following ambulatory surgery. The use of postoperative opioid medication increases the risk of opioid-related morbidity, particularly gastrointestinal, cardiorespiratory, and central nervous system depression [1–3]. Furthermore, several studies have shown that prescribing opioid analgesia to patients following surgery may be associated with increased long-term use [4–7]. This is of particular concern given the increase in opioid use and opioid-related deaths over the last decade [8–11].

These risks are further magnified in obese patients undergoing surgery. Obese patients are at increased risk of opioid-induced respiratory complications [12–16]. Additionally, specific comorbidities associated with obesity - namely diabetes, heart failure, and pulmonary disease - have been shown to correlate with prolonged opioid use following major surgery [5]. In the United States, up to 80% of opioid-naive patients who underwent a low-risk surgical procedure from 2004 to 2012 filled a prescription for an opioid, and these rates

* Correspondence: Michael.leitman@mssm.edu
[1]Icahn School of Medicine at Mount Sinai, New York, NY 10029, USA
[5]Department of Surgery, Icahn School of Medicine at Mount Sinai, One Gustave L. Levy Place, Box 1076, New York, NY 10029, USA
Full list of author information is available at the end of the article

increased over time [17]. Many of these prescriptions were found to be excessive or inappropriate [18, 19]. Several US studies have shown that patients often have leftover pills from their narcotic prescriptions following surgery, suggesting that such aggressive pain control protocols may be unnecessary [20, 21]. Regulations on prescription opioids are more stringent in Europe and other parts of the world, causing increased barriers to access to pain relief [22, 23]. However, while rates of opioid misuse are generally lower in Europe compared to the US, they have been increasing over the past few years [24].

The past decade has seen an increase in the prevalence of obesity and the number of ambulatory surgeries performed [25, 26]. However, postoperative pain management protocols are not well-described for obese patients in any field, bariatric surgery or otherwise. Despite the risks associated with postoperative opioid use and the evidence of over-prescription, few evidence-based academic or federal guidelines exist to date for the safe administration of opioid analgesia to obese patients following ambulatory surgery. A series of recommendations on postoperative pain management released by the American Pain Society does not specifically discuss special considerations for either obesity or ambulatory surgery [27]. Furthermore, the recent guidelines for prescribing opioids for chronic pain from the US Centers for Disease Control and Prevention makes only a brief mention of obesity, only to say that these patients are at increased risk of sleep apnea and therefore extra monitoring and careful titration should be used [28]. While there is a general recognition of the need to reduce the postoperative prescription of opioids to obese patients [14, 15, 29, 30], recommendations for alternative postoperative pain management methods have not translated into specific protocols for obese patients. Providers therefore face challenges in providing adequate pain control to obese patients while minimizing their risk of adverse events following surgery.

As such, there is a need to assess the attitudes and preferences of providers regarding their approach towards managing postoperative pain. This study surveys the preferences of providers in a large, urban network of academic health centers regarding their postoperative analgesic protocols of choice for their obese and non-obese patients following ambulatory surgery.

Methods
Setting
Providers caring for ambulatory surgery patients within a consortium of five medical centers in New York, NY from May through September 2015 were surveyed. These hospitals have a strong community presence and treat a diverse socioeconomic population with a wide adult age range. Providers surveyed were all of these hospitals with an appointment in a surgical department who have medication prescribing privileges. While all analgesic orders are generally reviewed by the attending surgeon, all providers in this study have the ability to independently propose and place orders for pain medication. At each participating hospital in this study, ambulatory surgery is defined as any surgery in which the patient is discharged on the same day as the operation. The participating hospitals are insured by the same medical liability company directed by a group of physicians focused on patient safety. This company regularly undertakes patient safety evaluations and quality initiatives aimed at identifying and mitigating patient risk.

Survey
For this pilot study, there was interest in evaluating the providers' baseline attitudes regarding use of opioid analgesia in patients with obesity, a population known to be at increased risk for respiratory complications. Threfore, a structured questionnaire was developed with the aim of eliciting current practice habits from these providers. Survey participants were asked to indicate their role (surgical attending, surgical resident, physician assistant, or nurse practitioner), specialty, and years in practice (years as an attending for surgical attending physicians, post-graduate year for residents, post-training years for physician assistants or nurse practitioners). They were asked to indicate whether there is a BMI at which they will not perform ambulatory surgery on a patient, and if so, to indicate the BMI. They were then asked to provide their most frequently prescribed postoperative analgesic to obese and non-obese patients based upon the predicted severity of pain: mild, moderate, or severe. Survey participants either completed paper versions of the survey during departmental meetings or received an electronic version through e-mail. Responses were recorded into an encrypted database with uniquely generated, de-identified respondent IDs linked to further protect respondent identity as well as to prevent duplicate submissions.

Primary analyses
The primary objective was to examine whether providers indicated different prescribing preferences for their obese vs. non-obese patients given the predicted severity of pain. Therefore, for each analgesic protocol indicated in the survey, the percent of providers that preferred the analgesic was calculated for both obese and non-obese patients for each pain severity level (mild, moderate, and severe). McNemar's tests for paired observations were performed to compare the prescribing preferences of the providers for their obese vs. non-obese patients. For

each pain severity level, the proportion of providers who indicated an opioid vs. a non-opioid protocol, as well as the proportion indicating each individual analgesic, were compared between obese and non-obese patients.

Secondary analyses

The secondary objective was to examine the relationship between provider experience and prescribing preferences. First, attending physician respondents were categorized by years in practice, with more experienced attending physicians defined as those with greater than 15 years in practice, and less experienced defined as 15 years or fewer. This designation was a pragmatic decision based on surveys routinely distributed throughout the medical community that group providers similarly [31–33]. The percentage of more and less experienced attending physicians who preferred each analgesic protocol was calculated for both obese and non-obese patients for each pain severity level. Fisher's exact tests were performed to compare the prescribing preferences of more vs. less experienced attending physicians. For each obesity status and pain severity level, the proportions of more vs. less experienced attending physicians who indicated an opioid vs. a non-opioid protocol, as well as the proportions indicating each individual analgesic, were compared. Second, the prescribing preferences of attending vs. resident physicians were examined. Fisher's exact tests were performed to compare the prescribing preferences of attending and resident physicians similarly to the comparison of more vs. less experienced attending physicians. For all analyses, p-values less than 0.05 were considered significant.

Results

Study population

A total of 452 providers, out of a possible 695, responded to the survey for an overall response rate of 65%. Of these, 260 (57.5%) were surgical attending physicians, 155 (34.3%) were surgical residents, and 24 (5.3%) were physician assistants or nurse practitioners. Of the surgical attending physicians, 113 (43.5%) had been in practice for greater than 15 years, and 116 (44.6%) less than or equal to 15 years. Of the surgical residents, 34 (21.9%) were PGY-1, 35 (22.6%) PGY-2, 27 (17.4%) PGY-3, 30 (19.4%) PGY-4, 16 (10.3%) PGY-5, and 9 (5.8%) PGY-6 or greater. The most represented subspecialties were general surgery (130, 28.8%), obstetrics and gynecology (80, 17.7%), and orthopedic surgery (53, 11.7%) (Table 1). 145 (32.1%) respondents indicated that there is a BMI over which they would not perform ambulatory surgery on an obese patient; of these, 109 (75.2%) indicated this BMI to be > 40, 24 (16.6%) from 36 to 40, 6 (4.1%) from 30 to 35, and

Table 1 Survey population: providers caring for ambulatory patients ($N = 452$)

	Number	Percent
Provider Type		
Surgical Attending	260	57.5
> 15 Years in Practice	113	43.5
< =15 Years in Practice	116	44.6
Not Reported	31	11.9
Surgical Resident	155	34.3
PGY-1	34	21.9
PGY-2	35	22.6
PGY-3	27	17.4
PGY-4	30	19.4
PGY-5	16	10.3
PGY-6 or Greater	9	5.8
Not Reported	4	2.6
Physician Assistant	22	4.9
Nurse Practitioner	2	0.4
Not Reported	13	2.9
Department/Specialty		
Department of Surgery		
General Surgery	130	28.8
Colorectal Surgery	15	3.3
Bariatric Surgery	13	2.9
Plastic Surgery	9	2
Vascular Surgery	9	2
Pediatric Surgery	3	0.7
Department of Obstetrics and Gynecology	80	17.7
Department of Orthopedic Surgery		
General Orthopedic Surgery	53	11.7
Podiatry	33	7.3
Department of Anesthesia	38	8.4
Department of Otolaryngology		
ENT/Head and Neck	25	5.5
Oral/Maxillofacial/Dental	3	0.7
Department of Urology	18	4
Department of Ophthalmology	16	3.5
Not Reported	7	1.5

2 (1.4%) < 30. The prevalence of obesity at the participating hospitals is 9–10%.

Prescribing preferences for obese vs. non-obese patients

Table 2 describes the preferred postoperative analgesics according to obesity status and pain level. Among providers who prescribe differently between obese and non-obese patients, there is a tendency to prescribe opioids

Table 2 Provider preferences for postoperative pain management for obese vs. non-obese patients. results of McNemar's paired tests

Obesity status	Obese, n (%)		Non-obese, n (%)		p-value
Pain Severity	Opioids	Non-opioids	Opioids	Non-opioids	
Mild pain	119 (26.4%)	333 (73.6%)	141 (31.1%)	311 (68.9%)	0.002
Moderate pain	329 (72.7%)	123 (27.3%)	348 (77.0%)	104 (23.0%)	0.011
Severe pain	398 (88.1%)	54 (11.9%)	423 (93.6%)	29 (6.4%)	< 0.001

less frequently to obese patients than to non-obese patients; this is consistent for all 3 pain severity levels.

For mild pain, 119 (26.4%) providers indicated an opioid as their analgesic of choice for obese patients compared to 141 (31.1%) providers for non-obese patients ($p = 0.002$). The most commonly listed analgesics for mild pain were acetaminophen, NSAIDs, and acetaminophen plus oxycodone. For moderate pain, 329 (72.7%) providers would prescribe an opioid to obese patients compared to 348 (77.0%) providers for non-obese patients ($p = 0.011$). For severe pain, 398 (88.1%) providers preferred an opioid for obese patients compared to 423 (93.6%) providers for non-obese patients ($p < 0.001$). For both moderate and severe pain, the most commonly preferred analgesics were acetaminophen plus oxycodone, acetaminophen plus codeine, and NSAIDs.

Prescribing preferences by physician experience

Table 3 compares the preferred postoperative analgesics according to obesity status and pain level between more experienced attending physicians (> 15 years of experience) and less experienced ones (<=15 years). 70 (62%) more experienced attending physicians indicated an opioid as their choice analgesic for obese patients with moderate pain compared to 86 (74.5%) less experienced ones ($p = 0.047$). There were no significant differences between the proportions of more vs. less experienced attending physicians who indicated an opioid as their analgesic of choice for obese patients with either mild or severe pain.

For non-obese patients with moderate pain, 75 (66.7%) more experienced attending physicians indicated an opioid as their choice analgesic compared to 93 (80.2%) less

Table 3 Physician preferences for postoperative pain management for obese vs. non-obese patients by experience and training. Results of fisher's exact tests

Pain severity	Physician characteristics	Obese, n (%)		p-value	Non-Obese, n (%)		p-value
		Opioid	Non-Opioid		Opioid	Non-Opioid	
Mild Pain	Experience as Attending			0.767			1
	> 15 years	29 (26.0%)	84 (74.0%)		36 (32.0%)	77 (68.0%)	
	≤15 years	33 (28.6%)	83 (71.4%)		37 (31.8%)	79 (68.2%)	
	Physician Status			0.799			0.713
	Attending	68 (26.2%)	192 (73.8%)		79 (30.2%)	181 (69.8%)	
	Resident	43 (27.5%)	112 (72.5%)		50 (32.2%)	105 (67.8%)	
Moderate Pain	Experience as Attending			**0.047**			**0.023**
	> 15 years	70 (62.0%)	43 (38.0%)		75 (66.7%)	38 (33.3%)	
	≤15 years	86 (74.4%)	30 (25.6%)		93 (80.2%)	23 (19.8%)	
	Physician Status			**0.002**			**< 0.001**
	Attending	177 (68.0%)	83 (32.0%)		186 (71.7%)	74 (28.3%)	
	Resident	129 (83.0%)	26 (17.0%)		135 (87.1%)	20 (12.9%)	
Severe Pain	Experience as Attending			0.3156			0.106
	> 15 years	96 (84.9%)	17 (15.1%)		102 (90.0%)	11 (10.0%)	
	≤15 years	104 (89.5%)	12 (10.5%)		111 (96.0%)	5 (4.0%)	
	Physician Status			0.358			0.155
	Attending	230 (88.4%)	30 (11.6%)		241 (92.6%)	19 (7.4%)	
	Resident	142 (91.8%)	13 (8.2%)		150 (96.6%)	5 (3.4%)	

experienced attending physicians ($p = 0.023$). Similarly to obese patients, there were no significant differences between the proportions of more vs. less experienced physicians who indicated an opioid as their analgesic of choice for non-obese patients with either mild or severe pain.

Table 3 also compares the preferred postoperative analgesics according to obesity status and pain level between attending and resident physicians. 177 (68.0%) attending physicians indicated an opioid as their choice analgesic for obese patients with moderate pain compared to 129 (83.0%) residents ($p = 0.002$). There were no significant differences between the proportions of attending vs. resident physicians who indicated an opioid as their analgesic of choice for obese patients with either mild or severe pain.

For non-obese patients with moderate pain, 186 (71.7%) attending physicians indicated an opioid as their choice analgesic compared to 135 (87.1%) resident physicians ($p < 0.001$). Similar to obese patients, there were no significant differences between the proportions of attending vs. resident physicians who indicated an opioid as their analgesic of choice for non-obese patients with either mild or severe pain.

Discussion

This study is one of the first to describe attitudes and preferences regarding opioid prescription to obese patients from the provider perspective. Most previous studies on this topic report data at the patient or the medical encounter level; i.e. how many patients received opioids, how many prescriptions for opioids were filled at pharmacies, or how many hospital visits included a prescription for opioids [34–37]. The prescribing preferences reported by providers in this study are consistent with a recognition of the unique risks of prescribing narcotic analgesia to postoperative obese patients. Fewer providers overall reported an opioid as their most frequently prescribed postoperative analgesic for their obese patients; this trend was consistent across all levels of pain severity. Of note, several providers in our study indicated tramadol as their analgesic of choice for obese patients for moderate pain. Tramadol is known to have a multi-modal mechanism of action including weak opioid receptor agonism and serotonin reuptake inhibition. It has demonstrated efficacy in treating moderate to severe postoperative pain and has been previously described as a potentially useful drug for patients who are at increased risk for respiratory complications, such as obese patients, due to its lower risk for respiratory depression compared to opioid analgesics [3, 38, 39].

However, the results from this study appear to confirm and contribute data toward the fact that providers may be overprescribing opioid analgesics to patients. Indeed, even for mild pain, about 30% of providers in this study stated their preference for an opioid analgesic. A notable result from this study was the finding that less experienced physicians – i.e., residents and attending physicians who have been in practice for 15 years or less – were more likely to prefer opioid medication for both their obese and non-obese patients with moderate pain compared to their more experienced counterparts. The results from this study may be suggestive of a difference in treatment priorities between younger and older physicians. It is possible that younger physicians are more concerned about preventing and treating their patients' postoperative pain, whereas older physicians are more worried about opioid-related complications. Several reports from the primary care literature have found that younger physicians are less confident in their understanding of opioids, less confident with managing pain, and more reluctant to prescribe opioids, seemingly in conflict with the results of this study [40, 41]. However, one dermatology study found that younger dermatologists are more likely to prescribe opioids to their patients after Mohs surgery, which is consistent with the findings from this study [42]. The high outright rates of opioid prescription found in this study, and the discrepancy between younger and older physicians, both highlight opportunities for improved physician education on postoperative pain management and further demonstrates the need for safe analgesic guidelines.

Given the heterogeneity in postoperative pain management approaches found amongst providers in this study, and the possible gaps in understanding regarding pain control and opioid prescription that it highlights, there remains a need for standardized postoperative analgesic protocols. Recommendations for postoperative analgesia that are focused on obese patients emphasize the need to limit opioid use and propose strategies such as preoperative doses of NSAIDs, opioid alternatives, and multimodal analgesia [29, 30, 43–49]. However, these recommendations have not been fully synthesized into standard evidence-based protocols. Guidelines that do exist lack attention to the unique requirements of obese patients. For example, a series of recommendations for management of postoperative pain released jointly by the American Pain Society, the American Society of Regional Anesthesia and Pain Medicine, and the American Society of Anesthesiologists' Committee on Regional Anesthesia includes strategies to reduce opioid requirements after surgery, but fails to discuss considerations specifically for obese patients [27]. As such, postoperative pain management continues to be driven by consensus rather than evidence, leading to variability in treatment and high rates of postoperative narcotic prescription to patients both with and without obesity.

This study has several limitations that are necessary to mention. First, all of the providers are employees of the participating hospitals within the consortium insured by the single medial liability company. All of these hospitals serve the New York City community. While this is a socioeconomically diverse community, the providers themselves may share common practices by virtue of being within a common academic setting. The results may not be generalizable to providers working in different settings, such as more rural communities or those in private/independent practices. Additionally, the survey relied on providers' subjective interpretations of mild, moderate, and severe pain. One way to address this would have been to design a study in which clinical vignettes are given to the providers, and they are asked to propose an analgesic protocol. However, the primary objective of this study was to assess providers' baseline attitudes and perceptions regarding postoperative analgesia for obese patients. It was felt that the more straightforward approach – i.e., asking directly about management with respect to pain severity – would avoid confounders such as age, demographics, and other comorbidities that, while allowing for a more standardized assessment of analgesic management, would detract from the primary question of pain control in obese vs. non-obese patients. Additionally, this was not meant to be an educational intervention, and there was concern that exposure to such vignettes would inadvertently lead to changes in patient care before a proper evaluation of baseline provider habits was assessed. Furthermore, providers were asked to identify a BMI above which they would not perform surgery. There is a risk that this oversimplifies the complexities involved in determining whether a patient is a candidate for surgery, including the patient's comorbidities and the type of procedure being done. However, this study focused specifically on ambulatory surgery, which is defined in this study as surgery in which the patient leaves the hospital on the same day. This was felt to be a sufficiently narrow clinical scope for the purposes of this survey. Lastly, it is possible that the design of the survey could contribute towards survey bias. Providers were asked to fill in their preferred analgesic protocol for obese and non-obese patients for different levels of severity side-by-side. It is possible that providers would reflexively assume that they should input different responses upon seeing this format, when in practice their analgesic management of obese vs. non-obese management is not different. However, the fact that there was such a heterogeneous set of responses, including a high rate of providers who preferred opioids for mild pain as mentioned previously, seems to under-line the initial motivation behind this study – that there are very few guidelines to aid in the management of these patients.

Conclusion

This study, which aimed to survey of the prescribing preferences of providers for the pain management in obese and non-obese patients after ambulatory surgery, found that while providers tend to favor opioid analgesics less for their obese patients, many providers still prefer opioid analgesics even in situations when they may not be necessary. Furthermore. less experienced physicians may be prescribing narcotics at higher rates to both obese and non-obese patients than more experienced physicians. These results emphasize the need to develop post-discharge analgesic protocols with specific consideration for patients with obesity in order to provide adequate pain control while minimizing the risk of opioid-related adverse events.

Authors' contributions

AB, IML, DD'A, and PS contributed to the analysis and interpretation of data in addition to the drafting of the manuscript. MB, RK, MR, CS, DLF, PK, DS, SM, IML, and PS contributed to the original conception and design of the study in addition to the acquisition of data. All authors were involved with editing of the manuscript and gave final approval for the manuscript to be published.

Competing interests

The authors declare that they have no competing interests.

Author details

[1]Icahn School of Medicine at Mount Sinai, New York, NY 10029, USA. [2]Hospitals Insurance Company, New York, NY, USA. [3]Montefiore Medical Center/Albert Einstein College of Medicine, Bronx, NY, USA. [4]Maimonides Medical Center, Brooklyn, NY, USA. [5]Department of Surgery, Icahn School of Medicine at Mount Sinai, One Gustave L. Levy Place, Box 1076, New York, NY 10029, USA.

References

1. Wheeler M, Oderda GM, Ashburn MA, Lipman AG. Adverse events associated with postoperative opioid analgesia: a systematic review. J Pain. 2002;3(3):159–80.
2. Oderda G. Challenges in the management of acute postsurgical pain. Pharmacotherapy. 2012;32(9 Suppl):6S–11S. https://doi.org/10.1002/j.1875-9114.2012.01177.x.
3. Pattinson KTS. Opioids and the control of respiration. Br J Anaesth. 2008; 100(6):747–58. https://doi.org/10.1093/bja/aen094.
4. Alam A, Gomes T, Zheng H, Mamdani MM, Juurlink DN, Bell CM. Long-term analgesic use after low-risk surgery: a retrospective cohort study. Arch Intern Med. 2012;172(5):425–30. https://doi.org/10.1001/archinternmed.2011.1827.
5. Clarke H, Soneji N, Ko DT, Yun L, Wijeysundera DN. Rates and risk factors for prolonged opioid use after major surgery: population based cohort study. BMJ. 2014;348:g1251. https://doi.org/10.1136/bmj.g1251. Accessed 30 Mar 2016

6. Raebel MA, Newcomer SR, Reifler LM, et al. Chronic use of opioid medications before and after bariatric surgery. JAMA. 2013;310(13):1369–76. https://doi.org/10.1001/jama.2013.278344.

7. Brummett CM, Waljee JF, Goesling J, et al. New persistent opioid use after minor and major surgical procedures in US adults. JAMA Surg. 2017;176(3): e170504. https://doi.org/10.1001/jamasurg.2017.0504.

8. Frenk SM, Porter KS, Paulozzi LJ. Prescription opioid analgesic use among adults: United States, 1999-2012. NCHS Data Brief. 2015;189:1–8.

9. Manchikanti L, Singh A. Therapeutic opioids: a ten-year perspective on the complexities and complications of the escalating use, abuse, and nonmedical use of opioids. Pain Physician. 2008;11(2 Suppl):S63–88.

10. Okie S. A flood of opioids, a rising tide of deaths. N Engl J Med. 2010; 363(21):1981–5. https://doi.org/10.1056/NEJMp1011512.

11. Volkow ND, Frieden TR, Hyde PS, Cha SS. Medication-assisted therapies- tackling the opioid-overdose epidemic. N Engl J Med. 2014;370(22):2063–6. https://doi.org/10.1056/NEJMp1402780.

12. Zammit C, Liddicoat H, Moonsie I, Makker H. Obesity and respiratory diseases. Int J Gen Med. 2010;3:335–43. https://doi.org/10.2147/IJGM.S11926.

13. Murugan AT, Sharma G. Obesity and respiratory diseases. Chron Respir Dis. 2008;5(4):233–42. https://doi.org/10.1177/1479972308096978.

14. Lloret-Linares C, Lopes A, Declèves X, et al. Challenges in the optimisation of post-operative pain management with opioids in obese patients: a literature review. Obes Surg. 2013;23(9):1458–75. https://doi. org/10.1007/s11695-013-0998-8.

15. Porhomayon J, Leissner KB, El-Solh AA, Nader ND. Strategies in postoperative analgesia in the obese obstructive sleep apnea patient. Clin J Pain. 2013;29(11):998–1005. https://doi.org/10.1097/AJP. 0b013e31827c7bc7.

16. Ahmad S, Nagle A, McCarthy RJ, Fitzgerald PC, Sullivan JT, Prystowsky J. Postoperative hypoxemia in morbidly obese patients with and without obstructive sleep apnea undergoing laparoscopic bariatric surgery. Anesth Analg. 2008;107(1):138–43. https://doi.org/10.1213/ane. 0b013e318174df8b.

17. Wunsch H, Wijeysundera DN, Passarella MA, Neuman MD. Opioids prescribed after low-risk surgical procedures in the United States, 2004- 2012. JAMA. 2016;315(15):1654. https://doi.org/10.1001/jama.2016.0130.

18. Hill MV, McMahon ML, Stucke RS, Barth RJ. Wide variation and excessive dosage of opioid prescriptions for common general surgical procedures. Ann Surg. 2017;265(4):709–14. https://doi.org/10.1097/SLA. 0000000000001993.

19. Waljee JF, Zhong L, Hou H, Sears E, Brummett C, Chung KC. The use of opioid analgesics following common upper extremity surgical procedures. Plast Reconstr Surg. 2016;137(2):355e–64e. https://doi.org/10.1097/01.prs. 0000475788.52446.7b.

20. Bates C, Laciak R, Southwick A, Bishoff J. Overprescription of postoperative narcotics: a look at postoperative pain medication delivery, consumption and disposal in urological practice. J Urol. 2011; 185(2):551–5. https://doi.org/10.1016/j.juro.2010.09.088.

21. Rodgers J, Cunningham K, Fitzgerald K, Finnerty E. Opioid consumption following outpatient upper extremity surgery. J Hand Surg Am. 2012;37(4): 645–50. https://doi.org/10.1016/j.jhsa.2012.01.035.

22. Cherny NI, Baselga J, de Conno F, Radbruch L. Formulary availability and regulatory barriers to accessibility of opioids for cancer pain in Europe: a report from the ESMO/EAPC opioid policy initiative. Ann Oncol. 2010;21(3):615–26. https://doi.org/10.1093/annonc/mdp581.

23. Cleary JF, Hutson P, Joranson D. Access to therapeutic opioid medications in Europe by 2011? Fifty years on from the single convention on narcotic drugs. Palliat Med. 2010;24(2):109–10. https://doi.org/10.1177/ 0269216309360103.

24. European Monitoring Centre for Drugs and Drug Addiction. 2016 EU Drug Markets Report: In-Depth Analysis. Office of the European Union; 2016. http://www.emcdda.europa.eu/publications/joint- publications/eu-drug-markets-2016-in-depth-analysis_en. Accessed 1 Mar 2018.

25. Ogden CL, Carroll MD, Fryar CD, Flegal KM. NCHS Data Brief No. 219 - Prevalence of Obesity Among Adults and Youth: United States, 2011– 2014. Washington, DC; 2015. https://www.cdc.gov/nchs/data/databriefs/ db219.pdf. Accessed 22 July 2017.

26. Cullen KA, Hall MJ, Golosinskiy A. National Health Statistics Reports: ambulatory surgery in the United States, 2006. Washington DC; 2009. https://www.cdc.gov/nchs/data/nhsr/nhsr011.pdf. Accessed 22 July 2017

27. Chou R, Gordon DB, de Leon-Casasola OA, et al. Management of Postoperative Pain: A Clinical Practice Guideline From the American Pain Society, the American Society of Regional Anesthesia and Pain Medicine, and the American Society of Anesthesiologists' Committee on Regional Anesthesia, Executive Commi. J Pain. 2016;17(2):131–57. https://doi.org/10.1016/j.jpain.2015.12.008.

28. Dowell D, Haegerich TM, Chou R. CDC guideline for prescribing opioids for chronic pain — United States, 2016. MMWR Recomm Reports. 2016; 65(1):1–49. https://doi.org/10.15585/mmwr.rr6501e1er.

29. Alvarez A, Singh PM, Sinha AC. Postoperative analgesia in morbid obesity. Obes Surg. 2014;24(4):652–9. https://doi.org/10.1007/s11695-014-1185-2.

30. Ebert TJ, Shankar H, Haake RM. Perioperative considerations for patients with morbid obesity. Anesthesiol Clin. 2006;24(3):621–36.

31. Hartz A, Lucas J, Cramm T, et al. Physician surveys to assess customary care in medical malpractice cases. J Gen Intern Med. 2002;17(7):546–55. https://doi.org/10.1046/J.1525-1497.2002.10740.X.

32. Meadow W, Bell A, Lantos J. Physicians' experience with allegations of medical malpractice in the neonatal intensive care unit. Pediatrics. 1997; 99(5):E10.

33. Ballard DW, Rauchwerger AS, Reed ME, et al. Emergency physicians' knowledge and attitudes of clinical decision support in the electronic health record: a survey-based study. Carpenter CR, ed. Acad Emerg Med. 2013;20(4):352–60. https://doi.org/10.1111/acem.12109.

34. Nissen LM, Tett SE, Cramond T, Williams B, Smith MT. Opioid analgesic prescribing and use - an audit of analgesic prescribing by general practitioners and the multidisciplinary pain Centre at Royal Brisbane Hospital. Br J Clin Pharmacol. 2001;52(6):693–8. https://doi.org/10.1046/J. 1365-2125.2001.01502.X.

35. Sites BD, Beach ML, Davis MA. Increases in the use of prescription opioid analgesics and the lack of improvement in disability metrics among users. Reg Anesth Pain Med. 2014;39(1):6–12. https://doi.org/10.1097/AAP. 0000000000000022.

36. Mazer-Amirshahi M, Mullins PM, Sun C, Pines JM, Nelson LS, Perrone J. Trends in opioid analgesic use in encounters involving physician trainees in U.S. emergency departments. Pain Med. 2016;17(12):2389–96. https://doi. org/10.1093/pm/pnw048.

37. Volkow ND, McLellan AT. Opioid abuse in chronic pain — misconceptions and mitigation strategies. Longo DL. N Engl J Med. 2016;374(13):1253–63. https://doi.org/10.1056/NEJMra1507771.

38. Scott LJ, Tramadol PCM. A review of its use in perioperative pain. Drugs. 2000;60(1):139–76.

39. Nossaman VE, Ramadhyani U, Kadowitz PJ, Nossaman BD. Advances in Perioperative Pain Management: Use of Medications with Dual Analgesic Mechanisms, Tramadol & Tapentadol. Anesthesiol Clin. 2010;28(4):647– 66. https://doi.org/10.1016/j.anclin.2010.08.009.

40. Jamison PDRN, Sheehan BAKA, Scanlan NPE, Matthews PDM, Ross MDEL. Beliefs and attitudes about opioid prescribing and chronic pain management: survey of primary care providers. J Opioid Manag. 2014;10(6): 375. https://doi.org/10.5055/jom.2014.0234.

41. Jamison RN, Scanlan E, Matthews MH, Jurcik DC, Ross EL. Attitudes of Primary Care Practitioners in Managing Chronic Pain Patients Prescribed Opioids for Pain: A Prospective Longitudinal Controlled Trial. Pain Med. 2015;17(1):n/a-n/a. https://doi.org/10.1111/pme.12871.

42. Harris K, Calder S, Larsen B, et al. Opioid prescribing patterns after Mohs micrographic surgery and standard excision. Dermatologic Surg. 2014;40(8): 906–11. https://doi.org/10.1097/DSS.0000000000000073.

43. Oderda GM, Evans RS, Lloyd J, et al. Cost of opioid-related adverse drug events in surgical patients. J Pain Symptom Manag. 2003;25(3): 276–83.

44. Oderda GM, Said Q, Evans RS, et al. Opioid-related adverse drug events in surgical hospitalizations: impact on costs and length of stay. Ann Pharmacother. 2007;41(3):400–6. https://doi.org/10.1345/aph.1H386.

45. Kessler ER, Shah M, Gruschkus SK, Raju A. Cost and quality implications of opioid-based postsurgical pain control using administrative claims data from a large health system: opioid-related adverse events and their impact on clinical and economic outcomes. Pharmacotherapy. 2013;33(4):383–91. https://doi.org/10.1002/phar.1223.

46. Oderda GM, Gan TJ, Johnson BH, Robinson SB. Effect of opioid-related adverse events on outcomes in selected surgical patients. J Pain Palliat Care Pharmacother. 2013;27(1):62–70. https://doi.org/10.3109/15360288. 2012.751956.

47. Maher DP, Wong W, White PF, et al. Association of increased postoperative opioid administration with non-small-cell lung cancer recurrence: a retrospective analysis. Br J Anaesth. 2014;113 Suppl:i88–94. https://doi.org/10.1093/bja/aeu192.

48. Quidley AM, Bland CM, Bookstaver PB, Kuper K. Perioperative management of bariatric surgery patients. Am J Health Syst Pharm. 2014;71(15):1253–64. https://doi.org/10.2146/ajhp130674.

49. Schug SA, Raymann A. Postoperative pain management of the obese patient. Best Pract Res Clin Anaesthesiol. 2011;25(1):73–81.

23

Longitudinal study assessing the one-year effects of supervision performance assessment and recognition strategy (SPARS) to improve medicines management in Uganda health facilities

Birna Trap[1]* [iD], Richard Musoke[2], Anthony Kirunda[2], Martin Olowo Oteba[3], Martha Embrey[4] and Dennis Ross-Degnan[5]

Abstract

Background: In late 2010, Uganda introduced a supervision, performance assessment, and recognition strategy (SPARS) to improve staff capacity in medicines management in government and private not-for-profit health facilities. This paper assesses the impact of SPARS in health facilities during their first year of supervision.

Methods: SPARS uses health workers trained as Medicines Management Supervisors (MMS) to supervise health facilities and address issues identified through indicatorbased performance assessment in five domains: stock management, storage management, ordering and reporting, prescribing quality, and dispensing quality. We used routine data generated during SPARS visits to 1222 health facilities to evaluate performance changes during the first year of supervision as well as the time until achieving an adequate score in this period. We also explored variables related to facilities, MMS, and intensity of implementation as predictors of performance improvement and time until achieving an adequate score.

Results: Health facilities received an average of 3.4 MMS visits during the first year of supervision, with an average of 88 days between visits; each MMS implemented a median of 28 visits per year. Overall SPARS scores (maximum of 25) improved by 2.3 points (22.3%) per visit from a mean baseline score of 10.3. The adjusted improvement in overall SPARS score was significantly higher in primary health care facilities (2.36) versus higher-level health facilities and hospitals (2.15) ($p = 0.001$). The incremental improvement was highest at visit 2, with decreasing but continuing positive gains in subsequent visits. The adjusted mean incremental improvement per visit was highest in the prescribing quality domain, followed by dispensing quality, ordering and reporting, stock management, and storage management. Adjusted improvement in SPARS scores varied by region, year of implementation, and facility ownership. After one year of SPARS, 22% of facilities achieved an adequate score of 18.75 (75% of maximum score).

(Continued on next page)

* Correspondence: birna.trap@gmail.com
[1]USAID/Uganda Health Supply Chain Program, Management Sciences for Health, Plot 15, Princess Anne Drive, BugolobiP.O. Box 71419, Kampala, Uganda
Full list of author information is available at the end of the article

(Continued from previous page)

Conclusions: SPARS was effective in building health facility capacity in medicines management, with a median overall improvement of almost 70% during the first year. The greatest improvements occurred in prescribing quality and at lower levels of care, although the highest level of performance was achieved in storage management. We recommend broad dissemination of the SPARS approach in all Ugandan health facilities as well as in other countries seeking a practical strategy to improve medicines management performance.

Keywords: Supportive supervision, Medicines management interventions, Multipronged intervention, Performance assessment, Public sector, Uganda, Supply chain, Medicines use, Medicines indicators

Background

In Uganda, the Ministry of Health's (MOH) Pharmacy Department implemented a new national strategy that reorganizes health services around patients' needs and coordinates relationships between essential medicines and health supplies (EMHS) and other health system components to increase responsiveness and produce better outcomes [1]. As part of this focus on responsiveness and accountability, facilities need to be able to optimize available resources and meet growing expectations for better performance in medicines management (MM).

Effective MM in health care delivery involves many stakeholders and systems, and requires the optimization of processes covering five domains: stock management, storage management, ordering and reporting, prescribing quality, and dispensing quality [2]. Barriers to effective MM are many, complex, and interconnected, which calls for a holistic health system improvement approach [3]. Previously, Uganda had implemented predominantly educational interventions in health facilities, though with limited and unsustainable impact [4–6]. In late 2010, Uganda's MOH began to pilot a Supervision, Performance Assessment and Recognition Strategy (SPARS) to improve MM in health facilities, an approach that uses supportive supervisory visits, indicator-based performance assessment, sharing performance findings with managers at all levels, and special recognition for good performance. This multi-pronged approach is based on evidence on best practices in achieving sustainable health system performance improvements [7–9]. The cornerstones of SPARS are the Medicines Management Supervisors (MMS), who in addition to supportive supervision, also provide managerial support to staff in the form of manuals and tools needed to standardize MM practices. The MMS use SPARS indicators measured during each visit to identify weak areas and focus attention using effective supportive supervision principles [2, 10–12]. The SPARS method is described in detail in the first article of this theme issue [2].

To assess the longitudinal impact of the SPARS program, which was rolled out nationally in 2012, we assessed performance results during the first year of supervision in government and private not-for-profit (PNFP) health facilities

initiated in the program from the end of 2010 through 2013. Facilities represented all levels of care and came from 45 districts, representing about half of Uganda's districts.

Methods

Study design

This was an indicator-based longitudinal prospective study assessing incremental changes in SPARS scores, both overall and by MM domain, from the initial MMS visit through to the last visit conducted during the first year of supervision in each facility.

Setting and context

Uganda had a 2013 population of close to 38 million with an annual growth rate of 3.2% per year [13]. In that year, health care services were provided in the then 116 districts through 6404 health facilities, of which 63% (4035) were public (comprising 48% [3074] government-owned and 15% [961] PNFP) and 37% (2369) were private for-profit [13]. Service levels range from health center 1 (HC1), which represents volunteer health teams rather than actual facilities, to national referral hospitals. Each level of health facility is intended to supervise the level below. Table 1 lists the number of government and PNFP facilities and service levels in Uganda.

When SPARS was introduced, the average availability of a basket of 22 vital items in public health facilities was 53% on the day of survey, and providers at only 1% of health facilities provided the correct treatment for simple cough and cold [4]. Moreover, less than 8% (31) of pharmacy posts in the public sector were filled [14], and the health services referral system was poorly implemented [15].

Government hospitals and HC4s order their medicines and supplies, while HC2s and HC3s receive pre-packed kits; PNFP facilities at all levels order their supplies. Government facilities provide EMHS free of charge, which resulted in US$2.40 per capita spending for EMHS in 2013/14; the supply is heavily dependent on donor funds, which covered 77% of EMHS costs in 2013/14 [14].

SPARS intervention and its components

MMS are health sector employees such as clinical officers, nurses, EMHS storekeepers, or pharmacy staff who

Table 1 Government and PNFP health facilities and services by level of care in Uganda in 2017

	HC1	HC2	HC3	HC4	General hospital	Regional referral hospital	National referral hospital
Total number	25,000	2354	1291	196	117	16	2
Population served	1000	5000	20,000	100,000	500,000	2 million	10 million
Service area	Village	Parish	Sub-county	Sub-district	District	Regional	National
Staffing	Village health workers	Nurses	Clinical officers, nurses	Doctors, clinical officers, nurses	Doctors, clinical officers, pharmacy technicians, nurses	Specialists, doctors, clinical officers, pharmacists nurses	Specialists, doctors, clinical officers, pharmacists nurses
Services	Preventive; health promotion; reproductive, maternal, newborn, child health	Preventive; promotion; outpatient curative; maternity; community outreach and emergencies	HC2 plus: inpatient health services; simple diagnostic/ laboratory services	HC3 plus: emergency surgery; blood transfusion; laboratory services	HC4 plus: service training; consultation; research	General hospital plus: specialist's services such as psychiatry, ear, nose, and throat, ophthalmology, dentistry, intensive care, radiology, pathology, and more complex surgery	Regional referral hospital plus: specialists' services; training and research

are trained to make SPARS supervisory visits along with their other duties. MMS are selected by district health officers. Each district has one MMS who supervises mainly higher-level facilities (HC4 and hospitals) and oversees two to five health sub-district (HSD) MMS, who supervise lower-level facilities (HC3 and HC2). MMS are given motorbikes for transportation; net-books and modems to submit facility performance assessment data to a central information platform; MM tools such as stock cards, dispensing logs, and manuals describing standard operating procedures; and job aids and recognition materials for health facilities. The MMS are reimbursed US$12 for each assessment report they submit.

The MMS carry out the following activities to implement SPARS:

- Inform facilities in advance about upcoming SPARS visits
- Orient facility staff on the visit's purpose and conduct the indicator-based performance assessment
- Discuss assessment findings with health facility staff to highlight indicators that have improved, to see if targets have been met, and to identify problems
- Follow up with mentoring and training sessions that focus on skills or procedures that need improvement
- Agree with the facility staff on tasks to complete for the next visit
- Debrief health facility staff and facility in-charge about the visit
- Fill out the SPARS supervisory book with SPARS indicator scores for the current visit and targets for the next visit

- Fill in the SPARS data collection electronic tool [2] and submit to the central database

District and HSD MMS are each expected to complete three and five supervisory visits per month, respectively. Optimally, after the initial assessment, MMS should visit facilities every 60 days until they achieve an acceptable SPARS score (see below); after that, the maintenance phase of the program calls for three (3) visits per facility per year.

Sampling and data sources

For this study, we randomly selected 45 of the 80 districts included in the SPARS implementation from the end of 2010 to mid-2013, representing 15, 13, 9, and 8 districts from the Western, Eastern, Northern, and Central regions, respectively. Data for this study were results from SPARS performance assessments extracted from the centralized data platform for all visits that occurred for a period of 1 year after the initial visit to each facility. The data for the performance assessments came from stock management records, receipt and issue vouchers, dispensing logs, and laboratory logs. MMS also observed staff practices and the facility environment, and conducted exit interviews to assess patient knowledge and medicine labeling.

Outcome variables

SPARS overall, domain scores and achievement of adequate scores

The 25 SPARS indicators are classified into five MM domains: dispensing quality (seven indicators); prescribing quality (five indicators); stock management (four indicators); storage management (five indicators); and ordering and reporting (four indicators). Each of the five domains is assigned a maximum score of 5, resulting in a maximum overall SPARS score of 25. Each indicator is weighted proportionally to its contribution to the domain score, with missing indicators removed from the weighted domain score calculation. We defined an "adequate" SPARS score to be 18.75, equal to 75% of the maximum score.

Assessment of change in SPARS and domain scores

The primary outcome measure in this study was the change in total SPARS score between each pair of successive visits that took place during the first year of follow-up in each facility; changes in individual domain scores were secondary outcomes. We also assessed the median number of visits per facility and the median number of days between visits in the follow-up year. Finally, we determined whether a facility achieved an adequate SPARS score of 18.75 at any time during the follow-up year, as well as the time it took for the facility to reach this score.

Predictor variables

We identified two categories of predictor variables. Facility characteristics, which were assessed for all study facilities from either administrative data or from SPARS visit records, included: level of care (HC2, HC3, HC4, or hospital); ownership (government or PNFP); region (Eastern, Western, Northern, Central); calendar year of the initial SPARS visit; number of SPARS visits in the follow-up year; number of health facility staff supervised in the initial visit (one or more than one); number of MMS supervising at the initial visit (one or more than one); and whether the MMS who conducted the initial visit was assigned to the facility (yes or no). Because of differences in staffing, supply ordering, and services delivered, we stratified facilities by level of care for all analyses, with HC4 and hospitals grouped together at the highest level of care.

For each visit, we also assessed key characteristics of the MMS who conducted the visit including: gender; level (district or HSD); professional training (doctor/clinical officer, pharmacist/dispenser, nurse/midwife, supply officer); and number of facilities assigned to the MMS. For 74.5% of visits, we linked results of a survey completed in 2013 that included data on age, highest level of education, number of years of work experience, frequency of meeting with the District Health Officer (DHO), whether the MMS received feedback from the DHO about reports, whether the MMS felt that there was sufficient time to provide adequate supportive supervision during a visit, and whether the MMS felt that health workers responded well to the supervision.

Imputation

Based on data from completed SPARS visits, we employed multiple imputation methods to impute values of missing survey predictors for use in regression models [16, 17]; we also imputed values for missing SPARS domain scores.

Statistical analysis

We used chi-square tests to compare characteristics of facilities and MMS by level of health facility. Mean, median, and interquartile ranges (IQR) of overall SPARS and domain scores were calculated by follow-up visit number and compared across level of care. We examined changes in baseline scores during the initial SPARS visits in the period from 2011 to 2013 in order to examine possible temporal changes in scores unrelated to the intervention. We used generalized linear models with clustering on facility and MMS to assess the association between each individual predictor variable and the outcomes of interest. Predictors that were statistically significant in bivariate analyses were considered for multivariate analyses using the same models. Based on the estimates from the final multivariate models, we calculated adjusted values of the change scores along with their means and 95% confidence intervals. We displayed time until reaching an adequate SPARS score by level of care with Kaplan–Meier survival curves and used Cox-proportional hazard models to assess the time until attainment of an adequate score and the predictors of this outcome. Multiple imputation of missing data and all statistical analyses were conducted using STATA version 13.1.

Results

Characteristics of health facilities and visits

MMS visited 1499 facilities between 2010 and 2013 in the 45 sample districts; due to lost or incomplete reports, 1384 facilities (92%) had an analyzable record available for their initial assessment, and 1222 (82%) had at least one follow-up visit in the 12 months after their initial visit and were included in the analysis. Overall, 85% were government and 15% were PNFP facilities, and the analyses included 681 HC2s (56%), 416 HC3s (34%) and 125 HC4s and general hospitals (10%) (Table 2).

Facilities were comparable across levels of care by region. Lower-level facilities had higher percentages of government ownership ($p = 0.002$) and fewer had started SPARS supervision in 2011 ($p < 0.001$). At the initial visit, a greater percentage of HC2s were supervised by only one MMS ($p < 0.001$) and higher-level facilities had a greater percentage of initial visits in which two or more health workers were supervised ($p < 0.001$). The designated MMS for a facility conducted the initial supervision in about two-thirds of facilities.

Table 2 Facility and visit characteristics

Study facilities	Total		HC2		HC3		HC4/hospital		χ^2
	No.	%	No.	%	No.	%	No.	%	p-value
	1222	100	681	100	416	100	125	100	
Region									
Central	250	21	133	20	92	22	25	20	0.343
Western	421	35	224	33	145	35	52	42	
Eastern	379	31	226	33	118	28	35	28	
Northern	172	14	98	14	61	15	13	10	
Ownership									
Government	1039	85	596	88	349	84	94	75	0.002
PNFP	183	15	85	13	67	16	31	25	
Year of initial visit									
2011	753	62	368	54	289	70	96	77	<0.001
2012	406	33	263	39	117	28	26	21	
2013	63	5	50	7	10	2	3	2	
Health workers supervised at initial visit									
One	280	23	223	33	45	11	12	10	<0.001
More than one	942	77	458	67	371	89	113	90	
MMS supervising during initial visit									
One	957	78	603	89	292	70	62	50	<0.001
More than one	265	22	78	12	124	30	63	50	
Designated MMS supervised initial visit[a]									
No	394	32	208	31	150	36	36	29	0.118
Yes	828	68	473	69	266	64	89	71	

[a]Designated MMS is the MMS assigned to a facility who was responsible for a majority of visits

Characteristics of medicines management supervisors

Of the 148 MMS included in the study, 84% (124) were male, 64% (95) were HSD level, 55% (81) supervised 10 facilities or fewer, and 59% (87) were trained as clinical officers (Table 3). A total of 111 of the 148 MMS (75%) included in the study completed the 2013 MMS characteristic survey. Of these, 42% (46) were age 36 to 45, 83% (92) had secondary or diploma level education, and 40% (45) had fewer than 10 years of experience. The majority of MMS completing the survey reported having a monthly or weekly meeting with the DHO, and 85% (92) received feedback from the DHO on their submitted reports. About two-thirds of MMS felt they had sufficient time for conducting supervision during visits, and two-thirds thought that health workers responded well to the supervision (Table 3).

Intensity of intervention implementation

In the 1222 health facilities, MMS carried out 4172 supervisory visits in the first year of supervision with an average of 3.4 visits per facility. The median number of visits per facility was 3 (IQR 2–4), and the median number of days between visits was 88 (IQR 61–132). The median number of visits per year per designated MMS was 28 (IQR 17–39) (Table 4).

Changes in SPARS scores over time, overall, by level of care, and by domain

The median overall SPARS score increased by 68.9% from 10.3 (IQR 8.7–11.7) at the initial visit to 17.4 (IQR 15.6–19.4) at visit 5 (Fig. 1). The median improvements in SPARS score declined with each succeeding visit during the first year. The mean overall SPARS scores were slightly higher in HC4s and hospitals and slightly lower in HC3s at all visits, but improvements in SPARS scores by visit were very similar across all levels of care (Fig. 2). The initial visit domain scores and the improvement over time differed by MM domain. Storage management had the highest mean score at the initial visit (baseline) of 2.8 (95% CI 2.75–2.85), while the prescribing quality domain had the lowest mean of 1.0 (0.93–1.00). By visit

Table 3 Medicines management supervisor and district health officer characteristics

Characteristics	No.	%
MMS study total	148	100
Gender		
Male	124	84
Female	24	16
Level		
District MMS	53	36
Sub district MMS	95	64
Regions		
Central	31	21.0
Western	56	37.8
Eastern	41	27.7
Northern	20	13.5
Facilities supervised		
1-10	81	54.7
11-15	47	31.7
16+	20	13.6
Professional training		
Clinical officer	87	59
Pharmacist/dispenser	15	10
Nurse	36	24
Supplies officer	10	7
MMS completing 2013 survey	111	75
Age group		
26-35	37	34
36-45	46	42
46+	26	24
Highest level of education		
Secondary/diploma/other	92	83
Bachelors/Master's degree	19	17
Number of years of work experience		
0-9	45	40
10+	66	60
Frequency of meetings with DHO		
Monthly/weekly	60	54
Quarterly/semi-annually	24	22
Irregularly/other	27	24
Received feedback from DHO about MMS report		
No	16	15
Yes	92	85
Sufficient time during visits to provide adequate supportive supervision		
No	38	35
Yes	71	65

Table 3 Medicines management supervisor and district health officer characteristics (Continued)

Characteristics	No.	%
Health workers respond well to supervision		
Some of them	40	37
Most/all of them	68	63

5, the mean domain scores were all above 3.0 except for prescribing quality at 2.8 (2.65–2.94); however, prescribing quality experienced the greatest absolute improvement during the course of follow-up (Fig. 3).

The average adjusted baseline SPARS score in the study facilities prior to any intervention in 2010 to 2011 was 10.25, which improved to 10.57 in 2012 and to 11.29 in 2013. This represented 0.32 and 1.04 point improvements in baseline scores in 2012 and 2013, respectively, unrelated to the SPARS intervention.

Improvement in SPARS scores by visit

Table 5 presents the average changes in SPARS scores by level of care, overall and by domain, adjusted for the predictors included in the multivariate models. Averaged over all visits in the first year of supervision, the adjusted improvement in SPARS score per visit was slightly but significantly higher in HC2s (2.2) compared to hospitals or HC4s (2.0). The adjusted mean improvement in SPARS scores was highest at visit 2 (i.e., following the initial supervision) at all facility levels, but the improvement was significantly higher in HC2s and HC3s (3.2 and 2.8, respectively) than in higher-level facilities (2.5). Across all the three levels of care, the adjusted mean improvements were lower at visit 3 (after two rounds of supervision) and lower still at visit 4. The numbers of facilities with a fifth supervisory visit in the first year were low at all levels of care, but among those with a fifth visit, changes in adjusted overall SPARS scores remained positive.

Across the five indicator domains, improvements in SPARS scores tended to follow a similar pattern with the largest improvements observed at visits 2 and 3, and

Table 4 Number of MMS visits within the first year of supervision, overall and by level of care

No. of visits	All facilities		HC2		HC3		HC4/hospitals	
	No.	%	No.	%	No.	%	No.	%
2	328	27	184	27	115	28	29	23
3	334	27	176	26	115	28	43	34
4	323	26	180	26	108	26	35	28
5	201	16	122	18	62	15	17	14
6	35	3	19	3	15	4	1	1
7	1	0	0	0	1	0	0	0
Total	1222	100	681	100	416	100	125	100

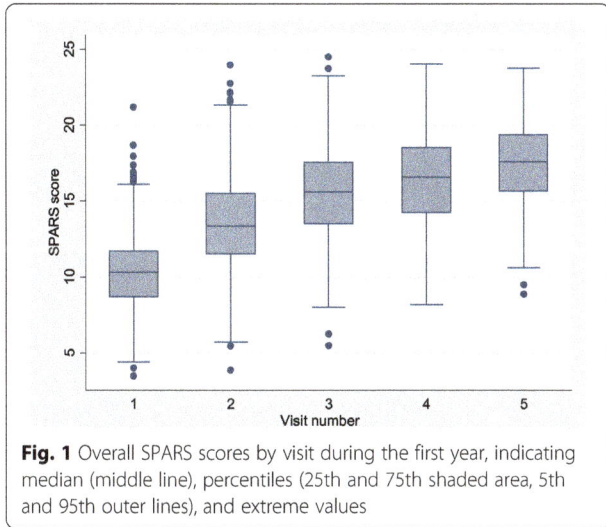

Fig. 1 Overall SPARS scores by visit during the first year, indicating median (middle line), percentiles (25th and 75th shaded area, 5th and 95th outer lines), and extreme values

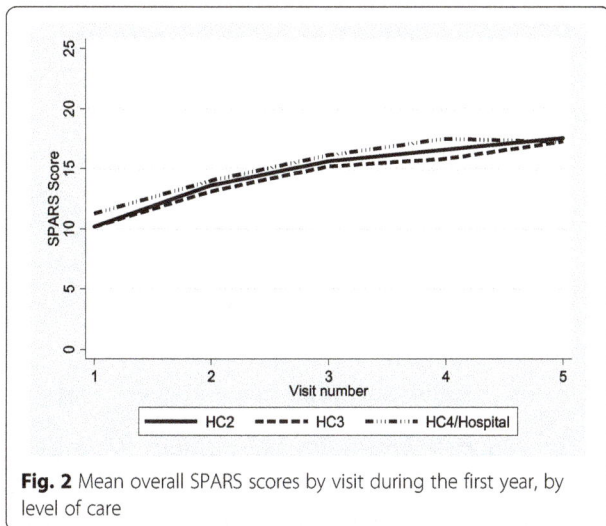

Fig. 3 Overall domain score by visits

smaller gains observed in later visits. Across all visits, average improvements in prescribing quality scores were notably lower in HC4s and hospitals (0.4) than in HC2s and HC3s (0.6 each). The average adjusted improvements in the first year in the prescribing domain were the highest of any domain. For HC4s and hospitals, the largest adjusted improvements in any domain were observed for ordering and reporting (0.5), with a particularly large gain observed after the first visit (0.7) (Table 5).

Predictors of improvement in SPARS and domain scores

In addition to the baseline score, the factors significantly associated with average visit-to-visit improvement in overall SPARS scores at all facilities in multivariate models included region, ownership, the number of MMS supervising a facility at the previous visit, MMS profession, and whether the MMS received feedback from the DHO (Table 6). Specifically, adjusting for the level of the

baseline SPARS score, significantly greater improvements were observed in the Northern (0.8 greater improvement, 95% CI [0.55, 1.01]), Western (0.5, [0.32, 0.72]), and Eastern (0.3, [0.13, 0.51]) regions compared to the Central region, with differences primarily in lower level health facilities. Greater changes were observed when more than one MMS supervised a facility (0.3, [0.02, 0.63]), driven primarily by performance in HC4 and hospitals (0.9, [0.21, 1.58]). MMS who were pharmacists or dispensers tended to be associated with higher overall improvements in SPARS scores compared to other professions, and facilities supervised by storekeepers experienced significantly lower improvements (− 0.7, [− 1.04, − 0.35]) than those supervised by pharmacists. Significantly greater improvement in overall SPARS scores occurred in facilities supervised by MMS who were supported by an engaged DHO who provided feedback on the SPARS reports to the MMS (0.6, [0.30, 0.95]).

Additional file 1 shows the factors that are significantly associated with improvements in the individual SPARS domain scores by level of care. Notably, improvements in the prescribing indicators were significantly higher when the MMS was a clinical officer or nurse in HC3, and at all facility levels, MMS who were trained as storekeepers had significantly lower impact on prescribing. Improvements in ordering and reporting and in stock management were higher when the MMS had a pharmaceutical background, and stock management improvements were significantly higher when the MMS received regular supervision and more than one health worker was supervised.

Time and number of visits to reach adequate score

A total of 273 (22%) out of 1222 facilities attained an adequate score of 18.75 in the first year of supervision (Fig. 4). A greater proportion of HC2s achieved an

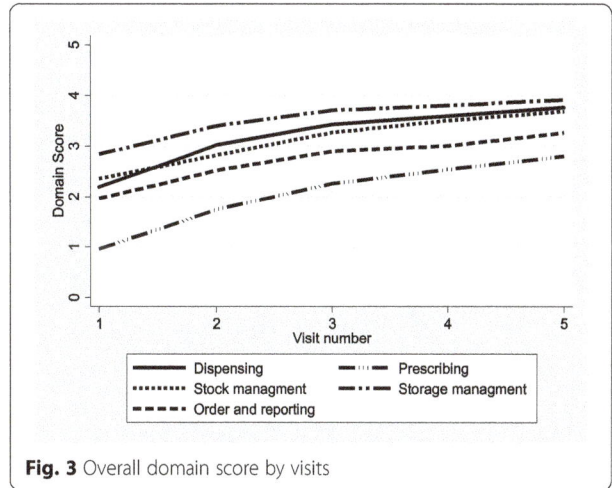

Fig. 2 Mean overall SPARS scores by visit during the first year, by level of care

Table 5 Adjusted [a] mean change in overall SPARS and domain scores by level of care and visit number during the first year of supervision

HC2			HC3		HC4/hospital		All facilities	
Observations		Adj. Diff. (95%CI)	Observations	Adj. Diff. (95%CI)	Observations	Adj. Diff. (95%CI)	Observations	Adj. Diff. (95%CI)
Total SPARS score								
All	1639	2.2 (2.14 - 2.27)	980	2.1 (2.04 - 2.19)	292	2.0 (1.87 - 2.11)	2911	2.2 (2.11 - 2.20)
2	679	3.2 (3.07 - 3.26)	416	2.8 (2.68 - 2.87)	125	2.5 (2.34 - 2.66)	1220	3.0 (2.90 - 3.02)
3	496	2.1 (1.97 - 2.19)	301	2.1 (1.87 - 2.25)	96	2.1 (1.85 - 2.42)	893	2.1 (2.01 - 2.15)
4	323	0.8 (0.72 - 0.95)	186	1.0 (0.75 - 1.16)	53	1.1 (0.91 - 1.28)	562	0.9 (0.82 - 0.97)
5	141	1.2 (1.03 - 1.33)	77	1.6 (1.31 - 1.93)	18	0.3 (-0.01 - 0.68)	236	1.3 (1.15 - 1.36)
Stock management								
All	1635	0.3 (0.31 - 0.36)	980	0.4 (0.34 - 0.40)	292	0.4 (0.29 - 0.42)	2907	0.4 (0.32 - 0.38)
2	679	0.4 (0.37 - 0.45)	416	0.5 (0.40 - 0.53)	125	0.4 (0.24 - 0.50)	1220	0.4 (0.38 - 0.47)
3	494	0.4 (0.36 - 0.43)	301	0.4 (0.31 - 0.42)	96	0.5 (0.40 - 0.56)	891	0.4 (0.37 - 0.42)
4	321	0.1 (0.10 - 0.18)	186	0.3 (0.20 - 0.32)	53	0.2 (0.04 - 0.35)	560	0.2 (0.16 - 0.21)
5	141	0.2 (0.15 - 0.34)	77	0.2 (0.04 - 0.35)	18	0.1 (-0.22 - 0.42)	236	0.2 (0.15 - 0.28)
Storage management								
All	1639	0.4 (0.34 - 0.38)	980	0.4 (0.33 - 0.39)	292	0.3 (0.23 - 0.30)	2911	0.3 (0.34 - 0.36)
2	679	0.6 (0.51 - 0.59)	416	0.5 (0.45 - 0.61)	125	0.4 (0.29 - 0.53)	1220	0.5 (0.50 - 0.57)
3	496	0.4 (0.29 - 0.43)	301	0.3 (0.21 - 0.34)	96	0.2 (0.05 - 0.29)	893	0.3 (0.28 - 0.34)
4	323	0.1 (0.03 - 0.11)	186	0.1 (0.06 - 0.23)	53	0.2 (0.12 - 0.35)	562	0.1 (0.08 - 0.14)
5	141	0.1 (-0.03 - 0.23)	77	0.2 (0.13 - 0.33)	18	-0.1 (-0.27 - 0.06)	236	0.1 (0.05 - 0.20)
Order reporting								
All	1639	0.4 (0.34 - 0.39)	980	0.3 (0.29 - 0.35)	292	0.5 (0.46 - 0.58)	2911	0.4 (0.35 - 0.38)
2	679	0.5 (0.42 - 0.52)	416	0.3 (0.29 - 0.41)	125	0.7 (0.62 - 0.83)	1220	0.5 (0.42 - 0.48)
3	496	0.4 (0.30 - 0.40)	301	0.4 (0.32 - 0.45)	96	0.5 (0.32 - 0.60)	893	0.4 (0.33 - 0.42)
4	323	0.2 (0.12 - 0.25)	186	0.1 (0.01 - 0.22)	53	0.2 (0.05 - 0.38)	562	0.2 (0.11 - 0.22)
5	141	0.3 (0.24 - 0.40)	77	0.5 (0.39 - 0.58)	18	0.3 (-0.02 - 0.58)	236	0.4 (0.30 - 0.44)
Prescribing quality								
All	1639	0.6 (0.59 - 0.62)	980	0.6 (0.52 - 0.60)	292	0.4 (0.38 - 0.45)	2911	0.6 (0.56 - 0.58)
2	679	0.8 (0.76 - 0.80)	416	0.7 (0.65 - 0.81)	125	0.5 (0.41 - 0.54)	1220	0.7 (0.70 - 0.75)
3	496	0.6 (0.60 - 0.66)	301	0.5 (0.49 - 0.57)	96	0.5 (0.44 - 0.58)	893	0.6 (0.56 - 0.60)
4	323	0.3 (0.26 - 0.33)	186	0.3 (0.24 - 0.37)	53	0.2 (0.12 - 0.35)	562	0.3 (0.27 - 0.32)
5	141	0.4 (0.33 - 0.43)	77	0.4 (0.35 - 0.51)	18	0.1 (-0.19 - 0.30)	236	0.4 (0.32 - 0.42)
Dispensing quality								
All	1639	0.5 (0.52 - 0.56)	980	0.5 (0.48 - 0.52)	292	0.4 (0.40 - 0.46)	2911	0.5 (0.51 - 0.53)
2	679	1.0 (0.95 - 0.98)	416	0.7 (0.68 - 0.73)	125	0.5 (0.48 - 0.56)	1220	0.8 (0.82 - 0.84)
3	496	0.3 (0.33 - 0.36)	301	0.5 (0.48 - 0.54)	96	0.5 (0.47 - 0.55)	893	0.4 (0.40 - 0.43)
4	323	0.1 (0.12 - 0.16)	186	0.1 (0.09 - 0.16)	53	0.2 (0.16 - 0.28)	562	0.1 (0.13 - 0.16)
5	141	0.1 (0.11 - 0.17)	77	0.3 (0.23 - 0.33)	18	0.0 (-0.08 - 0.1)	236	0.2 (0.15 - 0.20)

[a]Models adjusted for baseline SPARS scores and the significant predictors in the individual multivariate analyses, which are listed for each model in Table 6 and Appendix 1

adequate score earlier in the year, but the proportion of HC4s and hospitals performing at this level surpassed them by the end of the follow-up year; HC3s had the lowest proportion of adequately performing facilities. Of all facilities achieving an adequate score, the median

number of days to reach that level of performance was 234 (IQR 173–294).

Adjusting for whether a facility was above or below the baseline mean level of SPARS performance, factors that significantly influenced whether the facility reached

Table 6 Results of multivariable models showing factors significantly associated with average changes in the overall SPARS scores by level of care and in all facilities

	HC2		HC3		HC4/Hospital		All facilities	
	Observations	Adj. Diff. (95%CI)	Observations	Adj. Diff. (95%CI)	Observations	Adj. Diff. (95%CI)	Observations	Adj. Diff. (95%CI)
Region								
Central	290	—	208	-			554	-
Western	493	**0.3 (0.00, 0.55)**	285	**0.7 (0.42, 1.04)**			883	**0.5 (0.32, 0.72)**
Eastern	625	0.2 (-0.09, 0.43)	365	**0.5 (0.16, 0.76)**			1087	**0.3 (0.13, 0.51)**
Northern	231	**0.7 (0.35, 0.96)**	122	**0.9 (0.46, 1.29)**			383	**0.8 (0.55, 1.01)**
Ownership								
Government	1434	—					2472	—
PNFP	205	**-0.4 (-0.69, -0.13)**					435	-0.2 (-0.39, 0.01)
Number of MMS supervising a facility								
One MMS					196	—	2541	—
More than one MMS					96	**0.9 (0.21, 1.58)**	366	**0.3 (0.02, 0.63)**
Number of facilities MMS is designated								
1-10	578	—						
11-15	724	**0.2 (0.06, 0.44)**						
16+	337	**0.3 (0.05, 0.61)**						
Profession of responsible MMS								
Pharmacist/dispensers	135	—					302	—
Clinician	928	**-0.4 (-0.75, -0.01)**					1618	-0.2 (-0.47, 0.01)
Nurse/midwife	478	**-0.4 (-0.83, -0.06)**					789	-0.2 (-0.46, 0.05)
Storekeeper	98	**-0.8 (-1.33, -0.29)**					198	**-0.7 (-1.04, -0.35)**
Received feedback from DHO about MMS report								
No			162	—			414	—
Yes			818	**0.7 (0.32, 1.17)**			2493	**0.6 (0.30, 0.95)**
Baseline score	1639	**-0.2 (-0.29, -0.21)**	980	**-0.3 (-0.33, -0.21)**	292	**-0.2 (-0.3, -0.13)**	2907	**-0.3 (-0.28, -0.22)**

Figures in bold indicate adjusted differences with 95%CIs that did not include zero based on the multivariable models

an adequate score in the first year of SPARS supervision included: greater number of visits, region, MMS profession, and receiving feedback from the DHO (Additional file 2). Specifically, health facilities were significantly more likely to achieve an adequate score in the fourth visit or later (hazard ratio = 3.0 [2.29,3.93]) and facilities in the Northern (3.7 [2.28,6.16]), Western (2.5 [1.49,4.06]), and Eastern (2.2 [1.36,3.58]) regions reached this standard more rapidly than those in the Central region; facilities supervised by clinical officers reached an acceptable score significantly faster than those supervised by pharmacists (1.7 [1.20,2.51]), especially in HC2s; and facilities supervised by MMS that received

feedback from the DHO about their reports reached their goals significantly faster (2.3 [1.30,4.00]) than those supervised by MMS who did not receive DHO feedback.

Discussion

Improvement in SPARS scores over time

With an average of 22.3% increase in overall SPARS scores per visit during the first year of supervision, our study documents that SPARS is an effective multipronged intervention to improve MM in all levels of health care in both government and PNFP sectors. Almost one in four facilities reached an adequate score within the

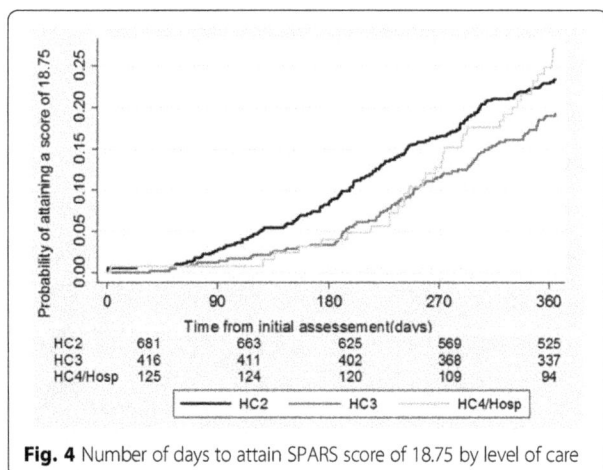

Fig. 4 Number of days to attain SPARS score of 18.75 by level of care

first year. The SPARS intervention was associated with the greatest improvements after the first supervisory visit, although the gains in SPARS scores continued to be positive but tapering in subsequent visits.

Comparison to other studies

Other studies of supervision interventions in low resource settings suggest a small positive effect of supervision [7, 8, 18], but most have not used a comprehensive intervention approach or estimated the relative improvement in performance between sequential visits. The observed improvements associated with the SPARS strategy of 22.3% per visit and 68.9% following four visits were very high, suggesting that multifaceted strategies may be more successful than supervision alone (7). A review of 30 interventions targeting prescribing practices demonstrated a median improvement relative to control of 18% (8). In comparison, we saw a 180% improvement in the prescribing quality domain during the first year of SPARS supervision. A supervisory intervention in Zimbabwe demonstrated a statistically significant improvement (7%) in supply chain management compared to control [19], while SPARS produced a 14% improvement (2.8 to 3.2) in the mean SPARS stock management score after the initial visit. The SPARS approach is more comparable to an intervention in the Philippines that combined supervision of midwives with follow-up visits using an indicator-based checklist for performance assessment at each visit [20]. The study found 24% improvement in scores following an average of 3.1 visits or a 7.7% score increase per visit compared to the SPARS score improvement of 22.3% per visit. The large magnitude of relative improvement in SPARS may be partly due to the low level of initial performance, but the continuing improvement in scores following subsequent visits suggests that SPARS may be an effective approach even after performance reaches a higher level.

Level of care

MM performance improved at all levels of care, independent of service complexity and staffing, but with considerable individual facility variation. In addition, similar to other studies, we found that level of care influenced intervention effect [7]. The highest impact occurred at the lowest level of care, HC2, followed by HC3, HC4, and hospitals. HC2 facilities have only one staff person, so that supervision in that level of care is consistently provided one-on-one; moreover, the services provided are simpler and fewer compared to higher levels of care.

Domains

The prescribing quality domain had the lowest initial mean scores, while storage management had the highest by almost three-fold. We observed improvements in all five domains, with the prescribing quality domain experiencing the largest incremental gain per visit followed by dispensing quality, ordering and reporting, stock management, and storage management. The improvement in all domains tended toward a score ceiling of 4 out of maximum 5 by the end of 1 year of visits.

Performance in the ordering and reporting domain proved to be the hardest to improve. Lower levels of care (HC2 and HC3) still received essential medicines kits; therefore, they did not submit orders and had no way to practice and maintain their related skills in this domain. Meanwhile, facilities that did place orders (HC4 and hospitals), were slow to adhere to a new order and delivery schedule introduced in 2010. However, following the initial SPARS visits to orient staff on the new practices, HC4s and hospitals experienced the largest initial improvement in ordering and reporting scores, demonstrating the usefulness of SPARS in accelerating the take up of the new order and delivery schedule. In addition, all facilities in the public and PNFP sectors are supposed to report monthly into Uganda's health management information system. However, no incentives exist for timely and accurate reporting, and no feedback is provided to facilities on their reporting performance. Therefore, we recommend incorporating SPARS indicators in this domain that assess reporting quality and accuracy, and then providing regular feedback on that performance to health facilities.

The prescribing domain had the lowest initial SPARS domain scores, but also the highest adjusted improvement of all the domains within 1 year. However, the average improvement per visit was notably lower in HC4s and hospitals. At these higher levels of care, the number of prescribers and prescribing complexity makes it more difficult to increase capacity in all prescribers.

We believe that the initial rapid improvement in dispensing quality is linked to the SPARS recognition component which assured that facilities received dispensing tools such as counting trays, dispensing envelopes, and also adequate shelving that facilitated appropriate storage and dispensing practices.

Regions

SPARS had the greatest impact on performance in facilities in the Northern region, especially in HC2s and HC3s. We think that previous civil unrest in the Northern region deprived the population of most health service improvement interventions; now, facilities in the area are eager to catch up and make full use of the opportunities offered. The reasons for variation in other regions are unclear.

Facility ownership

We found government facilities to be more responsive to the SPARS intervention, with PNFP facilities having a significantly lower average increase in SPARS score per visit—0.4 points lower than public facilities. One explanation could be that the MMS initially chose their target facilities, and although PNFP facilities fall under the DHOs' responsibility, MMS might have prioritized government facilities. Since then, the MOH has established and trained MMS from the four medical bureaus that oversee the PNFP facilities. Having dedicated PNFP MMS who can ensure sufficient supervision will especially benefit the HC2 PNFP facilities, which are typically weaker performers located in very remote areas.

Supervision by more than one supervisor

SPARS has a practical training component where district MMS lead HSD-MMS through five supervisory visits until they are prepared to carry out their own visits. Because the district MMS oversee higher-level facilities, those facilities often received supervision from more than one MMS, unlike the HC2 and HC3 facilities that HSD-MMS oversee alone. In addition, MOH staff members accompany district MMS on HC4 and hospital visits as part of their hierarchical oversight structure. Having more than one MMS at supervisory visits benefited the higher-level facilities, particularly, because their pharmaceutical management functions are more complex—more services, more staff members, and more medicines. Not only can the MMS support each other, but they can split tasks and interact with more staff members. Revised SPARS procedures should consider having two MMS visit the higher-level facilities during the first two visits.

Volume of facilities and supervisory visits

SPARS was designed to have MMS making five supervisory visits per month for 10 months a year, with each facility receiving about five MMS visits in the first year. After 1 year of regular supervision, we expected facilities to reach an adequate performance score; after this, the

frequency of visits could be reduced to a maintenance level, with four to 6 months between supervisory visits. In practice, we found that MMS made 28 visits per year with 88 days between supervisory visits, and each facility received an average of only 3.4 visits per year. Though the greatest performance increases occurred within the first three visits, only 22% of the facilities reached an adequate score within the first year. The impact was in line with our expectations, but because of the lower level of implementation intensity, it will take longer to reach national SPARS coverage and for the majority of facilities to achieve adequate scores. Other studies have confirmed our findings that effects increase with multiple supervision visits [20] and that the interval between visits had no observable impact [18]. It is important to recognize that all MMS have these responsibilities added to their normal duties; therefore, realistically, MMS were only able to dedicate three to 4 days per month to SPARS supervision. Our findings suggested that visiting one facility per day is an appropriate target for MMS. Two-thirds of them felt that they had sufficient time to assess performance and implement supportive supervision.

Surprisingly, we found that MMS with responsibility for a greater number of facilities had a higher impact in improving MM. HSD-MMS generally had more than 10 facilities to supervise, but because they were mostly HC2 facilities, it may have been easier to improve simpler MM practices.

MMS profession

The selection of MMS for the SPARS program is critical. The most important criteria are motivation, interest in the program, and being effective and supportive supervisors [21]. The supervisor's profession also influenced impact; MMS with a clinical background were more successful in changing the staff's prescribing behavior compared to pharmaceutical or storekeeping backgrounds; presumably they were viewed more as professional colleagues with an understanding of the complexity of diagnosing and prescribing according to standard treatment guidelines. On the other hand, MMS who were trained in pharmacy had more effect on performance in the stock management and ordering and reporting domains, where expertise in EMHS logistics gave them an advantage in explaining related standard operation practices. Storekeepers working as MMS who had a more limited logistics background were not as successful in improving performance in these domains. We concluded that MMS who were experienced had technical expertise in certain areas were better able to influence performance in those areas, which has been confirmed by other studies [10].

DHO engagement

As expected based on other evidence [7], having a dedicated and engaged DHO that is interested in SPARS and

MMS performance made a substantial difference in the improvements observed; therefore, we recommend finding ways to meaningfully engage the DHOs early and routinely in SPARS implementation in their districts.

Study limitations

The 45 randomly selected study districts were included because they were targeted by the US Agency for International Development health system strengthening program in Uganda. However, they represented more than half of the 89 districts in the country at the time of the study and were selected based on diversity, regional representation, poverty, and need. We believe they provided a good cross-sectional representation of Uganda's districts. As noted previously, the MMS chose facilities to target within the selected districts, which could have biased the study (e.g., the MMS could have given priority to government, better-performing, or closer facilities). However, we included over 80% of the facilities in the selected districts in the study, which limited the extent of this possible bias. The study facilities represented one-third of the government and PNFP facilities in Uganda, with government facilities slightly overrepresented (85% of the sample) compared to their actual proportion (76%) [13]. Despite the imbalance, we were still able to detect significant differences related to facility ownership.

Over the study period, new MMS joined the study, some left, and their overall level of experience increased—effects that might have influenced the degree and timing of impact; however, because this was a real-world study, we did not try to control for MMS longevity or experience. We saw wide variation between facilities in impact that may be due to unmeasured factors, such as MMS supportive supervisory skills [22] or facility staffing or resources. Another limitation related to the analysis of predictors of improvement was that we only had a 75% response rate for predictor data from MMS in the MMS survey despite several follow-up telephone calls. However, we were able to use multiple imputation methods to impute results for these missing surveys; results using only cases with complete data were essentially equivalent to those obtained using imputed data.

During the 12-month follow-up period, an almost equal number of facilities had two, three, and four supervisory visits, and only about half of the facilities had five or more visits as intended. This may have been linked to limitations on the number of visits that MMS could actually implement in a month. However, some facilities might have had more active MMS or have been located closer to the MMS place of work, which may have resulted in differential improvement.

Baseline SPARS scores improved slightly but significantly by 0.32 and 1.04 points in 2012 and 2013 compared to 2011, independent of the SPARS interventions.

SPARS was implemented in facilities in a phased manner in all intervention districts, and facilities implemented later in the study period would have known about SPARS prior to their first visit. Thus, we cannot rule out the possibility that some contamination from earlier SPARS facilities may have led to a slight improvement in MM over time in all facilities in the district. Alternatively, other external factors in the health system may have led to improvements in the performance areas measured by SPARS. Ideally, we would have had a control group of facilities outside of the SPARS districts, but such a design was not feasible in the context of SPARS implementation. However, the types of consistent improvements in performance that we observed are most likely due in large part to the intervention rather than to other unobserved factors.

These study data were collected almost 5 years ago. However, SPARS is still highly relevant in its current context; a few modifications were introduced at the end of 2017 including two new indicators linked to malaria testing and treatment and to data quality for health information systems. No other supervision models have superseded SPARS. However, because of its well-documented influence, the MOH has now adapted a SPARS approach for laboratory, tuberculosis, and HIV/AIDS management. Although pharmacists were found to be very successful as MMS's, it is not realistic to establish pharmacists at district level to implement SPARS in the near future in Uganda due to resource constraints. Steps have instead been taken to institute regional-level pharmacists to supervise MMS.

Despite these limitations, we believe that we have documented that SPARS is an effective strategy for improving MM at all levels of care within the government and PNFP sectors.

Conclusions

Building capacity in MM at public and PNFP sector health facilities is critical to ensure high quality health services that rely on medicines availability and appropriate use. This study showed that the SPARS approach effectively improved medicines management practices in Uganda, with an improvement in overall performance of nearly 70% during the first year of supervision. We recognize that SPARS will evolve and that the performance assessment tool will change as health facility staff members become more adept in their skills. However, this study demonstrates the benefit of combining intervention strategies to change behaviors and performance in a low-resource health setting. We recommend monitoring SPARS scores for an extended time to assess further gains and to ascertain the program's long-term cost-effectiveness.

Abbreviations

DHO: District Health Officer; EMHS: Essential medicines and health supplies; HC: Health center; HSD: Health sub-district; IQR : Interquartile range; MM: Medicines management; MMS: Medicines management supervisors; MOH: Ministry of Health; PNFP: Private not-for-profit; SPARS: Supervision, Performance Assessment and Recognition Strategy

Acknowledgements

This study was funded by the United States Agency for International Development (USAID). We thank the medicines management supervisors for undertaking SPARS visits and the district health officers and facility staff for their cooperation and implementation of the SPARS program. We gratefully acknowledge the input of Dr. Anita K. Wagner on earlier versions of the manuscript and Moses Lubale, who contributed to the data analysis.

Funding

This study was funded by the United States Agency for International Development (USAID). USAID did not have any role in the study design, data analysis, or writing of this paper or in the decision to submit the paper for publication (see acknowledgement).

Authors' contributions

BT conceived of, designed, and oversaw the study. She contributed substantially to the development of study methods, oversaw implementation, data analysis, and drafted the manuscript. AK and MO contributed to developing the study methods and implementation. RM and DRD contributed to data and statistical analysis. DRD and ME contributed to the interpretation, discussion, and writing of the manuscript. All authors read and approved the final version.

Competing interests

The authors declare that they have no competing interests.

Author details

[1]USAID/Uganda Health Supply Chain Program, Management Sciences for Health, Plot 15, Princess Anne Drive, BugolobiP.O. Box 71419, Kampala, Uganda. [2]Management Sciences for Health, Plot 15, Princess Anne Drive, BugolobiP.O. Box 71419, Kampala, Uganda. [3]Ministry of Health Uganda, Pharmacy Department, Plot 6/Lourdel Rd, P.O. Box 7272, Kampala, Uganda. [4]Management Sciences for Health, 4301 N. Fairfax Drive, Suite 400, Arlington, VA 22203, USA. [5]Harvard Medical School and Harvard Pilgrim Health Care Institute, 401 Park Drive Suite 401, Boston, MA 02215, USA.

References

1. Ministry of Health Uganda. National Medicines Policy, 25 July, 2015. [Cited 2017 Nov 19]. http://www.google.com/url?sa=t&rct=j&q=&esrc=s&source=web&cd=1&ved=0ahUKEwj-iM6slcrXAhWFzRQKHeHJAqAQFggoMAA&url=http%3A%2F%2Fhealth.go.ug%2Fdownload%2Ffile%2Ffid%2F589&usg=AOvVaw0sycl_K8H5yxLSquF7F9Gv

2. Trap B, Ladwar DO, Oteba MO, Embrey M, Khalid K, Wagner AK. Article 1: supervision, performance assessment, and recognition strategy (SPARS) - a multipronged intervention strategy for strengthening medicines management in Uganda: method presentation and facility performance at baseline. J Pharm Policy Pract. 2016;9(1):1–15. https://doi.org/10.1186/s40545-016-0070-x

3. Bigdeli M, Peters DH, and Wagner AK. Medicines in health systems. Advancing access, affordability and appropriate use. World Health Organ Alliance Health Policy Syst Res; 2014. ISBN 978 92 4 150762 2. http://www.who.int/alliance-hpsr/resources/publications/9789241507622/en/.

4. Ministry of Health Uganda. Uganda Pharmaceutical Sector Report 2010 [Internet]. 2010. [Cited 2017 Nov 19]. Available from: http://library.health.go.ug/publications/medical-products-technologies/pharmaceuticals-and-drugs/uganda-pharmaceutical-sector.

5. Ssengooba F, Rahman SA, Hongoro C, et al. Health sector reforms and human resources for health in Uganda and Bangladesh: mechanisms of effect. Hum Resour Health. 2007;5:3. https://doi.org/10.1186/1478-4491-5-3.

6. Kyabayinze DJ, Asiimwe C, Nakanjako D, et al. Programme level implementation of malaria rapid diagnostic tests (RDTs) use : outcomes and cost of training health workers at lower level health care facilities in Uganda. BMC Public Health. 2012;12(1):1. https://doi.org/10.1186/1471-2458-12-291.

7. Rowe AK, De Savigny D, Lanata CF, Victora CG. How can we achieve and maintain high-quality performance of health workers in low-resource settings? Lancet. 2005;366(9490):1026–35. https://doi.org/10.1016/S0140-6736(05)67028-6.

8. Ross-Degnan D, Laing R, Santoso B, Ofori-Adjei D, Lamoureux C, Hogerzeil H. Improving Pharmaceutical Use in Primary Care in Developing Counties: A Critical Review of Experience and Lack of Experience. Presented at the International Conference on Improving Use of Medicines, (Chiang Mai, Thailand, April); 1997. [Cited 2017 Nov 19]. Available from: http://www.google.com/url?sa=t&rct=j&q=&esrc=s&source=web&cd=1&ved=0ahUKEwia-8zBncrXAhWLuBQKHbfXCiIQFggkMAA&url=http%3A%2F%2Farchives.who.int%2Fprduc2004%2FResource_Mats%2FRossDegnanReviewV4.doc&usg=AOvVaw00Pp2dQtHiM6ez0Vn875uS

9. Trap R, Trap B, Wind HT, Holme HE. Performance based reward for immunization: experiences from GAVI. South Med Rev. 2011;4(1):40–7. https://doi.org/10.5655/smr.v4i1.69.

10. Marquez L, Kean L. Making supervision supportive and sustainable: new approaches to old problems. Maximising Access Qual Initiat MAQ Pap 1(4). 2002;1(4):1–28. https://doi.org/10.1111/j.1471-0528.2005.00718.x.

11. Tavrow P, Kim Y, Malianga L. Measuring the quality of supervisor – provider interactions in health care facilities in Zimbabwe. Int J Qual Heal Care. 2002; 14:57–66. https://doi.org/10.1093/intqhc/14.suppl_1.57.

12. Suh S, Moreira P, Ly M. Improving quality of reproductive health care in Senegal through formative supervision: results from four districts. Hum Resour Health. 2007;5(1):26. https://doi.org/10.1186/1478-4491-5-26.

13. Uganda Bureau of Statistics. Uganda Bureau of Statistics Statistical Abstract [Internet].2014. [Cited 2017 Nov 19]. Available from: http://www.ubos.org/onlinefiles/uploads/ubos/statistical_abstracts/Statistical%20Abstract2014.pdf.

14. Ministry of Health Uganda. Annual Pharmaceutical Sector Performance Report 2013-2014 [Internet]. 2015. [Cited 2017 Nov 19]. Available from: http://health.go.ug/content/report-pharmacy.

15. Peterson S, Nsungwa-Sabiiti J, Were W, Nsabagasani X, Magumba G, Nambooze J, Mukasa G. Coping with paediatric referral–Ugandan parents' experience. Lancet. 2004;363(9425):1955–6. https://doi.org/10.1016/S0140-6736(04)16411-8.

16. Horton NJ, Kleinman KP. Much ado about nothing. Am Stat. 2007;61(1):79–90. https://doi.org/10.1198/000313007X172556.

17. Royston P, White I. Multiple imputation by chained equations (MICE): implementation in Stata. J Stat Softw. 2011;45(4) https://doi.org/10.18637/jss.v045.i04.

18. Bosch-Capblanch X, Garner P. Primary health care supervision in developing countries. Trop Med Int Heal. 2008;13(3):369–83. https://doi.org/10.1111/j.1365-3156. 2008.02012.x.

19. Trap B, Todd CH, Moore H, Laing R. The impact of supervision on stock management and adherence to treatment guidelines: a randomized controlled trial. Health Policy Plan. 2001;16(3):273–80.

20. Loevinsohn BP, Guerrero ET, Gregorio SP. Improving primary health care through systematic supervision: a controlled field trial. Health Policy Plan. 1995;10(2):144–53. https://doi.org/10.1093/heapol/10.2.144.

21. Henry R, Nantongo L, Wagner AK, Embrey M, Trap B. Competency in supportive supervision: a study of public sector medicines management supervisors in Uganda. J. Pharm. Policy Pract. 2017;10(1) https://doi.org/10.1186/s40545-017-0121-y.

22. Blick, et al. Evaluating inter-rater reliability of indicators to assess performance of medicines management in health facilities in Uganda. J Pharm Policy Pract. 2018;11:11. https://doi.org/10.1186/s40545-018-0137-y.

Permissions

All chapters in this book were first published in JPPP, by BioMed Central; hereby published with permission under the Creative Commons Attribution License or equivalent. Every chapter published in this book has been scrutinized by our experts. Their significance has been extensively debated. The topics covered herein carry significant findings which will fuel the growth of the discipline. They may even be implemented as practical applications or may be referred to as a beginning point for another development.

The contributors of this book come from diverse backgrounds, making this book a truly international effort. This book will bring forth new frontiers with its revolutionizing research information and detailed analysis of the nascent developments around the world.

We would like to thank all the contributing authors for lending their expertise to make the book truly unique. They have played a crucial role in the development of this book. Without their invaluable contributions this book wouldn't have been possible. They have made vital efforts to compile up to date information on the varied aspects of this subject to make this book a valuable addition to the collection of many professionals and students.

This book was conceptualized with the vision of imparting up-to-date information and advanced data in this field. To ensure the same, a matchless editorial board was set up. Every individual on the board went through rigorous rounds of assessment to prove their worth. After which they invested a large part of their time researching and compiling the most relevant data for our readers.

The editorial board has been involved in producing this book since its inception. They have spent rigorous hours researching and exploring the diverse topics which have resulted in the successful publishing of this book. They have passed on their knowledge of decades through this book. To expedite this challenging task, the publisher supported the team at every step. A small team of assistant editors was also appointed to further simplify the editing procedure and attain best results for the readers.

Apart from the editorial board, the designing team has also invested a significant amount of their time in understanding the subject and creating the most relevant covers. They scrutinized every image to scout for the most suitable representation of the subject and create an appropriate cover for the book.

The publishing team has been an ardent support to the editorial, designing and production team. Their endless efforts to recruit the best for this project, has resulted in the accomplishment of this book. They are a veteran in the field of academics and their pool of knowledge is as vast as their experience in printing. Their expertise and guidance has proved useful at every step. Their uncompromising quality standards have made this book an exceptional effort. Their encouragement from time to time has been an inspiration for everyone.

The publisher and the editorial board hope that this book will prove to be a valuable piece of knowledge for researchers, students, practitioners and scholars across the globe.

List of Contributors

Lita Araujo
Pharmaceutical Business and Administrative Sciences, MCPHS University, 179 Longwood Avenue, Boston, MA 02115, USA

Michael Montagne
School of Pharmacy, MCPHS University, 179 Longwood Avenue, Boston, MA, USA

Lindsey Rorden and Richard Laing
Department of Global Health, Boston University School of Public Health, Boston, MA, USA

Abhishek Sharma
Department of Global Health, Boston University School of Public Health, Boston, MA, USA
Center for Global Health and Development, Boston University School of Public Health, Boston, MA, USA
Precision Health Economics, Boston, MA, USA

Margaret Ewen
Health Action International, Amsterdam, The Netherlands

Eyerusalem Berhanemeskel, Gebremedhin Beedemariam and Teferi Gedif Fenta
Departement of Pharmaceutics and Social Pharmacy, School of Pharmacy, College of Health Sciences, Addis Ababa University, Ethiopia, Addis Ababa, Ethiopia

Charles Newman
University of Birmingham, Medical School, Birmingham, UK

Vamadevan S. Ajay and Dorairaj Prabhakaran
Centre for Chronic Disease Control, New Delhi, India

Ravi Srinivas
Research and Information Systems for Developing Countries (RIS), New Delhi, India

Sandeep Bhalla
Public Health Foundation of India, New Delhi, India

Amitava Banerjee
University of Birmingham Centre for Cardiovascular Sciences, Birmingham, UK

School of Health, University of Central Lancashire, Preston, UK

Rasmus Borup, Susanne Kaae and Janine Traulsen
Department of Pharmacy, University of Copenhagen, Universitetsparken 2, 2100 Copenhagen, Denmark

Timo Minssen
Centre for Information and Innovation Law, University of Copenhagen, Studiestræde, 1455 Copenhagen, Denmark

Chia-Ying Lee and Xiaohan Chen
Johns Hopkins University Bloomberg School of Public Health, Center for Drug Safety and Effectiveness, 624 N. Broadway, Room 644, Baltimore, MD 21205, USA

Jodi B. Segal
Johns Hopkins University Bloomberg School of Public Health, Center for Drug Safety and Effectiveness, 624 N. Broadway, Room 644, Baltimore, MD 21205, USA
Division of General Internal Medicine, Johns Hopkins University School of Medicine, 624 N. Broadway, Room 644, Baltimore, MD 21205, USA

Robert J. Romanelli
Palo Alto Medical Foundation Research Institute, Palo Alto, CA, USA

Louise E. Curley, Janice Moody, Rukshar Gobarani, Trudi Aspden, Maree Jensen, Maureen McDonald, John Shaw and Janie Sheridan
School of Pharmacy, Faculty of Medical and Health Sciences, University of Auckland, Auckland 1142, New Zealand

Bvudzai Priscilla Magadzire
School of Public Health, University of the Western Cape, Bellville 7535, South Africa

Bruno Marchal
School of Public Health, University of the Western Cape, Private Bag X17, Bellville 7535, South Africa
Department of Public Health, Institute of Tropical Medicine, Antwerp, Belgium

Kim Ward
School of Pharmacy, University of the Western Cape, Bellville, South Africa

Niranjan Konduri, Emily Delmotte and Edmund Rutta
Program, Management Sciences for Health, 4301 N. Fairfax Dr. Suite 400, Arlington, VA 22203, USA

Gemma L. Buckland-Merrett, Catherine Kilkenny and Tim Reed
Health Action International, Overtoom 60 (2), 1054 HK Amsterdam, The Netherlands

Susanne Kaae
Department of Pharmacy, Section for Social and Clinical Pharmacy, Faculty of Health and Medical Sciences, University of Copenhagen, Universitetsparken 2, 2100 København Ø, Denmark

Admir Malaj and Iris Hoxha
Faculty of Pharmacy, University of Medicine Tirana, Albania, Fakulteti Farmacise, Rr. Dibres 371, 1000 Tirana, Albania

Warren A. Kaplan, Paul G. Ashigbie and Veronika J. Wirtz
Department of Global Health, Boston University School of Public Health, Crosstown Center, Room CT-363, 801 Massachusetts Avenue, Boston, Massachusetts 02118, USA

Mohamad I. Brooks
Department of Global Health, Boston University School of Public Health, Crosstown Center, Room CT-363, 801 Massachusetts Avenue, Boston, Massachusetts 02118, USA
Pathfinder International, 9 Galen Street, Suite 217, Watertown 02472, Massachusetts, USA

Raewyn Rees
School of Interprofessional Health Studies, Faculty of Health and Environmental Sciences, Auckland University of Technology, Auckland, New Zealand

Ali Seyfoddin
School of Interprofessional Health Studies, Faculty of Health and Environmental Sciences, Auckland University of Technology, Auckland, New Zealand
Drug Delivery Research Group, School of Science, Faculty of Health and Environmental Sciences, Auckland University of Technology, Auckland, New Zealand

Jeromie Ballreich and Taruja Karmarkar
Department of Health Policy and Management, Johns Hopkins Bloomberg School of Public Health, 624 N. Broadway, Baltimore, MD 21205, USA

Center for Drug Safety and Effectiveness, Johns Hopkins Bloomberg School of Public Health, Baltimore, MD, USA

Mariana Socal
Department of Health Policy and Management, Johns Hopkins Bloomberg School of Public Health, 624 N. Broadway, Baltimore, MD 21205, USA
Center for Drug Safety and Effectiveness, Johns Hopkins Bloomberg School of Public Health, Baltimore, MD, USA
Department of International Health, Johns Hopkins Bloomberg School of Public Health, Baltimore, MD, USA

Gerard Anderson
Department of Health Policy and Management, Johns Hopkins Bloomberg School of Public Health, 624 N. Broadway, Baltimore, MD 21205, USA
Center for Drug Safety and Effectiveness, Johns Hopkins Bloomberg School of Public Health, Baltimore, MD, USA
Division of General Internal Medicine, Johns Hopkins Medicine, Baltimore, MD, USA
Department of International Health, Johns Hopkins Bloomberg School of Public Health, Baltimore, MD, USA

G. Caleb Alexander
Center for Drug Safety and Effectiveness, Johns Hopkins Bloomberg School of Public Health, Baltimore, MD, USA
Department of Epidemiology, Johns Hopkins Bloomberg School of Public Health, Baltimore, MD, USA
Division of General Internal Medicine, Johns Hopkins Medicine, Baltimore, MD, USA

Lindsey M. Philpot, Priya Ramar and Raphael Mwangi
Robert D. and Patricia E. Kern Mayo Clinic Center for the Science of Health Care Delivery, Mayo Clinic College of Medicine, 200 1st Street SW, Rochester, MN 55905, USA

Muhamad Y. Elrashidi and Jon O. Ebbert
Robert D. and Patricia E. Kern Mayo Clinic Center for the Science of Health Care Delivery, Mayo Clinic College of Medicine, 200 1st Street SW, Rochester, MN 55905, USA
Primary Care Internal Medicine, Mayo Clinic College of Medicine, Rochester, MN, USA

Frederick North
Primary Care Internal Medicine, Mayo Clinic
College of Medicine, Rochester, MN, USA

Paul Tern
University of Cambridge, School of Clinical
Medicine, Cambridge, UK
Polygeia (Global Health Student Think-Tank),
Cambridge, UK

Fawz Kazzazi
University of Cambridge, School of Clinical
Medicine, Cambridge, UK
Polygeia (Global Health Student Think-Tank),
Cambridge, UK
Leckhampton House, 37 Grange Road, Cambridge
CB3 9BJ, UK

Cleo Pollard
King's College London, London, UK
Polygeia (Global Health Student Think-Tank),
Cambridge, UK

Alejandro Ayuso-Garcia and Jack Gillespie
University of Cambridge, Cambridge, UK

Inesa Thomsen
Imperial College London, MRC London Institute of
Medical Sciences, London, UK
Polygeia (Global Health Student Think-Tank),
Cambridge, UK

Denis Kibira
WHO Collaborating Centre for Pharmaceutical
Policy and Regulation, Utrecht Institute for
Pharmaceutical Sciences (UIPS), Utrecht University,
Universiteitsweg 99, 3584 CG Utrecht, the
Netherlands
Coalition for Health Promotion and Social
Development (HEPS-Uganda), Plot 351A, Balintuma
Road, Namirembe Hill, Kampala, Uganda

Freddy Eric Kitutu
Makerere University, School of Public Health and
Pharmacy Department, College of Health Sciences,
Kampala, Uganda
Uppsala University, Department of Women's and
Children's Health, International Maternal and Child
Health, SE-751 85 Uppsala, Sweden

Gemma Buckland Merrett
Health Action International, Overtoom 60 (2), 1054
HK Amsterdam, The Netherlands.

Aukje K. Mantel-Teeuwisse
WHO Collaborating Centre for Pharmaceutical
Policy and Regulation, Utrecht Institute for
Pharmaceutical Sciences (UIPS), Utrecht University,
Universiteitsweg 99, 3584 CG Utrecht, the
Netherlands

Victor Basopo and Paschal N. Mujasi
School of Management, Universitat Pompeu Fabra,
Balmes 132, 08001 Barcelona, Spain

Joel Lexchin
School of Health Policy and Management, York
University, 4700 Keele St., Toronto, ON M3J 1P3,
Canada
University Health Network, 200 Elizabeth St.,
Toronto, ON M5G 2C4, Canada

Akram Hernández-Vásquez
Universidad Privada del Norte, Lima, Peru

Christoper A. Alarcon-Ruiz
Facultad de Medicina, Universidad Ricardo Palma,
Lima, Peru

Guido Bendezu-Quispe
Universidad Peruana Cayetano Heredia, Lima, Peru

Daniel Comandé
Institute for Clinical Effectiveness and Health Policy
(IECS), Buenos Aires, Argentina

Diego Rosselli
Departamento de Epidemiología Clínica y
Bioestadística, Facultad de Medicina, Pontificia
Universidad Javeriana, Bogotá, Colombia

Christine Årdal
Norwegian Institute of Public Health, Postboks
4404 Nydalen, 0403 Oslo, Norway

Enrico Baraldi
Uppsala University, 751 20 Uppsala, Sweden

Ursula Theuretzbacher
Center for Anti-Infective Agents, Vienna, Austria

Kevin Outterson
Boston University, 765 Commonwealth Avenue,
Boston, MA 02215, USA

Jens Plahte
Norwegian Institute of Public Health, Postboks
4404 Nydalen, 0403 Oslo, Norway

Francesco Ciabuschi
Uppsala University, 751 20 Uppsala, Sweden

John-Arne Røttingen
Norwegian Institute of Public Health, University of Oslo, Postboks 4404 Nydalen, 0403, Boks 1072 Blindern, 0316 Oslo, Norway

Anthony H. Bui, Michael L. Brodman and Meg A. Rosenblatt
Icahn School of Medicine at Mount Sinai, New York, NY 10029, USA

David L. Feldman
Icahn School of Medicine at Mount Sinai, New York, NY 10029, USA
Hospitals Insurance Company, New York, NY, USA

I. Michael Leitman
Icahn School of Medicine at Mount Sinai, New York, NY 10029, USA
Department of Surgery, Icahn School of Medicine at Mount Sinai, One Gustave L. Levy Place, New York, NY 10029, USA

Debra D'Angelo, Donna Somerville, Santosh Mudiraj and Patricia Kischak
Hospitals Insurance Company, New York, NY, USA

Peter Shamamian
Montefiore Medical Center/Albert Einstein College of Medicine, Bronx, NY, USA

Ronald N. Kaleya
Maimonides Medical Center, Brooklyn, NY, USA

Birna Trap
USAID/Uganda Health Supply Chain Program, Management Sciences for Health, Plot 15, Princess Anne Drive, Bugolobi Kampala, Uganda

Richard Musoke and Anthony Kirunda
Management Sciences for Health, Plot 15, Princess Anne Drive, Bugolobi Kampala, Uganda

Martin Olowo Oteba
Ministry of Health Uganda, Pharmacy Department, Plot 6/Lourdel Rd, Kampala, Uganda

Martha Embrey
Management Sciences for Health, 4301 N. Fairfax Drive, Suite 400, Arlington, VA 22203, USA

Dennis Ross-Degnan
Harvard Medical School and Harvard Pilgrim Health Care Institute, 401 Park Drive Suite 401, Boston, MA 02215, USA

Index